MRI, ARTHROSCOPY, AND SURGICAL ANATOMY OF THE JOINTS

MRI, ARTHROSCOPY, AND SURGICAL ANATOMY OF THE JOINTS

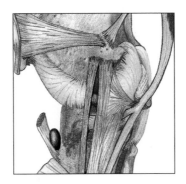

DAVID W. STOLLER, MD

Director
Marin Radiology and National Orthopaedic Imaging Associates
San Francisco, California

Director
California Advanced Imaging

Assistant Clinical Professor of Radiology
University of California at San Francisco
San Francisco, California

SALVADOR BELTRAN
Medical Illustrator

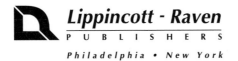

Lippincott - Raven
P U B L I S H E R S
Philadelphia • New York

Acquisitions Editor: James Ryan
Developmental Editor: Delois Patterson
Manufacturing Manager: Dennis Teston
Production Manager: Cassie Moore
Cover Designer: Jeane Norton
Indexer: Kathrin Unger
Compositor: Lippincott–Raven Desktop Division
Printer: Worzalla Publishers

Printed in the United States of America

9 8 7 6 5 4 3 2 1

Library of Congress Cataloging-in-Publication Data

Stoller, David W.
    MRI, arthroscopy, and surgical anatomy of the joints / David W. Stoller,
with 14 contributors.
       p. cm.
    Includes bibliographical references and index.
    ISBN 0-7817-1666-7 (hardcover)
    1. Joints—Atlases.   2. Joints—Magnetic resonance imaging—Atlases.
3. Arthroscopy—Atlases.   4. Anatomy, Surgical and topographical—Atlases.
I. Title.
    [DNLM: 1. Joints—anatomy and histology atlases.   2. Magnetic Resonance
Imaging atlases.   3. Arthroscopy atlases.   4. Diagnostic Imaging atlases.
WE 17 S875ma 1998]
QM131.S76   1998
DNLM/DLC
for Library of Congress   98-22297
                                             CIP

To my cherished son, Griffin, and my lovely wife, Marcia,
for their extraordinary love and support,
and to both our families, for understanding
and accommodating the sacrifices of personal time

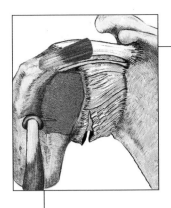

CONTRIBUTORS

JAVIER BELTRAN, MD

Chairman, Department of Radiology
Hospital for Joint Diseases
Professor of Radiology
New York University
New York, New York

SALVADOR BELTRAN, MD

Biocommunication Studio Gat Blau
Barcelona, Spain

GORDON A. BRODY, MD

Chief, Hand Surgery
Sports, Orthopedic and Rehabilitation
Medicine Associates
Menlo Park, California
Clinical Associate Professor of Orthopaedics
Stanford University School of Medicine
Palo Alto, California

W. DILWORTH CANNON, JR., MD

Professor of Clinical Orthopedics and
Director of Sports Medicine
University of California at San Francisco
San Francisco, California

SCOTT DYE, MD

San Francisco Sports Medicine
Ralph K. Davies Medical Center
Clinical Professor of Orthopaedic Surgery
University of California at San Francisco
San Francisco, California

RICHARD D. FERKEL, MD

Clinical Instructor of Orthopedic Surgery
University of California, Los Angeles, Center
for Health Sciences
Chief of Arthroscopy
Wadsworth VA Hospital
Los Angeles, California
Attending Surgeon and Director of
Fellowship
Southern California Orthopedic Institute
Van Nuys, California

RUSSELL C. FRITZ, MD

Medical Director
National Orthopaedic Imaging Associates
Assistant Clinical Professor of Radiology
University of California at San Francisco
San Francisco, California

ROBERT J. GILBERT, MD

Chairman, Department of Orthopaedic
Surgery
California Pacific Medical Center
Clinical Professor of Orthopedic Surgery
University of California at San Francisco
San Francisco, California

JAMES M. GLICK, MD

Associate Clinical Professor of
Orthopedics
University of California at San Francisco
San Francisco, California

CHARLES P. HO, MD, PHD

Medical Director, Bayside and Sandhill Imaging
Centers
Clinical Assistant Professor of Radiology
Stanford University School of Medicine
Palo Alto, California
Medical Director
National Orthopaedic Imaging Associates
San Francisco, California

LOUIS KEPPLER, MD

Chief Orthopaedic Surgeon for the Cleveland
Indians
Senior Partner, Huron Orthopaedics
Cleveland, Ohio

DAVID M. LICHTMAN, MD

Professor of Orthopedic Surgery
Chief, Division of Orthopaedic Surgery
Baylor College of Medicine
Houston, Texas

MATHIAS MASEM, MD

Clinical Instructor in Orthopaedic Surgery
University of California at San Francisco
San Francisco, California
Chief, Department of Orthopaedic Surgery
Summit Hospital Medical Center
Oakland, California

DAVID W. STOLLER, MD

Director, California Advanced Imaging/
Raytel Medical Imaging
Director, Marin Radiology and National Orthopedic
Imaging Associates
Assistant Clinical Professor of Radiology
University of California at San Francisco
San Francisco, California

EUGENE M. WOLF, MD

Department of Orthopedics
California Pacific Medical Center
San Francisco, California

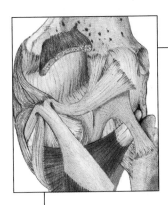

FOREWORD

The impetus for recent advances in the application of magnetic resonance imaging and arthroscopy to the diagnosis and management of orthopaedic injuries is grounded in a fundamental understanding of anatomy. When an orthopaedic surgeon approaches a problem, experience and knowledge of surgical anatomy are the basis for planning an appropriate surgical approach, for visualizing the internal pathology and surrounding structures, and for dissection of the area through suitable planes. The use of MRI enables the surgeon to have a global view (both intra- and extra-articular) of pathology in and around the joint, allowing a more refined treatment strategy and planning of precise surgical procedures based on accurate assessment and diagnosis. Use of MRI as a diagnostic tool allows the surgeon to look at different anatomic structures in a given area, any of which may be causing the symptoms which brought about the need for treatment. If the treatment plan is for open surgery, these areas may not be visible through the incision. If arthroscopic surgery is performed, the extra-articular tissues cannot be visualized. The advent of MRI, therefore, has promoted more precise surgical treatment and a more accurate approach to the injured area.

Dr. Stoller is to be congratulated for assembling a superb group of orthopaedic collaborators, each highly respected in his respective area of specialization. This atlas, *MRI, Arthroscopy, and Surgical Anatomy of the Joints* represents the first successful integration of the combined knowledge of advanced imaging in orthopaedics, using both arthroscopy and anatomic dissection as the gold standard. Particularly impressive is the incorporation of new concepts of articular anatomy as refined and validated by meticulous correlation between MR studies with arthroscopy and surgical dissection. Each of the six chapters of the book (which systematically examines all of the appendicular joints) includes a section on the orthopaedic perspective, which provides important insights into the clinical applications of arthroscopy and descriptions of surgical anatomy. The coverage of normal MR anatomy is extremely comprehensive and the sophisticated labeling of the MR images adds immeasurably to their usefulness. The use of high resolution techniques allows the depiction of superficial and deep capsular structures, once thought not visible by advanced imaging techniques. Each MR image is accompanied by orientation bars and an inset reference image to show the image location.

The color illustrations, developed and rendered by Drs. Stoller and Beltran, represent an insightful collection of detailed orthopaedic anatomic illustrations incorporating the latest breakthroughs in arthroscopic and surgical anatomy. The high level of detail in these outstanding renderings bridges the gap between traditional anatomy references and currently available reports of clinical research. Color illustrations such as these—depicting and explaining such concepts as the biceps labral complex, the inferior glenohumeral ligament complex, the tibial slip, and the popliteofibular ligament—are not available in any other single anatomy atlas resource.

In the second edition of *Magnetic Resonance Imaging in Orthopaedics and Sports Medicine,* Dr. Stoller provided orthopaedic surgeons and radiologists with the most comprehensive MRI text available. This text—*MRI, Arthroscopy, and Surgical Anatomy of the Joints*—too, will become an indispensable reference for radiologists, orthopaedic surgeons, and any specialists involved in the diagnosis and treatment of musculoskeletal injuries.

J. Richard Steadman, M.D.
Clinical Professor of Orthopaedic Surgery
University of Texas Southwestern Medical School
Director, Steadman–Hawkins Clinic
Vail, Colorado
Chairman, Medical Group for the
United States Ski Team

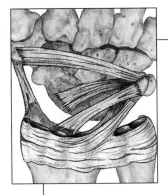

PREFACE

The creation of this atlas *MRI, Arthroscopy, and Surgical Anatomy of the Joints* represents a special collaboration between the fields of Radiology and Orthopaedics. This atlas is an extension of many of the concepts developed in the second edition of *MRI in Orthopaedics and Sports Medicine,* combined with an extensive database of MR images, arthroscopy, and surgical dissections performed on over two hundred anatomic specimens during the last six years.

Each of the six chapters in the atlas is divided into four sections (1) an orthopaedic perspective, (2) normal MR anatomy, (3) color anatomic illustrations, and (4) a correlative presentation using material from MR, arthroscopy, and gross anatomic dissections.

In each chapter, the orthopaedic perspective is based on the tenets of the orthopaedist who performed the arthroscopic and surgical dissections, providing continuity between the overview and specific arthroscopic and surgical concepts. For example, Dr. Dye's perspective on the superficial layers of the knee is reflected in his surgical dissection of the arciform fascia and intermediate oblique layers in the anterior exposure of the knee as well as in the meticulous dissection of the medial structures of the knee, including the semimembranosus branches, the posterior oblique ligament, and the medial collateral ligament.

In the second section, phased array coils were used to obtain images for all six joints and normal MR anatomy was then labeled in three separate planes.

The color illustrations for each joint represent the marriage of current anatomic concepts with information based on our experience with MR, arthroscopy, and surgical dissections. This collaboration is especially evident in the following instances:

- in the shoulder chapter, in the discussion and illustrations of the biceps labral complex and capsulolabral anatomy
- in the elbow chapter, in the illustrations depicting the lateral ulnar collateral ligament and the medial collateral ligament complex
- in the wrist chapter, in the depiction of the volar carpal and dorsal carpal ligaments
- in the hip chapter, in the detailed depiction of the capsular and ligamentous anatomy

    • in the knee chapter, in the depiction of the posteromedial structures and the posterolateral anatomy, including current concepts such as the depiction of the popliteofibular ligament

    • in the ankle chapter, in incorporating Dr. Ferkel's concepts of soft tissue impingement sites and in showing the relationships among the posterior ankle ligaments (the inferior tibiofibular ligament, the transverse tibiofibular ligament, and the tibial slip).

The final section of each chapter correlating MR, arthroscopy, and surgical perspectives provides a direct comparison between anatomy and arthroscopy with dissection. The mastery of the orthopaedists collaborating on the book is especially evident in this section, which directly compares anatomic structures from all three modalities.

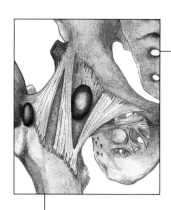

ACKNOWLEDGMENTS

I would like to acknowledge the contributions of the following individuals whose work is much appreciated.

Salvador Beltran, MD, an exceptionally talented illustrator whose genius made possible the rendering of anatomic concepts developed from MR, arthroscopy, and surgical anatomic study into color illustrations.

David M. Lichtman, MD, for Figure 3-59E demonstrating the intrinsic scapholunate ligament complex, and for modifications of illustrations showing the ligaments of the ulnar side of the carpus (from Lichtman, DM and Alexander, AH. *The Wrist and its Disorders,* Second Edition. W.B. Saunders, 1997.) **Richard D. Ferkel, MD,** for Figure 6-78D, E, and F; Figure 6-79E; Figure 6-81D and E; Figure 6-84 B and E; Figure 6-85E; Figure 6-87B; Figure 6-89A, B, C, and D; Figure 6-90A, B, and C; Figure 6-91A and B; Figure 6-92A and B; Table 6-1; and for illustrations for the orthopaedic perspective section of Chapter 6 from his text, *Arthroscopic Surgery of the Foot and Ankle* (Lippincott-Raven Publishers, 1996). **S.J. Snyder** and **S.L. Kollias** for adaptation of their classification of variations in labral anatomy into types A and B (from Detrisac's work as described in Andrews, JR and Timmerman, LA. *Diagnostic and Operative Arthroscopy.* W.B. Saunders, 1997.)

Chris G. Goumas, MD, for his invaluable assistance and collaboration in MR imaging of cadaveric joint specimens. **Carolin Elmquist, RT,** for her dedication and superior performance as Chief Technologist in performing MR examinations and filming of all anatomic joint specimens. **Gregory Ondera** and **William Vogler** of Insight Surgical Productions for their meticulous and professional camera work in recording all arthroscopic and surgical procedures used in this atlas. **Geneva Wright, RT; Diar Shipman,** and **Morry Blumenfeld, PhD,** of General Electric, for their support of the educational endeavors requisite to the development of the basic science and clinical research material. **Tom Shubert,** of MRI Devices, for the development of prototype phased array coils which greatly facilitated high resolution joint imaging. **Al Smoot,** of Stryker, for use of both his time and equipment to record arthroscopic and surgical procedures.

I would also like to express my appreciation to **Lauri Hafvenstein,** who was the initial force behind the preparation of the color arthroscopic and surgical dissections as converted from electronic to print media. Her interest in this project was a cornerstone for its successful completion. Thanks also go to **Kevin Taylor,** for careful quality control and preparation of the color arthroscopic and surgical dissection images. Kevin was instrumental in the development of the CD-ROM version of the atlas.

Thanks also go to **Katherine Pitcoff,** who served as West Coast editor, for superb development of the manuscript for presentation to the publishers; **Alicia Amodio** for meticulous typing of the manuscript; **Andrea Weisfield** for administrative activities required for the exchange of information and material with the publisher; and **Karma Raines** for assistance in preparing MR images for labeling.

I would also like to acknowledge the contribution of the Palo Alto Clinic and California Advanced Imaging for use of their MR facilities. Thanks also go to Kodak for their donation of laser camera film and Image Enhancement for use of their equipment in post image processing.

The staff of Lippincott-Raven Publishers, notably **Jim Ryan,** Editor-in-Chief; **Carol Field,** Director of Development; **Delois Patterson,** Senior Development Editor; **Cassie Moore,** Associate Director, Production; **Diana Andrews,** Creative Director; and **Vicky Alex,** Vice President of Medical Worldwide Sales and Marketing also deserve acknowledgment for their support of this project and appreciation of the necessary quality required to bring this textbook to completion.

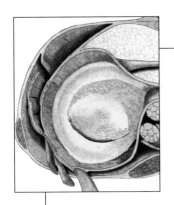

CONTENTS

MRI, ARTHROSCOPY, AND SURGICAL ANATOMY OF THE JOINTS

C H A P T E R 1

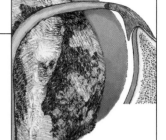

THE SHOULDER

David W. Stoller
Eugene M. Wolf
Salvador Beltran
Javier Beltran

SHOULDER ARTHROSCOPY AND
DISSECTION
MR NORMAL ANATOMY

COLOR ANATOMIC ILLUSTRATIONS
MR, ARTHROSCOPY, AND
SURGICAL DISSECTION

—————— SHOULDER ARTHROSCOPY ——————

ANATOMIC LANDMARKS FOR SHOULDER ARTHROSCOPY include the anterior acromion, the coracoacromial ligament, the coracoid, and the distal clavicle. Arthroscopy of the shoulder begins with the posterior portal as the standard portal. The posterior portal is created 1 cm medial and 2 cm distal to the posterolateral corner of the acromion. The anterior portal is located inferior and lateral to the coracoid. The posterior and anterior portals are commonly used standard portals in shoulder arthroscopy. A superior portal (the Neviaser portal) is an accessory portal located in the lateral aspect or corner of the supraspinatus fossa. This portal can be used to access the biceps labral complex. The lateral portal (lateral to the acromial edge) is used for bursoscopy.

The glenohumeral joint is entered by palpating the posterior rim of the glenoid and puncturing the joint capsule. A 4 mm arthroscope is placed into a 5 mm cannula. An additional portal is created for outflow through a retrograde cannula. The arthroscope has a 30° angle, which allows the examiner to look down at the glenoid from the biceps tendon, at 12 o'clock, to the most inferior portion of the labrum, at the 6 o'clock position. Frequently there is a sublabral foramen, which is located above the kidney bean-shaped indentation, the equator, of the anterior glenoid. The biceps tendon contributes to the posterior labrum at the biceps labral complex. The inferior glenohumeral ligament (IGL) consists of an anterior band (AB), which is contiguous with the anterior labrum, the axillary pouch (AP), and the posterior band (PB).

The inferior sling created by the IGL is key to the stability of the glenohumeral joint. The labrum deepens the glenoid by approximately 50% and is firmly attached to the glenoid rim. Bankart lesions, glenoid avulsions of the labrum, occur from six o'clock to two or three o'clock, where the gleno-humeral ligament labral complex is avulsed. SLAP lesions (superior labrum from anterior to posterior lesions) occur at the biceps labral complex at the level of the superior glenoid. Although SLAP lesions are rare from a symptomatic standpoint, they represent a common intraarticular finding. The biceps and labrum may split (SLAP Types III and IV) so that there is a bucket handle tear extending superiorly into the biceps tendon. The junction between the articular cartilage and labrum may be difficult to visualize.

There is normally a bare spot where the rotator cuff inserts on the humeral head. A transverse band or capsular ligament reinforces the rotator cuff as it runs from the posterior end, under the infraspinatus, to the rotator cuff interval anteriorly. This represents the rotator cable-crescent complex, as described by Burkart. The rotator cable is a thickening of the coracohumeral ligament, which extends from the biceps tendon across the supraspinatus and infraspinatus insertions to the inferior border of the infraspinatus. The rotator crescent, which lies within the avascular zone of the cuff, spans from the rotator cable to the greater tuberosity.

A switching stick is used to gain access to the joint from an anterior approach by switching from a posterior to an anterior portal. The middle glenohumeral ligament (MGL) crosses anterior to the subscapularis tendon. The subscapularis bursa extends medially along the anterior face of the scapula. The foramen of Weitbrecht, an opening in the subscapularis bursa, is located between the MGL and the superior glenohumeral ligament (SGL). The foramen of Rouviere communicates with the subscapularis bursa between the MGL and the IGL. Thus, these two foramina are located anterior and posterior to the MGL. The tendinous bands of the SGL run from a point on the lesser tuberosity to the glenoid, just anterior to the biceps and contiguous with the superior labrum. The equator of the glenoid, located at a nine o'clock position, determines whether labral detachment is normal or abnormal. Superior to the equator there may be a communication between the joint underneath the labrum and the MGL. For example, a Type 3 biceps labral complex (BLC), with a meniscoid superior labrum, is associated with a sublabral foramen. A Type 3 BLC may be more susceptible to developing a bucket handle tear, because of its meniscoid morphology.

The subacromial space is anterior to the acromion. Anatomically the subacromial space is primarily deltoid in location. The acromial surface is covered by fat and synovium. In the impingement syndrome, the coracoacromial (CA) ligament becomes eroded and frayed. The CA ligament, composed of two bands that run medially, drifts down anteriorly and medially toward the coracoid. Kissing lesions, with erosion of the CA ligament or acromial side of the cuff, are common, since the CA ligament is compressed between the rotator cuff and the acromion above. The rotator cuff has a synovial covering on both its bursal and articular surfaces.

SURGICAL DISSECTION OF THE SHOULDER

The acromion and location of the posterior portal are identified prior to surgical dissection. The acromion is primarily located posterior to the glenohumeral joint, and the infraspinatus and teres minor are located underneath the posterior margin of the deltoid. The skin is split down to the deltoid muscle, and the deltoid is removed from the lateral border of the acromion. (In clinical practice, deltoid fibers cannot be surgically cut without damaging the function of the deltoid muscle.) The acromioclavicular (AC) joint is then resected, including the distal clavicle and facet on the anterior acromion. The conoid and trapezoid components of the coracoclavicular ligament are divided. Although the coracoclavicular ligament is not part of the acromioclavicular joint, it functions to hold the clavicle in contact with the acromion.

A deltoid splitting approach is usually used to open the subacromial bursa. The lateral extent of the subacromial bursa is a critical surgical landmark, because the axillary nerve is always distal to the bursa. Normally, the subacromial bursa extends laterally, superior to the surface of the supraspinatus and superior infraspinatus tendons, to the level of the greater tuberosity. The posterior boundary of the subacromial bursa extends to the supraspinatus muscle and tendon and the superior aspect of the infraspinatus muscle and tendon. The anterior surface of the bursa is adjacent to the inferior surfaces of the acromion, the coracoacromial ligament, and the origin of the midportion of the deltoid muscle. Anteromedially, the subacromial bursa is adjacent to the deep surface of the acromioclavicular joint. The deltoid split is carried out to the inferior extent of the subacromial bursa. The axillary nerve is not located underneath the subacromial bursa. The subacromial-subdeltoid bursa is primarily situated underneath the deltoid muscle.

The deltoid split is an important part of the mini-open approach. The deltoid is divided into three parts with an anterior and posterior raphe. The cut coracoclavicular ligament remnant can be seen because the distal clavicle is resected. The coracoacromial ligament is a bifid ligament that originates from the lateral edge of the body and tip of the coracoid and inserts along the inferior surface of the acromion. The insertion is broad and extends along the undersurface of the anterior acromion and lateral acromion and terminates on the undersurface of the posterolateral acromion. In subacromial decompression, the coracoacromial ligament is cut from the anterior margin of the acromion to reduce compressive forces. The anterior lip of the acromion is removed with a burr on the undersurface. A fibrofatty area covers the surface of the acromion. Spurring is seen in the end stages of impingement. Cartilage metaplasia and endochondral bone formation may produce thickening on the inferior surface of the acromion.

The pectoralis major is removed to expose the biceps tendon. The biceps tendon is not readily palpable underneath the transverse ligament and deltoid. The origin of the tendon and the long head of the biceps is on the superior glenoid (the supraglenoid tubercle). The biceps tendon exits the joint in a hiatus between the subscapularis and supraspinatus tendons and runs in the intertubercular groove underneath the transverse humeral ligament. At the level of the superior pole of the glenoid, four separate attachments of the biceps tendon can be identified. These attachments include (1) the supraglenoid tubercle, (2) the posterior superior labrum, (3) the anterior superior labrum, and (4) an extraarticular attachment to the lateral edge of the base of the coracoid process. The BLC corresponds to the superior one-third of the glenoid. Superior to the epiphyseal line, or equator, of the glenoid, mobility of the anterior labrum or communication with the subscapularis bursa is normal. There are three different types of attachment of the BLC to the glenoid:

Type 1: The BLC is firmly adherent to the superior pole of the glenoid and there is no sublabral foramen in the anterosuperior quadrant.

- **Type 2:** The BLC is attached several millimeters medial to the sagittal plane of the glenoid and the superior pole of the glenoid continues its hyaline cartilage surface medially under the labrum. This configuration has a small sulcus at the superior pole of the glenoid that may be continuous with a sublabral foramen and communicate with the subscapularis bursa.

- **Type 3:** The labrum is meniscoid in shape and has a large sulcus that projects under the labrum and over the cartilaginous pole of the glenoid.

The rotator cuff includes the tendons of the supraspinatus, infraspinatus, teres minor, and subscapularis muscles. The rotator cuff becomes conjoined as the individual tendons blend together at the level of the glenoid and approach their insertion on the greater tuberosity. The supraspinatus inserts on the superior facet of the greater tuberosity, posterior to the biceps tendon. The rotator cuff is split in the area of the rotator cuff interval, which corresponds to the superior glenohumeral ligament. There is a plane between the supraspinatus and infraspinatus muscles. The capsule and rotator cuff muscles are static stabilizers that compress the humeral head onto the glenoid. In multidirectional instability, improvement in rotator cuff function prior to surgical reduction of capsular volume is key in successful rehabilitation. The joint capsule is adherent to the cuff in its lateral one-third. The subscapularis tendon inserts onto the lesser tuberosity, medial to the bicipital groove. Like all rotator cuff muscles, the subscapularis has a conjoined insertion. Only the superior portion of the subscapularis tendon is intraarticular. The subscapularis tendon is located on the anterior aspect of the anterior joint capsule, whereas the subscapularis bursa is found on the posterior aspect of the subscapularis muscle. This bursa extends from the glenohumeral joint to below the base of the coracoid process. Superiorly the subscapularis tendon is primarily tendinous; inferiorly it is primarily muscular. Removal of the subscapularis tendon from the lesser tuberosity is the standard open approach for visualization of the glenohumeral joint.

The superior glenohumeral ligament has its origin on the humeral neck of the medial aspect of the intertubercular groove (the lesser tuberosity). In a plane perpendicular to the middle glenohumeral ligament, the superior glenohumeral ligament curves anteriorly and superiorly and inserts on the anterior superior glenoid labrum and the base of the coracoid process. Fibers of the superior glenohumeral ligament may join directly with the middle glenohumeral ligament or the anterior band of the IGL, adjacent to the anterior superior glenoid articular surface. The coracohumeral ligament, an extraarticular structure, crosses over the middle portion of the superior glenohumeral ligament. The coracohumeral ligament has its origin on the medial aspect of the greater tuberosity and courses anteromedially to insert on the coracoid process.

The origin of the MGL is on the anterior humeral neck, medial to the lesser tuberosity. It inserts medially on the superior half of the bony glenoid and scapular neck. The MGL extends anteriorly and medially from the lesser tuberosity towards its glenoid attachment and creates a plane between the anterior band of the IGL or anterior labrum and the subscapularis muscle and tendon. The MGL crosses the posterior surface of the intraarticular portion of the subscapularis tendon. The anterior capsule and foramen of Weitbrecht are anterior to the MGL and subscapularis tendon. The foramen of Rouviere is posterior to the MGL. It is normal for the articular cartilage of the glenoid to get thinner towards the center of the glenoid fossa. The concavity of the articular cartilage is further accentuated as it extends onto the glenoid labrum. The glenoid is 3½ cm long and 2 cm wide. The Bankart lesion occurs from nine o'clock to six o'clock, where glenohumeral ligament labral avulsions occur. This area of labral tearing produces instability.

The IGL is composed of an anterior band, an axillary pouch, and a posterior band. The axillary pouch originates from the anatomic neck of the humerus on the inferior one-third of the humeral head and inserts along the inferior two-thirds of the glenoid. Axillary pouch fibers insert into the peripheral border of the labrum and the edge of the glenoid articular cartilage. The anterior band may vary in thickness, from a thin leading edge of the IGL to a thick redundant band. The anterior and posterior bands extend superiorly to join the labrum. The MGL attaches to the biceps labral complex. The SGL courses from the superior humeral anatomic neck to the edge of the superior pole of the glenoid, just anterior to the biceps tendon. The labrum and cartilage produce thickening both at the edge of the glenoid and deep in the glenoid concavity, which is congruent with the convexity of the humeral head.

SHOULDER: CORONAL OBLIQUE

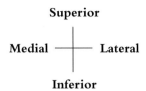

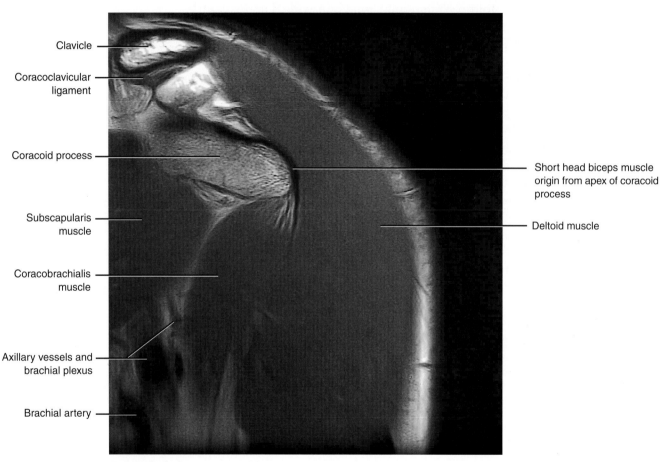

Clavicle

Coracoclavicular ligament

Coracoid process

Subscapularis muscle

Coracobrachialis muscle

Axillary vessels and brachial plexus

Brachial artery

Short head biceps muscle origin from apex of coracoid process

Deltoid muscle

FIGURE 1-1

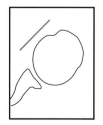

SHOULDER: CORONAL OBLIQUE

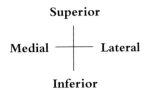

Superior

Medial — | — **Lateral**

Inferior

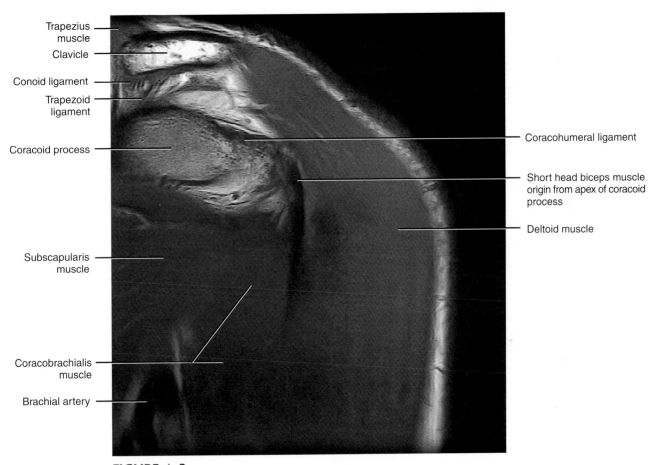

Trapezius muscle

Clavicle

Conoid ligament

Trapezoid ligament

Coracoid process

Subscapularis muscle

Coracobrachialis muscle

Brachial artery

Coracohumeral ligament

Short head biceps muscle origin from apex of coracoid process

Deltoid muscle

FIGURE 1-2

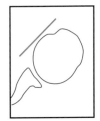

SHOULDER: CORONAL OBLIQUE

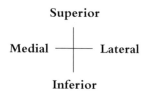

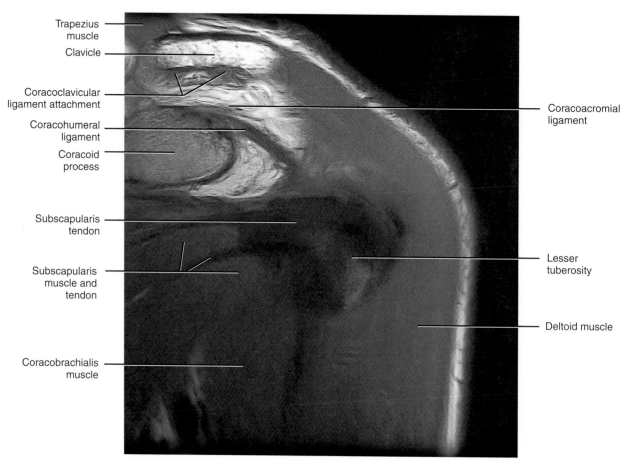

FIGURE 1-3

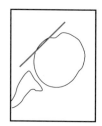

SHOULDER: CORONAL OBLIQUE

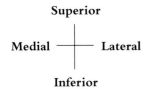

Superior

Medial ——┼—— Lateral

Inferior

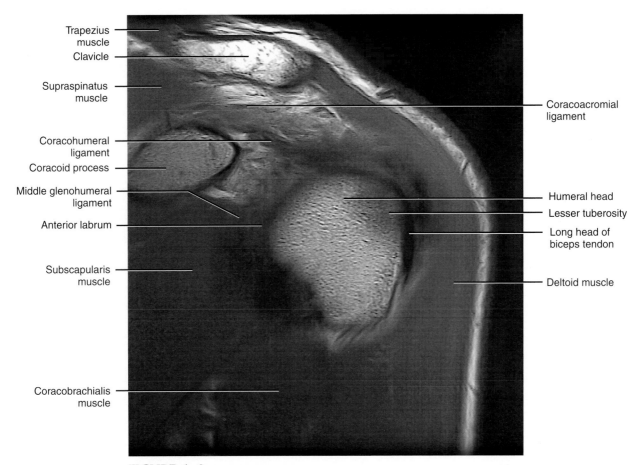

Trapezius muscle

Clavicle

Supraspinatus muscle

Coracoacromial ligament

Coracohumeral ligament

Coracoid process

Middle glenohumeral ligament

Anterior labrum

Humeral head

Lesser tuberosity

Long head of biceps tendon

Subscapularis muscle

Deltoid muscle

Coracobrachialis muscle

FIGURE 1-4

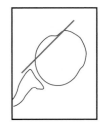

SHOULDER: CORONAL OBLIQUE

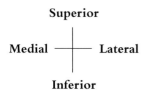

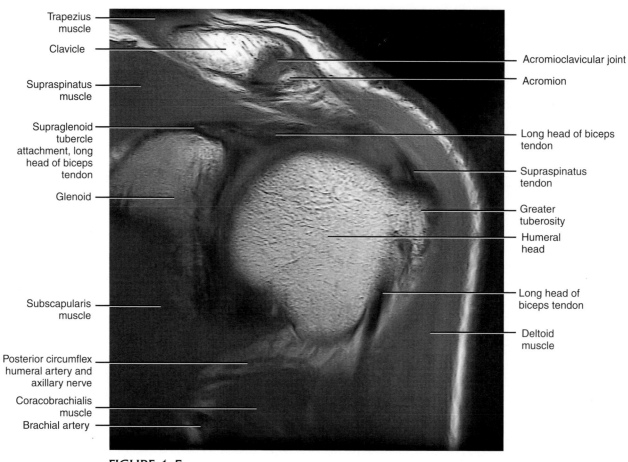

Trapezius muscle

Clavicle

Supraspinatus muscle

Supraglenoid tubercle attachment, long head of biceps tendon

Glenoid

Subscapularis muscle

Posterior circumflex humeral artery and axillary nerve

Coracobrachialis muscle

Brachial artery

Acromioclavicular joint

Acromion

Long head of biceps tendon

Supraspinatus tendon

Greater tuberosity

Humeral head

Long head of biceps tendon

Deltoid muscle

FIGURE 1-5

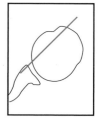

SHOULDER: CORONAL OBLIQUE

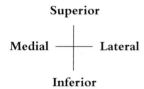

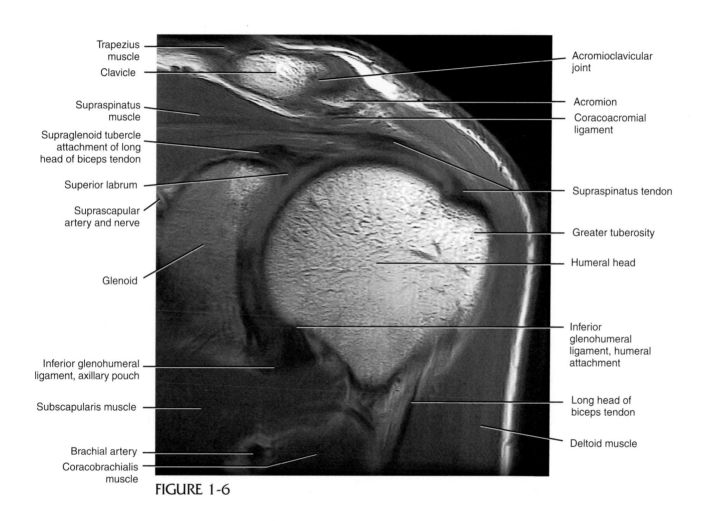

Trapezius muscle

Clavicle

Supraspinatus muscle

Supraglenoid tubercle attachment of long head of biceps tendon

Superior labrum

Suprascapular artery and nerve

Glenoid

Inferior glenohumeral ligament, axillary pouch

Subscapularis muscle

Brachial artery

Coracobrachialis muscle

Acromioclavicular joint

Acromion

Coracoacromial ligament

Supraspinatus tendon

Greater tuberosity

Humeral head

Inferior glenohumeral ligament, humeral attachment

Long head of biceps tendon

Deltoid muscle

FIGURE 1-6

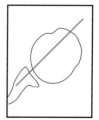

SHOULDER: CORONAL OBLIQUE

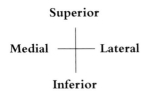

Superior

Medial ——|—— Lateral

Inferior

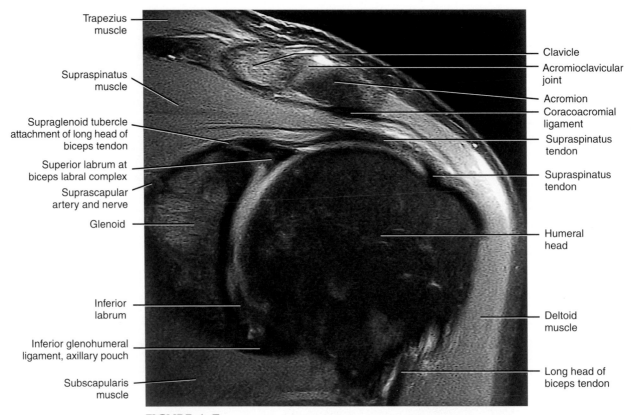

Trapezius muscle

Supraspinatus muscle

Supraglenoid tubercle attachment of long head of biceps tendon

Superior labrum at biceps labral complex

Suprascapular artery and nerve

Glenoid

Inferior labrum

Inferior glenohumeral ligament, axillary pouch

Subscapularis muscle

Clavicle

Acromioclavicular joint

Acromion

Coracoacromial ligament

Supraspinatus tendon

Supraspinatus tendon

Humeral head

Deltoid muscle

Long head of biceps tendon

FIGURE 1-7

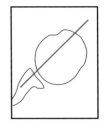

SHOULDER: CORONAL OBLIQUE

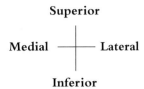

Superior

Medial —|— **Lateral**

Inferior

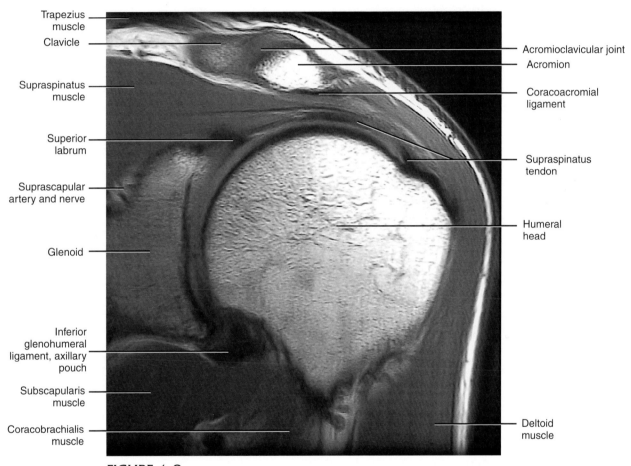

Trapezius muscle

Clavicle

Supraspinatus muscle

Superior labrum

Suprascapular artery and nerve

Glenoid

Inferior glenohumeral ligament, axillary pouch

Subscapularis muscle

Coracobrachialis muscle

Acromioclavicular joint

Acromion

Coracoacromial ligament

Supraspinatus tendon

Humeral head

Deltoid muscle

FIGURE 1-8

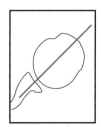

SHOULDER: CORONAL OBLIQUE

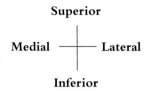

Superior

Medial ⎯⎯⊢⎯⎯ Lateral

Inferior

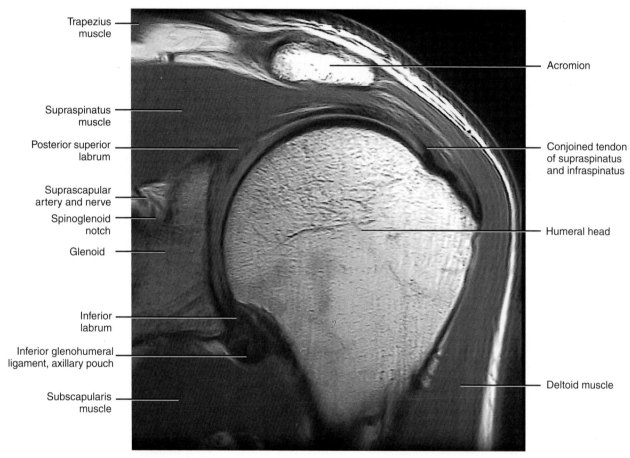

Trapezius muscle

Supraspinatus muscle

Posterior superior labrum

Suprascapular artery and nerve

Spinoglenoid notch

Glenoid

Inferior labrum

Inferior glenohumeral ligament, axillary pouch

Subscapularis muscle

Acromion

Conjoined tendon of supraspinatus and infraspinatus

Humeral head

Deltoid muscle

FIGURE 1-9

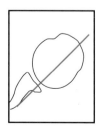

SHOULDER: CORONAL OBLIQUE

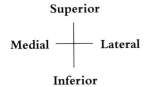

Superior

Medial ——|—— **Lateral**

Inferior

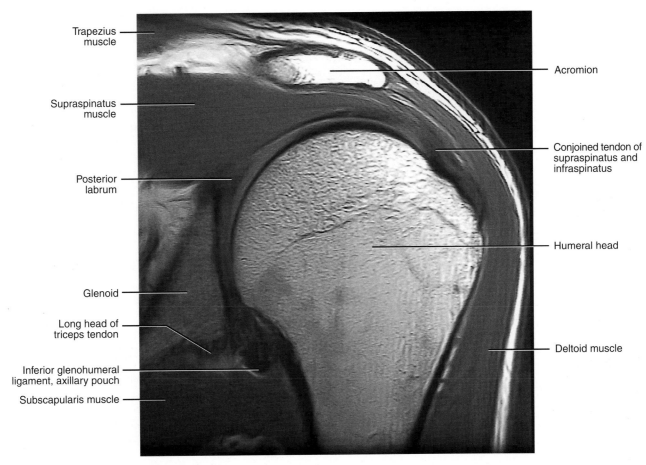

Trapezius muscle

Supraspinatus muscle

Posterior labrum

Glenoid

Long head of triceps tendon

Inferior glenohumeral ligament, axillary pouch

Subscapularis muscle

Acromion

Conjoined tendon of supraspinatus and infraspinatus

Humeral head

Deltoid muscle

FIGURE 1-10

SHOULDER: CORONAL OBLIQUE

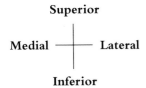

Superior

Medial —┼— Lateral

Inferior

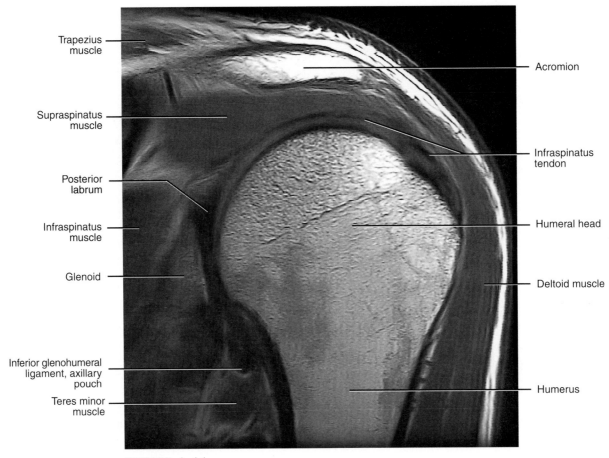

Trapezius muscle

Supraspinatus muscle

Posterior labrum

Infraspinatus muscle

Glenoid

Inferior glenohumeral ligament, axillary pouch

Teres minor muscle

Acromion

Infraspinatus tendon

Humeral head

Deltoid muscle

Humerus

FIGURE 1-11

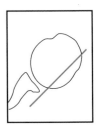

SHOULDER: CORONAL OBLIQUE

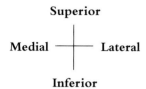

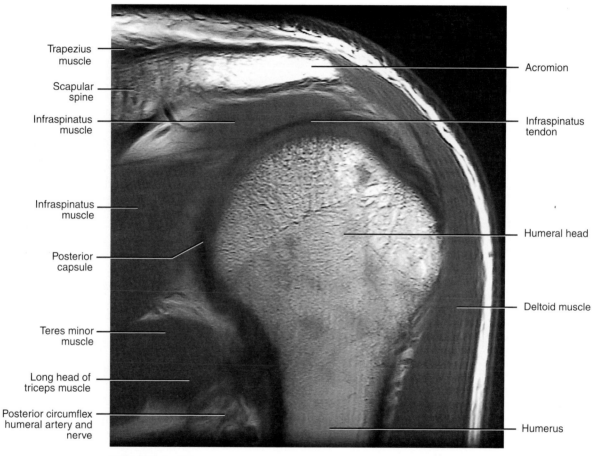

Trapezius muscle

Scapular spine

Infraspinatus muscle

Infraspinatus muscle

Posterior capsule

Teres minor muscle

Long head of triceps muscle

Posterior circumflex humeral artery and nerve

Acromion

Infraspinatus tendon

Humeral head

Deltoid muscle

Humerus

FIGURE 1-12

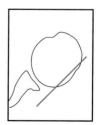

SHOULDER: CORONAL OBLIQUE

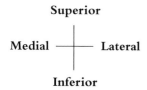

Superior

Medial ─── Lateral

Inferior

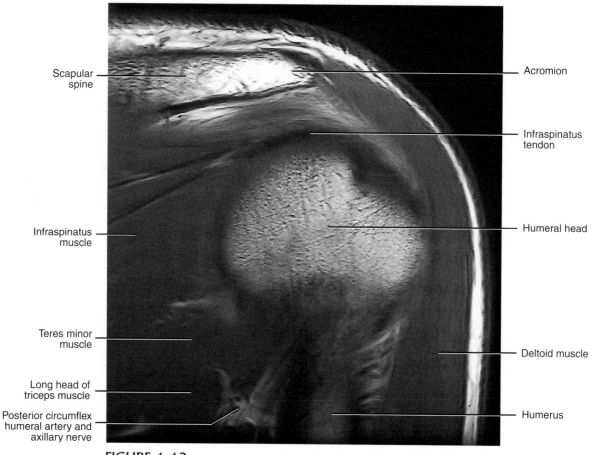

Scapular spine

Acromion

Infraspinatus tendon

Infraspinatus muscle

Humeral head

Teres minor muscle

Long head of triceps muscle

Deltoid muscle

Posterior circumflex humeral artery and axillary nerve

Humerus

FIGURE 1-13

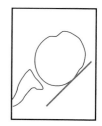

SHOULDER: CORONAL OBLIQUE

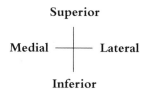

Superior

Medial ——+—— Lateral

Inferior

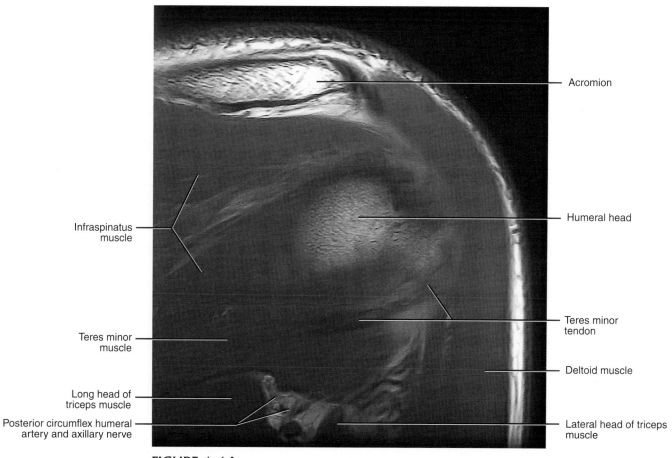

Acromion

Humeral head

Infraspinatus
muscle

Teres minor
tendon

Deltoid muscle

Teres minor
muscle

Long head of
triceps muscle

Posterior circumflex humeral
artery and axillary nerve

Lateral head of triceps
muscle

FIGURE 1-14

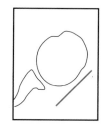

SHOULDER: AXIAL

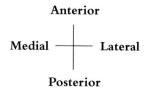

Anterior

Medial ──┼── **Lateral**

Posterior

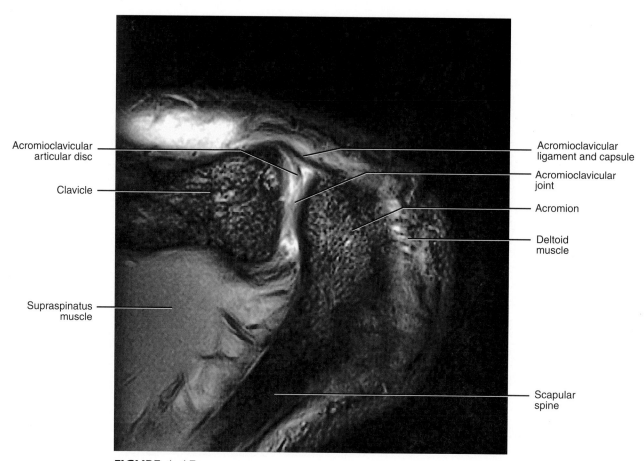

Acromioclavicular
articular disc

Clavicle

Supraspinatus
muscle

Acromioclavicular
ligament and capsule

Acromioclavicular
joint

Acromion

Deltoid
muscle

Scapular
spine

FIGURE 1-15

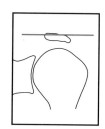

SHOULDER: AXIAL

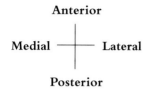

Anterior

Medial ——|—— Lateral

Posterior

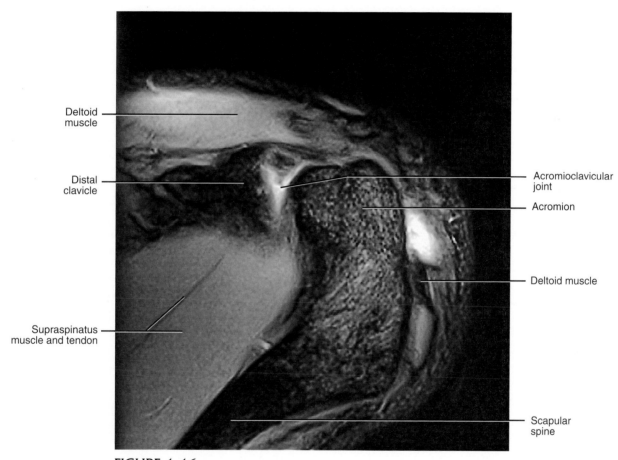

Deltoid muscle

Distal clavicle

Supraspinatus muscle and tendon

Acromioclavicular joint

Acromion

Deltoid muscle

Scapular spine

FIGURE 1-16

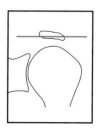

SHOULDER: AXIAL

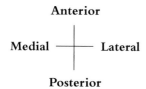

Anterior

Medial —|— Lateral

Posterior

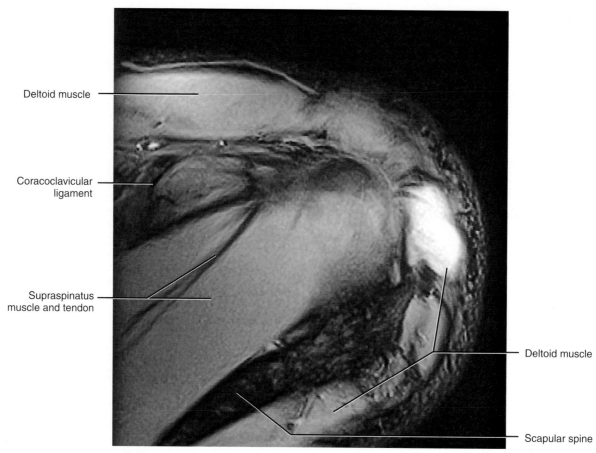

Deltoid muscle

Coracoclavicular
ligament

Supraspinatus
muscle and tendon

Deltoid muscle

Scapular spine

FIGURE 1-17

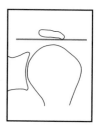

SHOULDER: AXIAL

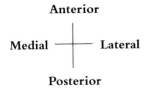

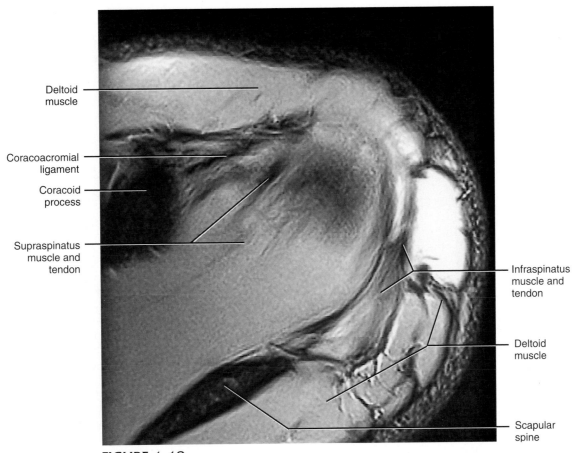

Deltoid muscle

Coracoacromial ligament

Coracoid process

Supraspinatus muscle and tendon

Infraspinatus muscle and tendon

Deltoid muscle

Scapular spine

FIGURE 1-18

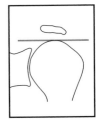

SHOULDER: AXIAL

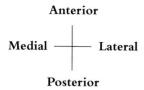

Anterior

Medial —|— **Lateral**

Posterior

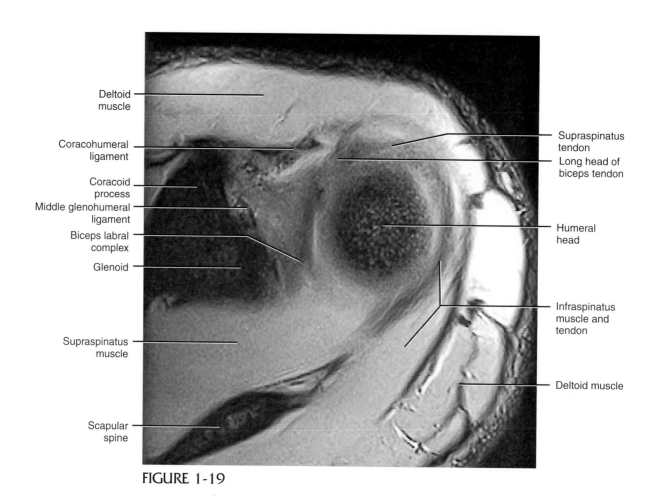

Deltoid muscle

Coracohumeral ligament

Coracoid process

Middle glenohumeral ligament

Biceps labral complex

Glenoid

Supraspinatus muscle

Scapular spine

Supraspinatus tendon

Long head of biceps tendon

Humeral head

Infraspinatus muscle and tendon

Deltoid muscle

FIGURE 1-19

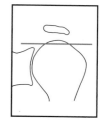

SHOULDER: AXIAL

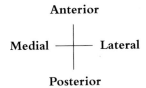

Anterior

Medial — Lateral

Posterior

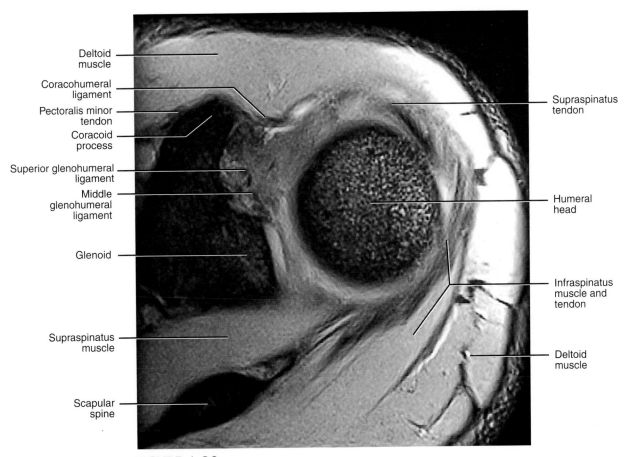

Deltoid muscle

Coracohumeral ligament

Pectoralis minor tendon

Coracoid process

Superior glenohumeral ligament

Middle glenohumeral ligament

Glenoid

Supraspinatus muscle

Scapular spine

Supraspinatus tendon

Humeral head

Infraspinatus muscle and tendon

Deltoid muscle

FIGURE 1-20

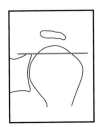

SHOULDER: AXIAL

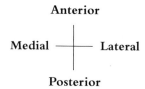

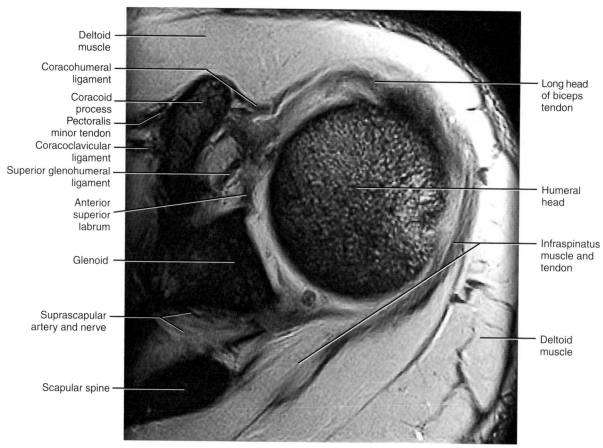

Deltoid muscle

Coracohumeral ligament

Coracoid process

Pectoralis minor tendon

Coracoclavicular ligament

Superior glenohumeral ligament

Anterior superior labrum

Glenoid

Suprascapular artery and nerve

Scapular spine

Long head of biceps tendon

Humeral head

Infraspinatus muscle and tendon

Deltoid muscle

FIGURE 1-21

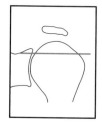

SHOULDER: AXIAL

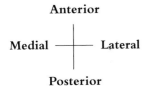

Anterior

Medial ──┼── Lateral

Posterior

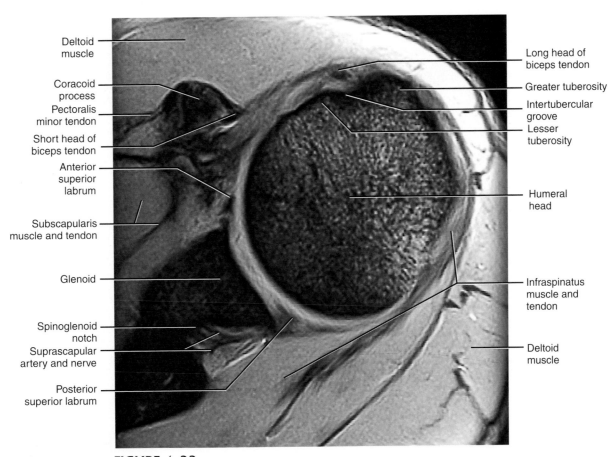

Deltoid muscle

Coracoid process

Pectoralis minor tendon

Short head of biceps tendon

Anterior superior labrum

Subscapularis muscle and tendon

Glenoid

Spinoglenoid notch

Suprascapular artery and nerve

Posterior superior labrum

Long head of biceps tendon

Greater tuberosity

Intertubercular groove

Lesser tuberosity

Humeral head

Infraspinatus muscle and tendon

Deltoid muscle

FIGURE 1-22

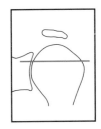

SHOULDER: AXIAL

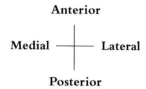

Anterior

Medial ——┼—— Lateral

Posterior

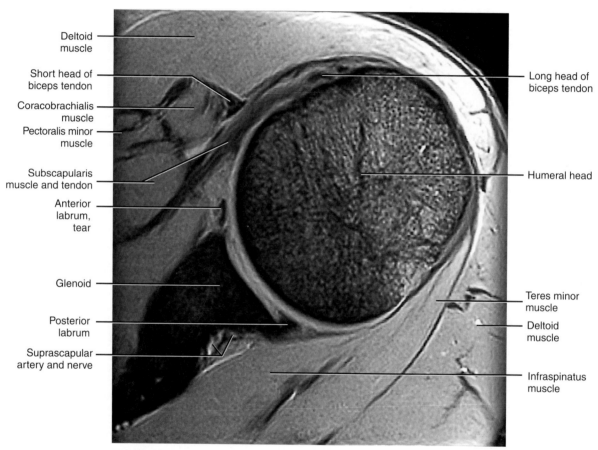

Deltoid
muscle

Short head of
biceps tendon

Coracobrachialis
muscle

Pectoralis minor
muscle

Subscapularis
muscle and tendon

Anterior
labrum,
tear

Glenoid

Posterior
labrum

Suprascapular
artery and nerve

Long head of
biceps tendon

Humeral head

Teres minor
muscle

Deltoid
muscle

Infraspinatus
muscle

FIGURE 1-23

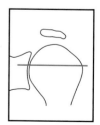

SHOULDER: AXIAL

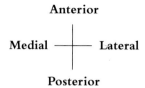

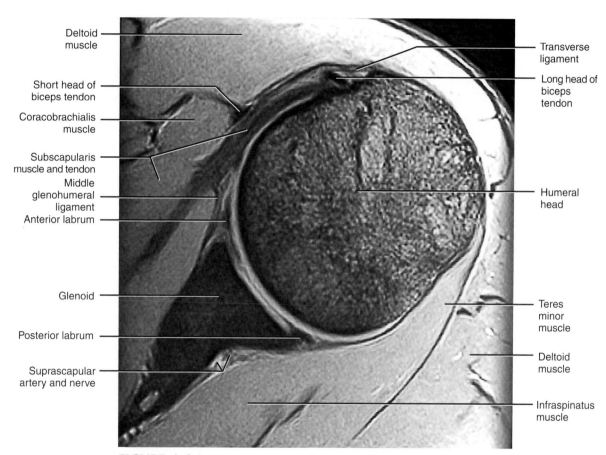

Deltoid muscle

Short head of biceps tendon

Coracobrachialis muscle

Subscapularis muscle and tendon

Middle glenohumeral ligament

Anterior labrum

Glenoid

Posterior labrum

Suprascapular artery and nerve

Transverse ligament

Long head of biceps tendon

Humeral head

Teres minor muscle

Deltoid muscle

Infraspinatus muscle

FIGURE 1-24

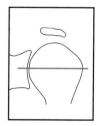

SHOULDER: AXIAL

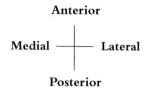

Anterior

Medial ———+——— Lateral

Posterior

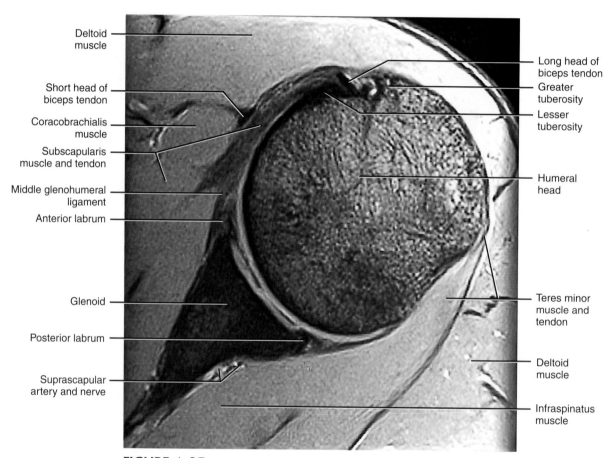

Deltoid muscle

Short head of biceps tendon

Coracobrachialis muscle

Subscapularis muscle and tendon

Middle glenohumeral ligament

Anterior labrum

Glenoid

Posterior labrum

Suprascapular artery and nerve

Long head of biceps tendon

Greater tuberosity

Lesser tuberosity

Humeral head

Teres minor muscle and tendon

Deltoid muscle

Infraspinatus muscle

FIGURE 1-25

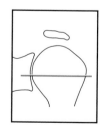

SHOULDER: AXIAL

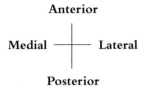

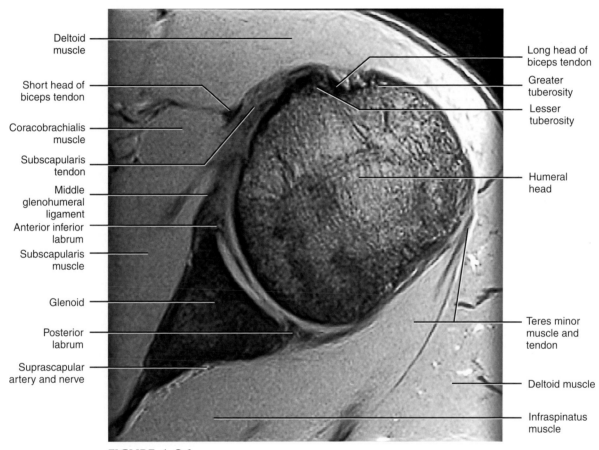

Deltoid muscle

Short head of biceps tendon

Coracobrachialis muscle

Subscapularis tendon

Middle glenohumeral ligament

Anterior inferior labrum

Subscapularis muscle

Glenoid

Posterior labrum

Suprascapular artery and nerve

Long head of biceps tendon

Greater tuberosity

Lesser tuberosity

Humeral head

Teres minor muscle and tendon

Deltoid muscle

Infraspinatus muscle

FIGURE 1-26

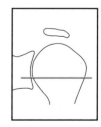

SHOULDER: AXIAL

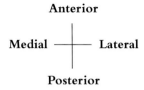

Anterior

Medial —|— Lateral

Posterior

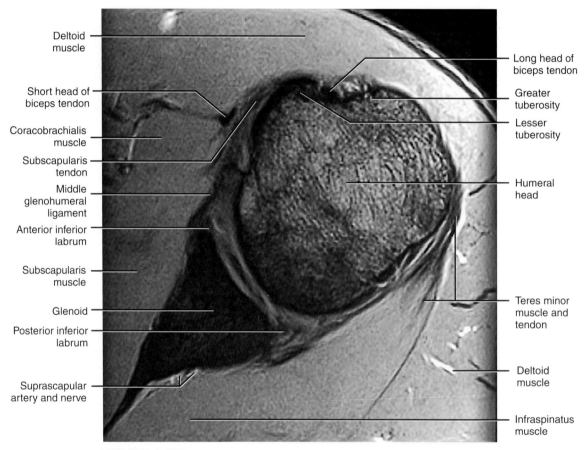

Deltoid muscle

Short head of biceps tendon

Coracobrachialis muscle

Subscapularis tendon

Middle glenohumeral ligament

Anterior inferior labrum

Subscapularis muscle

Glenoid

Posterior inferior labrum

Suprascapular artery and nerve

Long head of biceps tendon

Greater tuberosity

Lesser tuberosity

Humeral head

Teres minor muscle and tendon

Deltoid muscle

Infraspinatus muscle

FIGURE 1-27

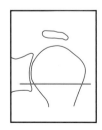

SHOULDER: AXIAL

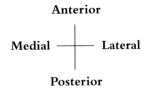

Anterior

Medial ─┼─ Lateral

Posterior

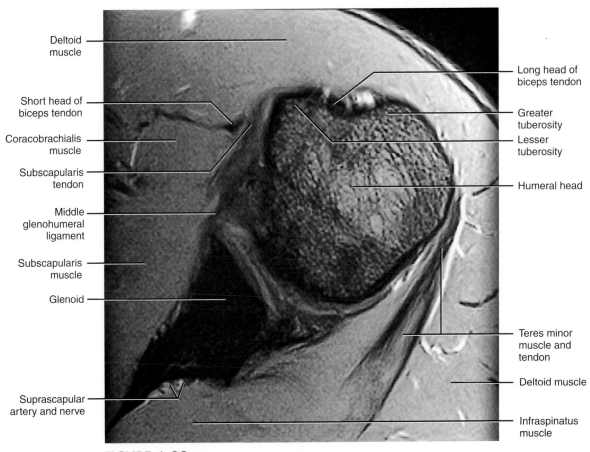

Deltoid muscle

Short head of biceps tendon

Coracobrachialis muscle

Subscapularis tendon

Middle glenohumeral ligament

Subscapularis muscle

Glenoid

Suprascapular artery and nerve

Long head of biceps tendon

Greater tuberosity

Lesser tuberosity

Humeral head

Teres minor muscle and tendon

Deltoid muscle

Infraspinatus muscle

FIGURE 1-28

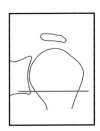

SHOULDER: AXIAL

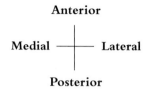

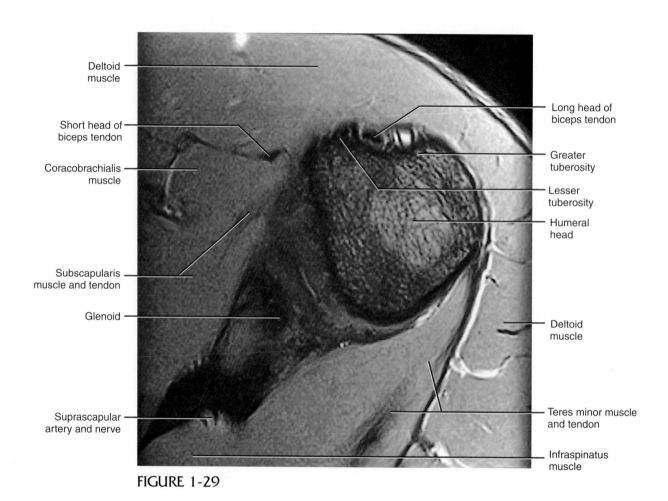

Deltoid muscle

Short head of biceps tendon

Coracobrachialis muscle

Subscapularis muscle and tendon

Glenoid

Suprascapular artery and nerve

Long head of biceps tendon

Greater tuberosity

Lesser tuberosity

Humeral head

Deltoid muscle

Teres minor muscle and tendon

Infraspinatus muscle

FIGURE 1-29

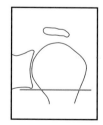

SHOULDER: AXIAL

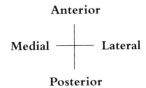

Anterior

Medial ─── **Lateral**

Posterior

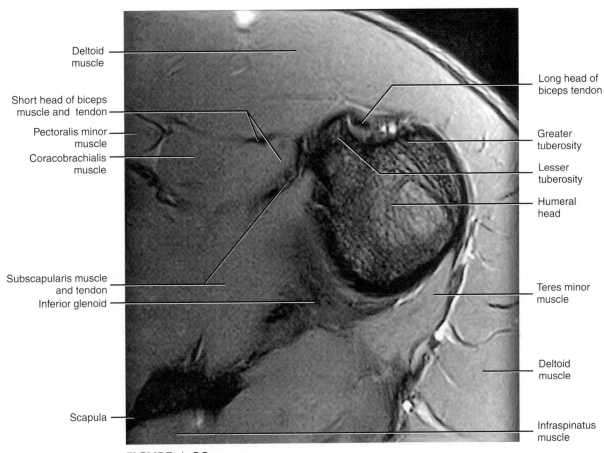

Deltoid muscle

Short head of biceps muscle and tendon

Pectoralis minor muscle

Coracobrachialis muscle

Subscapularis muscle and tendon

Inferior glenoid

Scapula

Long head of biceps tendon

Greater tuberosity

Lesser tuberosity

Humeral head

Teres minor muscle

Deltoid muscle

Infraspinatus muscle

FIGURE 1-30

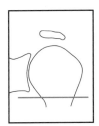

SHOULDER: SAGITTAL OBLIQUE

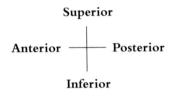

Superior

Anterior ─┼─ Posterior

Inferior

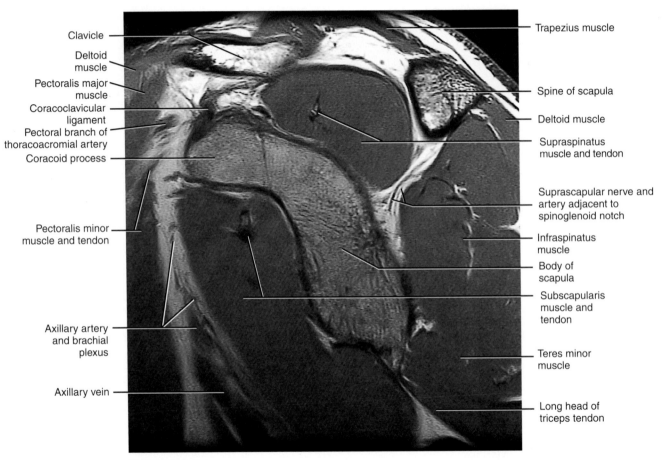

Clavicle

Deltoid muscle

Pectoralis major muscle

Coracoclavicular ligament

Pectoral branch of thoracoacromial artery

Coracoid process

Pectoralis minor muscle and tendon

Axillary artery and brachial plexus

Axillary vein

Trapezius muscle

Spine of scapula

Deltoid muscle

Supraspinatus muscle and tendon

Suprascapular nerve and artery adjacent to spinoglenoid notch

Infraspinatus muscle

Body of scapula

Subscapularis muscle and tendon

Teres minor muscle

Long head of triceps tendon

FIGURE 1-31

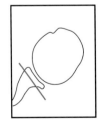

SHOULDER: SAGITTAL OBLIQUE

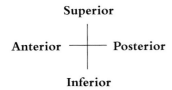

Superior

Anterior ——┼—— **Posterior**

Inferior

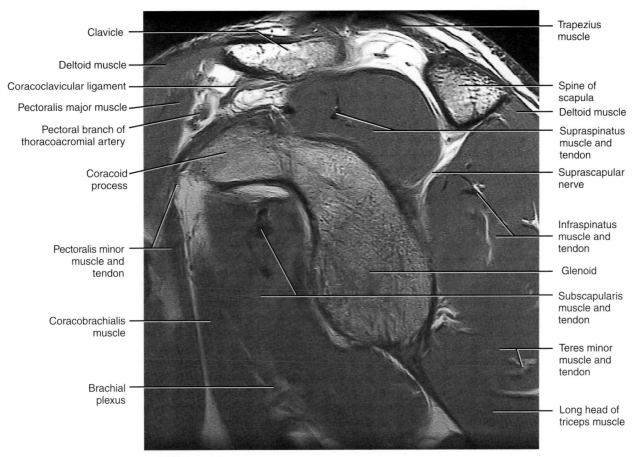

Clavicle

Deltoid muscle

Coracoclavicular ligament

Pectoralis major muscle

Pectoral branch of
thoracoacromial artery

Coracoid
process

Pectoralis minor
muscle and
tendon

Coracobrachialis
muscle

Brachial
plexus

Trapezius
muscle

Spine of
scapula

Deltoid muscle

Supraspinatus
muscle and
tendon

Suprascapular
nerve

Infraspinatus
muscle and
tendon

Glenoid

Subscapularis
muscle and
tendon

Teres minor
muscle and
tendon

Long head of
triceps muscle

FIGURE 1-32

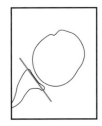

SHOULDER: SAGITTAL OBLIQUE

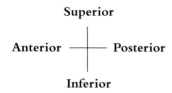

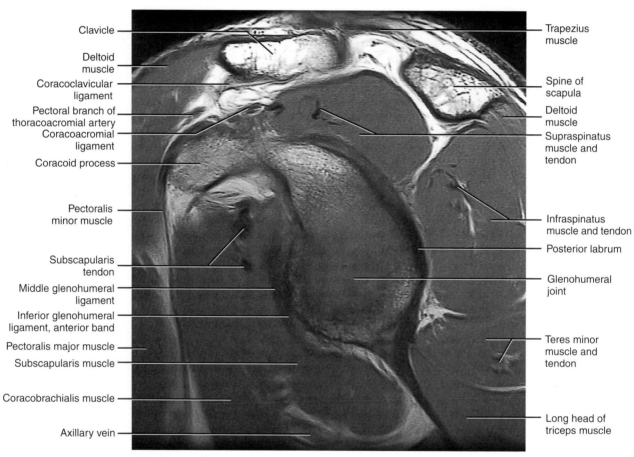

Clavicle

Deltoid muscle

Coracoclavicular ligament

Pectoral branch of thoracoacromial artery

Coracoacromial ligament

Coracoid process

Pectoralis minor muscle

Subscapularis tendon

Middle glenohumeral ligament

Inferior glenohumeral ligament, anterior band

Pectoralis major muscle

Subscapularis muscle

Coracobrachialis muscle

Axillary vein

Trapezius muscle

Spine of scapula

Deltoid muscle

Supraspinatus muscle and tendon

Infraspinatus muscle and tendon

Posterior labrum

Glenohumeral joint

Teres minor muscle and tendon

Long head of triceps muscle

FIGURE 1-33

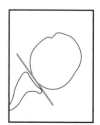

SHOULDER: SAGITTAL OBLIQUE

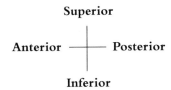

Superior

Anterior ─┼─ Posterior

Inferior

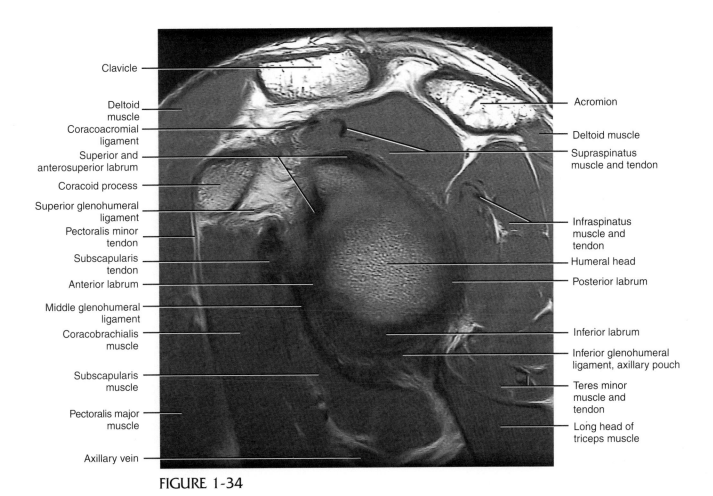

Clavicle

Deltoid muscle

Coracoacromial ligament

Superior and anterosuperior labrum

Coracoid process

Superior glenohumeral ligament

Pectoralis minor tendon

Subscapularis tendon

Anterior labrum

Middle glenohumeral ligament

Coracobrachialis muscle

Subscapularis muscle

Pectoralis major muscle

Axillary vein

Acromion

Deltoid muscle

Supraspinatus muscle and tendon

Infraspinatus muscle and tendon

Humeral head

Posterior labrum

Inferior labrum

Inferior glenohumeral ligament, axillary pouch

Teres minor muscle and tendon

Long head of triceps muscle

FIGURE 1-34

SHOULDER: SAGITTAL OBLIQUE

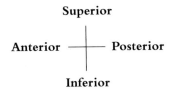

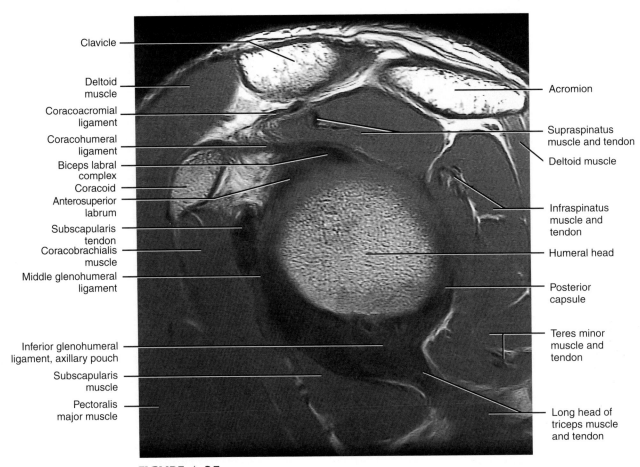

Clavicle

Deltoid muscle

Coracoacromial ligament

Coracohumeral ligament

Biceps labral complex

Coracoid

Anterosuperior labrum

Subscapularis tendon

Coracobrachialis muscle

Middle glenohumeral ligament

Inferior glenohumeral ligament, axillary pouch

Subscapularis muscle

Pectoralis major muscle

Acromion

Supraspinatus muscle and tendon

Deltoid muscle

Infraspinatus muscle and tendon

Humeral head

Posterior capsule

Teres minor muscle and tendon

Long head of triceps muscle and tendon

FIGURE 1-35

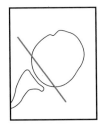

SHOULDER: SAGITTAL OBLIQUE

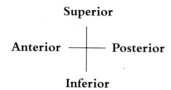

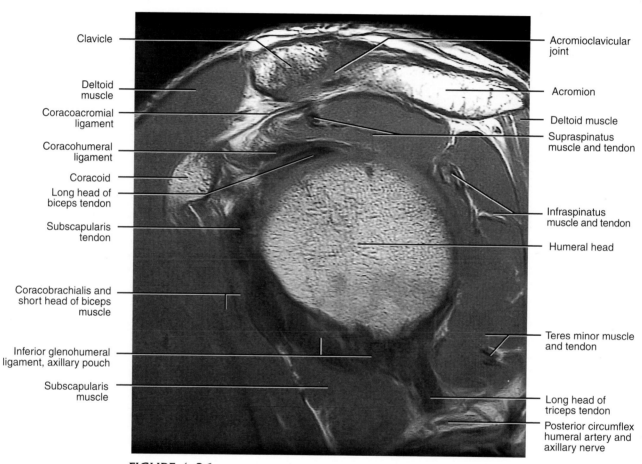

Clavicle

Deltoid muscle

Coracoacromial ligament

Coracohumeral ligament

Coracoid

Long head of biceps tendon

Subscapularis tendon

Coracobrachialis and short head of biceps muscle

Inferior glenohumeral ligament, axillary pouch

Subscapularis muscle

Acromioclavicular joint

Acromion

Deltoid muscle

Supraspinatus muscle and tendon

Infraspinatus muscle and tendon

Humeral head

Teres minor muscle and tendon

Long head of triceps tendon

Posterior circumflex humeral artery and axillary nerve

FIGURE 1-36

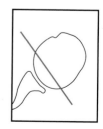

SHOULDER: SAGITTAL OBLIQUE

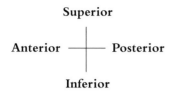

Superior

Anterior ——|—— Posterior

Inferior

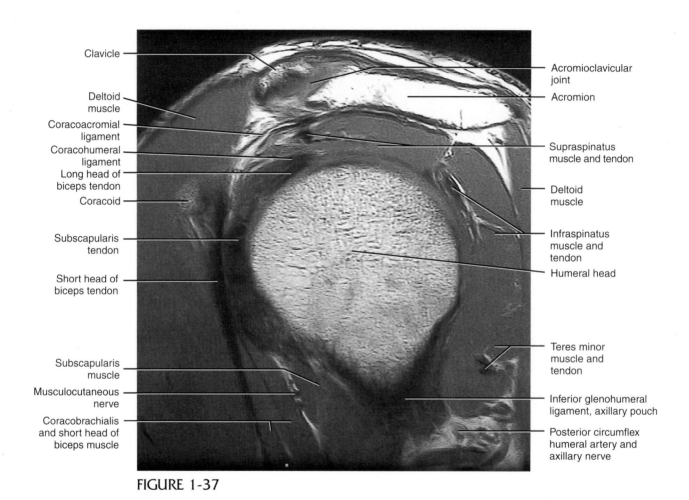

Clavicle

Deltoid muscle

Coracoacromial ligament

Coracohumeral ligament

Long head of biceps tendon

Coracoid

Subscapularis tendon

Short head of biceps tendon

Subscapularis muscle

Musculocutaneous nerve

Coracobrachialis and short head of biceps muscle

Acromioclavicular joint

Acromion

Supraspinatus muscle and tendon

Deltoid muscle

Infraspinatus muscle and tendon

Humeral head

Teres minor muscle and tendon

Inferior glenohumeral ligament, axillary pouch

Posterior circumflex humeral artery and axillary nerve

FIGURE 1-37

SHOULDER: SAGITTAL OBLIQUE

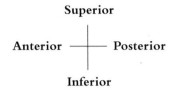

Superior

Anterior ——|—— Posterior

Inferior

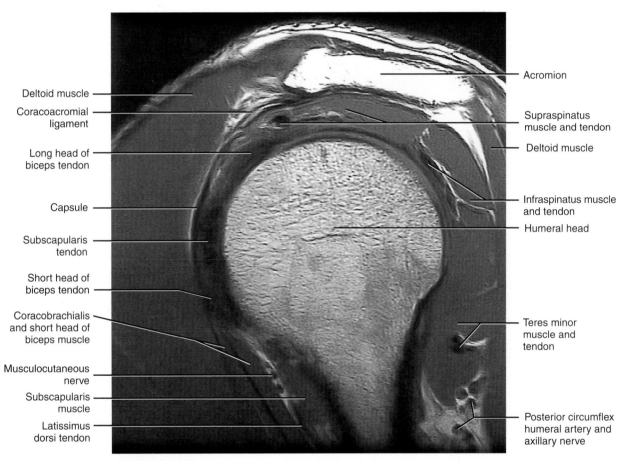

Deltoid muscle

Coracoacromial ligament

Long head of biceps tendon

Capsule

Subscapularis tendon

Short head of biceps tendon

Coracobrachialis and short head of biceps muscle

Musculocutaneous nerve

Subscapularis muscle

Latissimus dorsi tendon

Acromion

Supraspinatus muscle and tendon

Deltoid muscle

Infraspinatus muscle and tendon

Humeral head

Teres minor muscle and tendon

Posterior circumflex humeral artery and axillary nerve

FIGURE 1-38

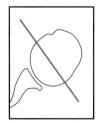

SHOULDER: SAGITTAL OBLIQUE

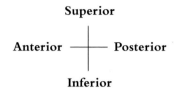

Superior

Anterior ——|—— Posterior

Inferior

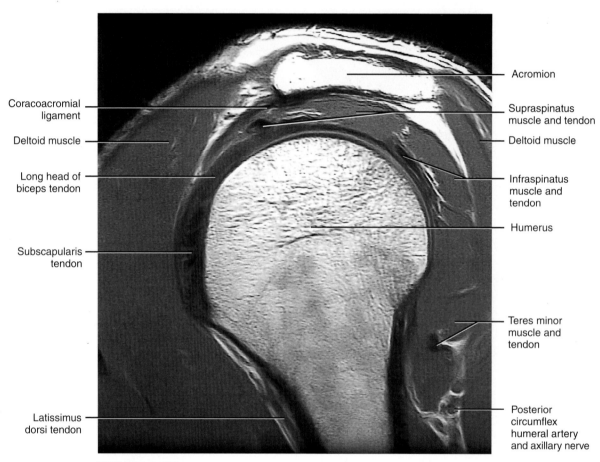

Coracoacromial ligament

Deltoid muscle

Long head of biceps tendon

Subscapularis tendon

Latissimus dorsi tendon

Acromion

Supraspinatus muscle and tendon

Deltoid muscle

Infraspinatus muscle and tendon

Humerus

Teres minor muscle and tendon

Posterior circumflex humeral artery and axillary nerve

FIGURE 1-39

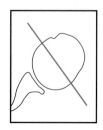

SHOULDER: SAGITTAL OBLIQUE

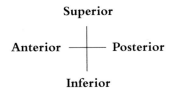

Superior

Anterior —|— **Posterior**

Inferior

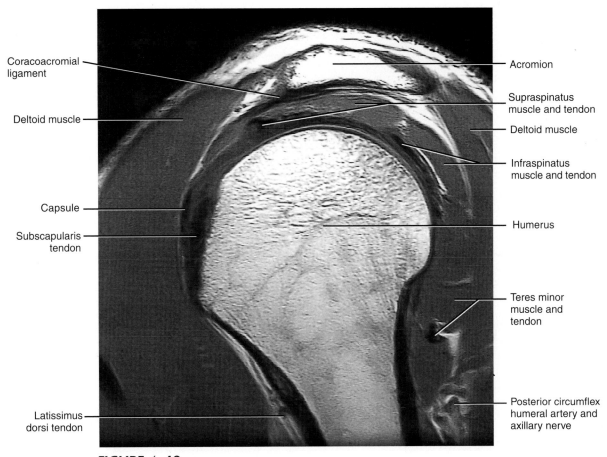

Coracoacromial ligament

Deltoid muscle

Capsule

Subscapularis tendon

Latissimus dorsi tendon

Acromion

Supraspinatus muscle and tendon

Deltoid muscle

Infraspinatus muscle and tendon

Humerus

Teres minor muscle and tendon

Posterior circumflex humeral artery and axillary nerve

FIGURE 1-40

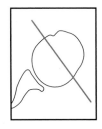

SHOULDER: SAGITTAL OBLIQUE

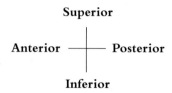

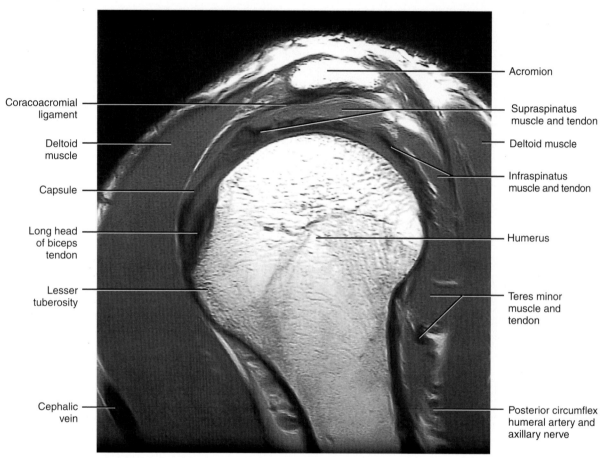

Coracoacromial ligament

Deltoid muscle

Capsule

Long head of biceps tendon

Lesser tuberosity

Cephalic vein

Acromion

Supraspinatus muscle and tendon

Deltoid muscle

Infraspinatus muscle and tendon

Humerus

Teres minor muscle and tendon

Posterior circumflex humeral artery and axillary nerve

FIGURE 1-41

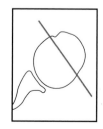

SHOULDER: SAGITTAL OBLIQUE

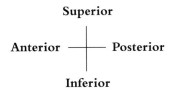

Superior

Anterior —— Posterior

Inferior

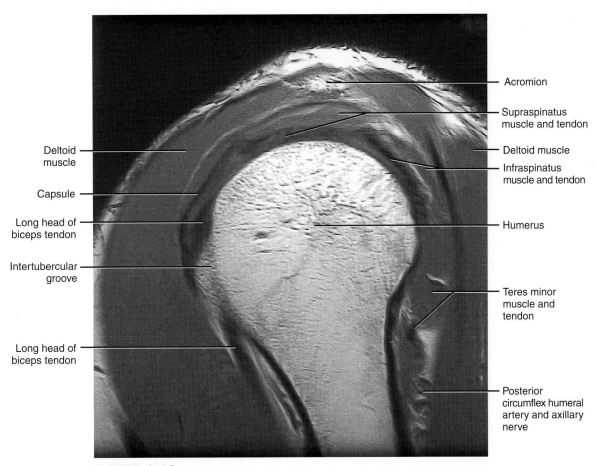

Deltoid muscle

Capsule

Long head of biceps tendon

Intertubercular groove

Long head of biceps tendon

Acromion

Supraspinatus muscle and tendon

Deltoid muscle

Infraspinatus muscle and tendon

Humerus

Teres minor muscle and tendon

Posterior circumflex humeral artery and axillary nerve

FIGURE 1-42

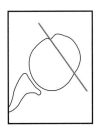

SHOULDER: SAGITTAL OBLIQUE

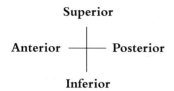

Superior

Anterior —— Posterior

Inferior

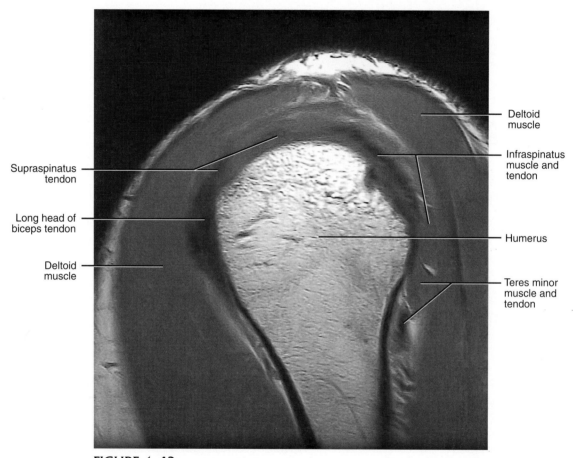

Supraspinatus
tendon

Long head of
biceps tendon

Deltoid
muscle

Deltoid
muscle

Infraspinatus
muscle and
tendon

Humerus

Teres minor
muscle and
tendon

FIGURE 1-43

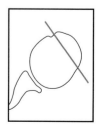

SHOULDER: SAGITTAL OBLIQUE

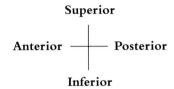

Superior

Anterior —|— Posterior

Inferior

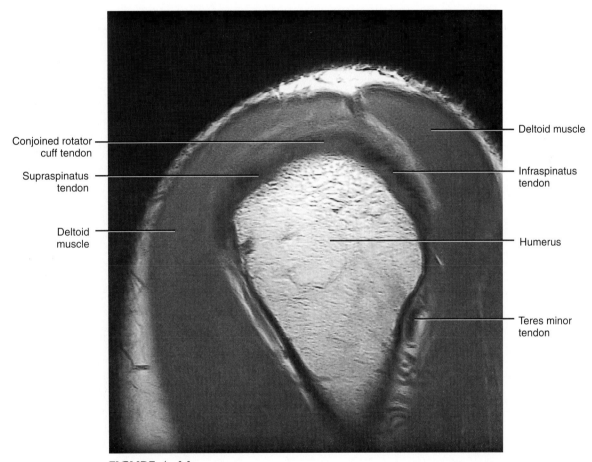

Conjoined rotator cuff tendon

Supraspinatus tendon

Deltoid muscle

Deltoid muscle

Infraspinatus tendon

Humerus

Teres minor tendon

FIGURE 1-44

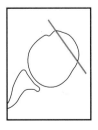

SHOULDER: SAGITTAL OBLIQUE

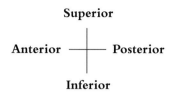

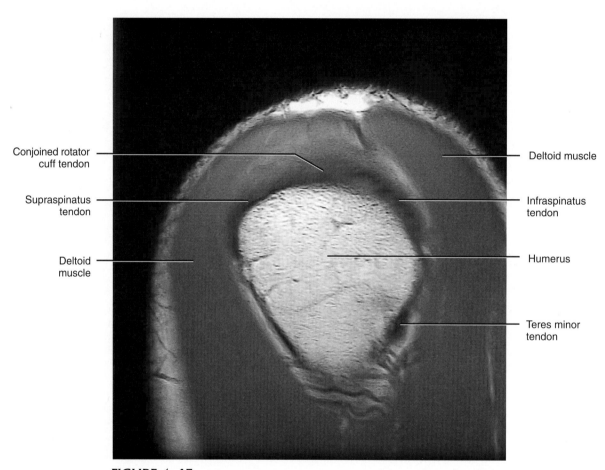

Conjoined rotator cuff tendon

Supraspinatus tendon

Deltoid muscle

Deltoid muscle

Infraspinatus tendon

Humerus

Teres minor tendon

FIGURE 1-45

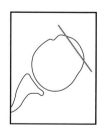

SHOULDER: SAGITTAL OBLIQUE

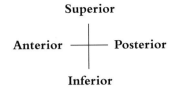

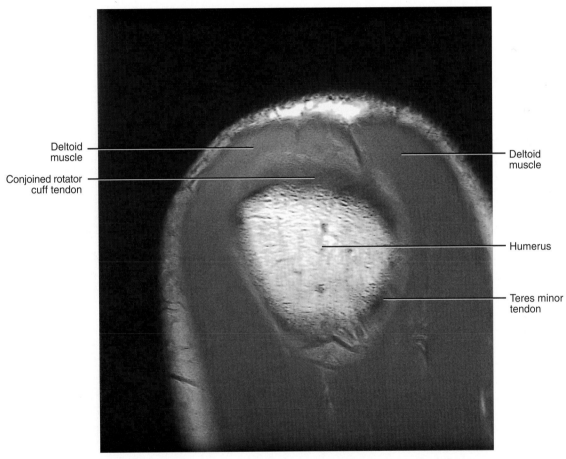

Deltoid muscle

Conjoined rotator cuff tendon

Deltoid muscle

Humerus

Teres minor tendon

FIGURE 1-46

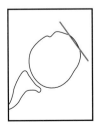

SHOULDER: SAGITTAL OBLIQUE

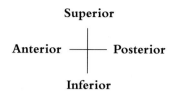

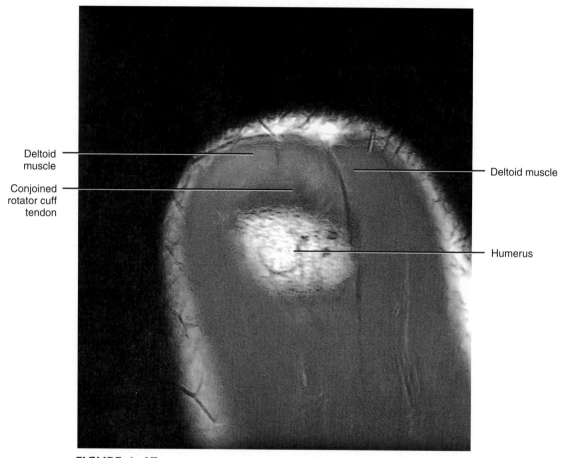

Deltoid muscle

Conjoined rotator cuff tendon

Deltoid muscle

Humerus

FIGURE 1-47

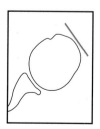

SHOULDER: ROTATOR CUFF, ANTERIOR VIEW

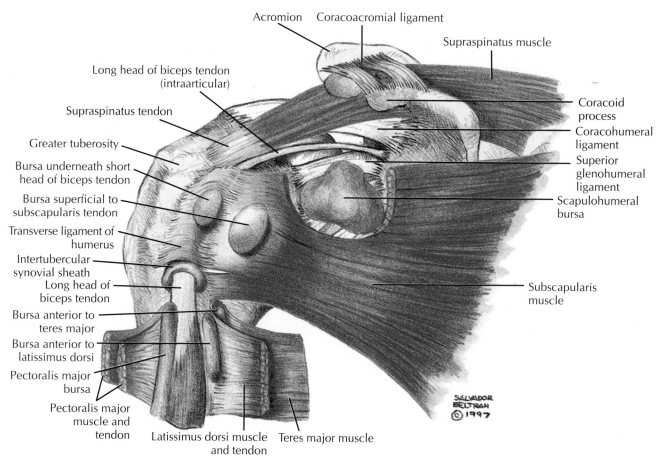

A

FIGURE 1-48A

The rotator cuff. Anterior **(A)** and posterior **(B)** views of the rotator cuff tendons. The supraspinatus, infra-spinatus, teres minor, and subscapularis muscles and tendons function primarily to centralize the humeral head, limiting superior translation during abduction. The supraspinatus, infraspinatus, and teres minor tendons insert on the greater tuberosity, whereas the subscapularis tendon inserts on the lesser tuberosity. For related MR, arthroscopy, and surgical anatomy images see Figures 1-64 through 1-68.

SHOULDER: ROTATOR CUFF, POSTERIOR VIEW

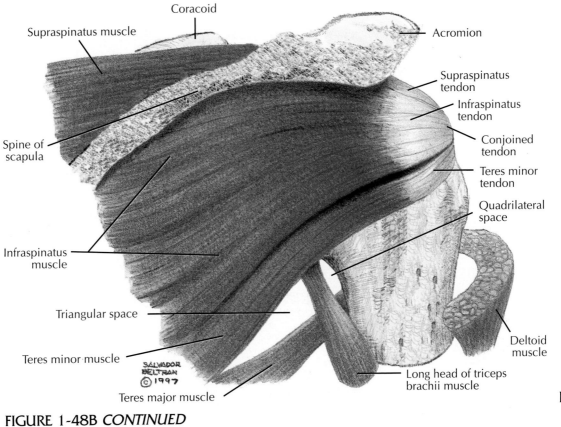

Coracoid

Supraspinatus muscle

Acromion

Supraspinatus tendon

Infraspinatus tendon

Conjoined tendon

Teres minor tendon

Spine of scapula

Quadrilateral space

Infraspinatus muscle

Triangular space

Deltoid muscle

Teres minor muscle

SALVADOR
BELTRAN
© 1997

Long head of triceps brachii muscle

Teres major muscle

B

FIGURE 1-48B *CONTINUED*

For related MR, arthroscopy, and surgical anatomy images see Figures 1-64 through 1-68.

SHOULDER: GLENOHUMERAL LIGAMENTS, ANTERIOR VIEW

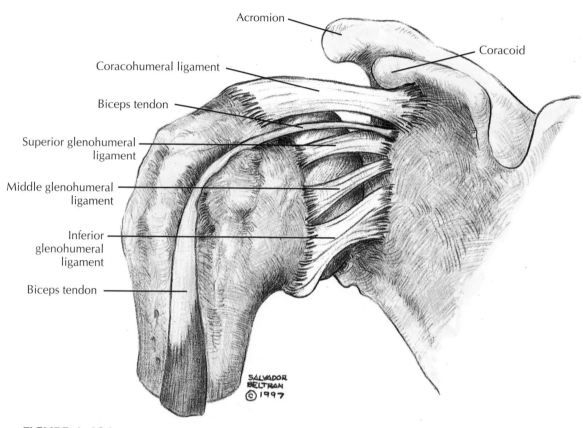

A

FIGURE 1-49A

Normal anatomy of the glenohumeral ligaments in anterior **(A)** and lateral **(B)** views. The coracohumeral ligament, which originates on the lateral aspect of the base of the coracoid inferior to the origin of the coracoacromial ligament, courses in a horizontal direction to its insertion on the greater tuberosity on the lateral aspect of the bicipital groove. The superior glenohumeral ligament originates from the upper pole of the glenoid cavity and the base of the coracoid process and is attached to the middle glenohumeral ligament, the biceps tendon, and the labrum. It inserts just superior to the lesser tuberosity in the region of the bicipital groove. The middle glenohumeral ligament attaches to the anterior aspect of the anatomic neck of the humerus, medial to the lesser tuberosity. It arises from the upper half of the glenoid and scapular neck. The inferior glenohumeral ligament consists of anterior and posterior bands and an axillary pouch that attaches to the inferior two-thirds of the entire circumference of the glenoid by means of the labrum. The long head of the biceps tendon attaches to the supraglenoid tubercle, the posterosuperior labrum, the anterosuperior glenoid labrum, and the base of the coracoid process. For related MR, arthroscopy, and surgical anatomy images see Figures 1-72 through 1-77.

SHOULDER: GLENOHUMERAL LIGAMENTS, LATERAL VIEW

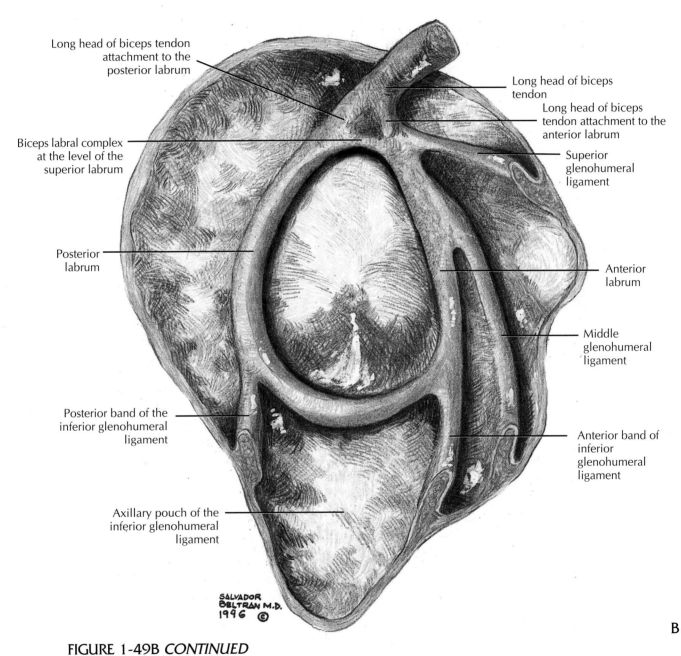

Long head of biceps tendon attachment to the posterior labrum

Biceps labral complex at the level of the superior labrum

Posterior labrum

Posterior band of the inferior glenohumeral ligament

Axillary pouch of the inferior glenohumeral ligament

Long head of biceps tendon

Long head of biceps tendon attachment to the anterior labrum

Superior glenohumeral ligament

Anterior labrum

Middle glenohumeral ligament

Anterior band of inferior glenohumeral ligament

SALVADOR BELTRAN M.D. 1996 ©

B

FIGURE 1-49B *CONTINUED*

For related MR, arthroscopy, and surgical anatomy images see Figures 1-72 through 1-77.

SHOULDER: BICEPS LABRAL COMPLEX TYPE 1, ANTERIOR VIEW

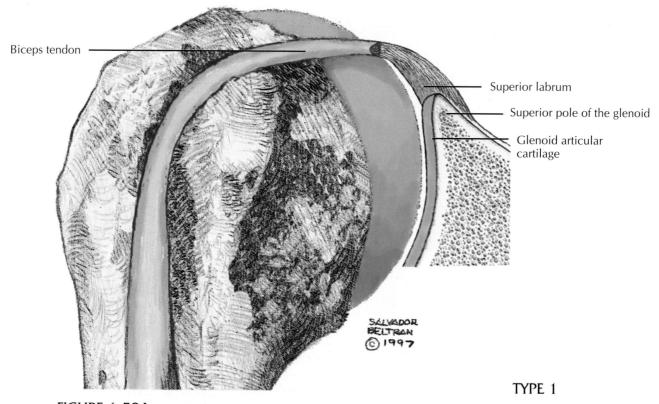

A

TYPE 1

FIGURE 1-50A

There are three different types of attachment of the biceps labral complex (BLC) to the glenoid. **(A)** A Type 1 BLC is firmly adherent to the superior pole of the glenoid and there is no associated sublabral foramen in the anterosuperior quadrant. **(B)** A Type 2 BLC is attached several millimeters medial to the sagittal plane of the glenoid, and the superior pole of the glenoid continues its hyaline cartilage surface medially underneath the labrum. This configuration has a small sulcus at the superior pole of the glenoid that may be continuous with a sublabral foramen and communicate with the subscapularis bursa. The sulcus, which is present at the level of the superior glenoid and biceps labral complex, however, should never be mistaken for a sublabral foramen. The sublabral foramen, when present, is located anterior to the BLC in the anterosuperior quadrant. **(C)** In a Type 3 BLC the labrum is meniscoid in shape and has a large sulcus that projects under the labrum and over the cartilaginous pole of the glenoid. The large sulcus created by the meniscoid labrum usually continues anteriorly as a sublabral foramen. For related MR, arthroscopy, and surgical anatomy images see Figures 1-69 through 1-71 and Figures 1-78 through 1-81.

SHOULDER: BICEPS LABRAL COMPLEX TYPE 2 AND 3, ANTERIOR VIEW

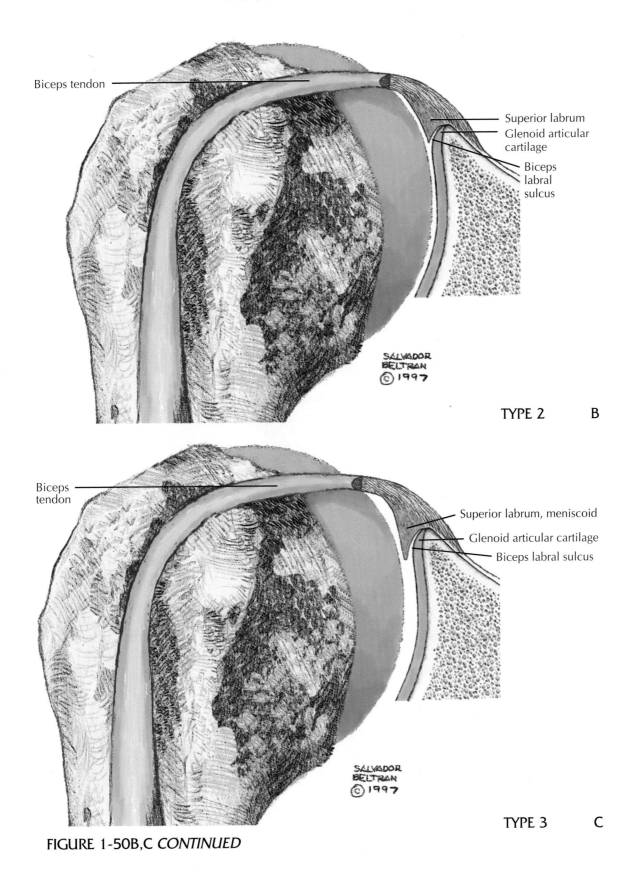

Biceps tendon

Superior labrum

Glenoid articular cartilage

Biceps labral sulcus

SALVADOR BELTRAN © 1997

TYPE 2   B

Biceps tendon

Superior labrum, meniscoid

Glenoid articular cartilage

Biceps labral sulcus

SALVADOR BELTRAN © 1997

TYPE 3   C

FIGURE 1-50B,C *CONTINUED*

SHOULDER: TYPE A LABRUM, AXIAL VIEW

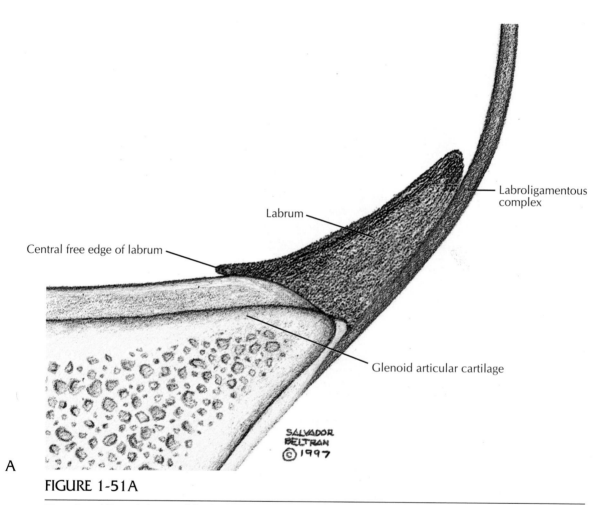

A

FIGURE 1-51A

Type A and B variations in labral anatomy as illustrated in the axial or transverse view. **(A)** The labrum in Type A has a detached free edge overhanging the glenoid articular surface but is well-attached peripherally. This variation is usually present in the superior quadrant, but may be seen anteriorly or posteriorly.

SHOULDER: TYPE B LABRUM, AXIAL VIEW

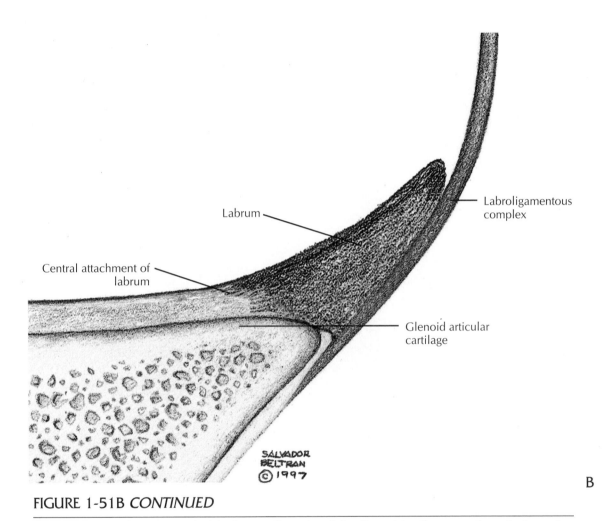

Labroligamentous
complex

Labrum

Central attachment of
labrum

Glenoid articular
cartilage

SALVADOR
BELTRAN
© 1997

B

FIGURE 1-51B *CONTINUED*

(B) The Type B labrum is attached both centrally and peripherally and is adherent to the articular surface without a free edge.

SHOULDER: SUBLABRAL FORAMEN, LATERAL VIEW

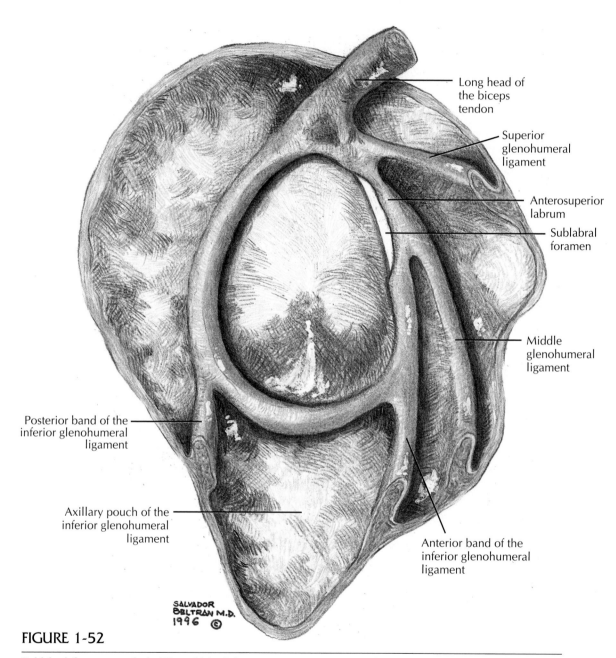

Long head of
the biceps
tendon

Superior
glenohumeral
ligament

Anterosuperior
labrum

Sublabral
foramen

Middle
glenohumeral
ligament

Posterior band of the
inferior glenohumeral
ligament

Axillary pouch of the
inferior glenohumeral
ligament

Anterior band of the
inferior glenohumeral
ligament

SALVADOR
BELTRAN M.D.
1996 ©

FIGURE 1-52

Sublabral foramen or hole. The sublabral foramen represents a normal variation with a relative lack of attachment or separation of the labrum from the glenoid rim in the anterosuperior quadrant superior to the
glenoid equator. For related MR, arthroscopy, and surgical anatomy image see Figure 1-84.

SHOULDER: BUFORD COMPLEX, LATERAL VIEW

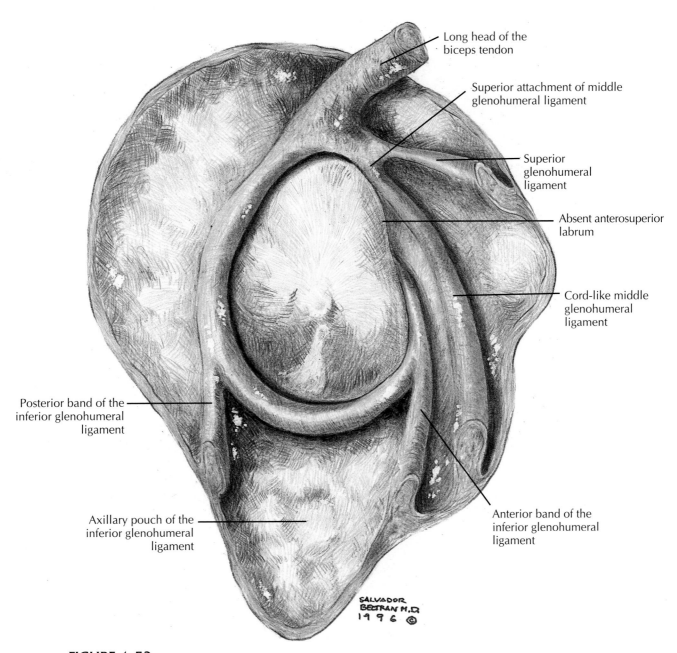

Long head of the
biceps tendon

Superior attachment of middle
glenohumeral ligament

Superior
glenohumeral
ligament

Absent anterosuperior
labrum

Cord-like middle
glenohumeral
ligament

Posterior band of the
inferior glenohumeral
ligament

Axillary pouch of the
inferior glenohumeral
ligament

Anterior band of the
inferior glenohumeral
ligament

FIGURE 1-53

Buford complex. The Buford complex consists of three elements: (1) a cord-like middle glenohumeral ligament, (2) a middle glenohumeral ligament that attaches directly to the superior labrum anterior to the biceps (at the base of the biceps anchor), and (3) an absent anterosuperior labrum. For related MR,
arthroscopy, and surgical anatomy image see Figure 1-85.

SHOULDER: BANKART LESION, LATERAL VIEW

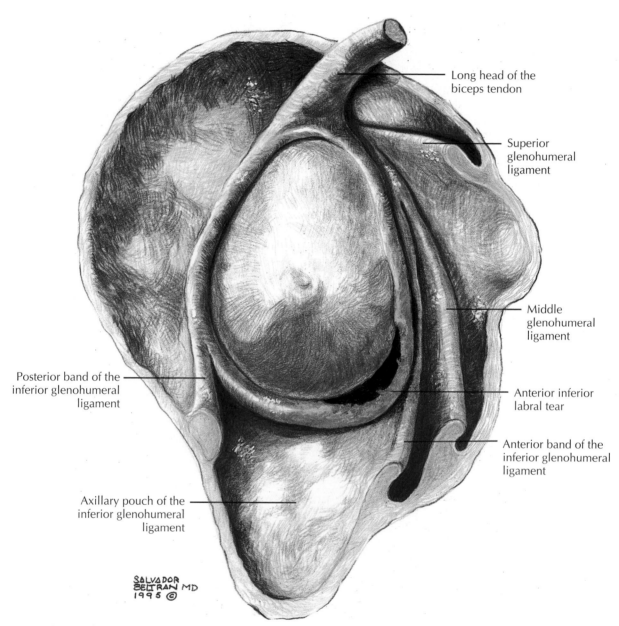

Long head of the
biceps tendon

Superior
glenohumeral
ligament

Middle
glenohumeral
ligament

Anterior inferior
labral tear

Anterior band of the
inferior glenohumeral
ligament

Posterior band of the
inferior glenohumeral
ligament

Axillary pouch of the
inferior glenohumeral
ligament

SALVADOR
BELTRAN MD
1995 ©

A

FIGURE 1-54A

Bankart lesion on lateral **(A)** and axial **(B)** views. Avulsion of the inferior glenohumeral ligament labral complex from the glenoid rim is known as a Bankart lesion. A Bankart lesion involves detachment of the anterior labrum and inferior glenohumeral ligament complex from the anterior inferior glenoid rim. A Bankart lesion may involve labral avulsion without a bony inferior glenoid rim fracture. The scapular periosteum is torn in the Bankart lesion. For related MR, arthroscopy. and surgical anatomy image see Figure 1–86.

SHOULDER: BANKART LESION, AXIAL VIEW

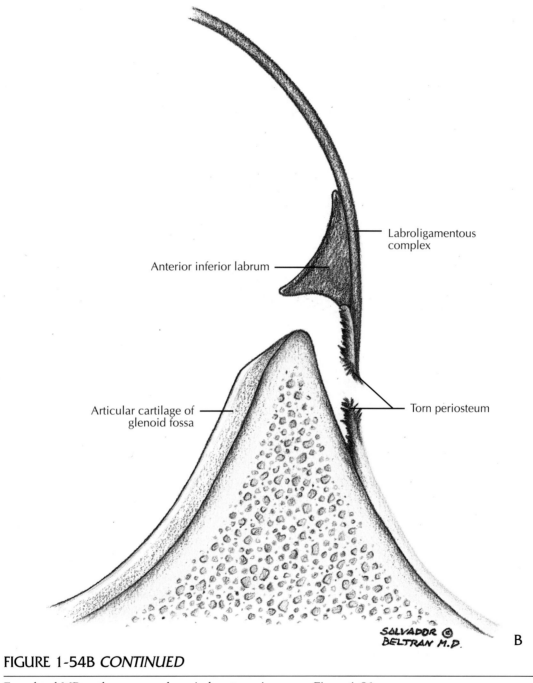

FIGURE 1-54B *CONTINUED*

For related MR, arthroscopy. and surgical anatomy image see Figure 1-86.

SHOULDER: NORMAL ANTERIOR LABRUM, AXIAL VIEW

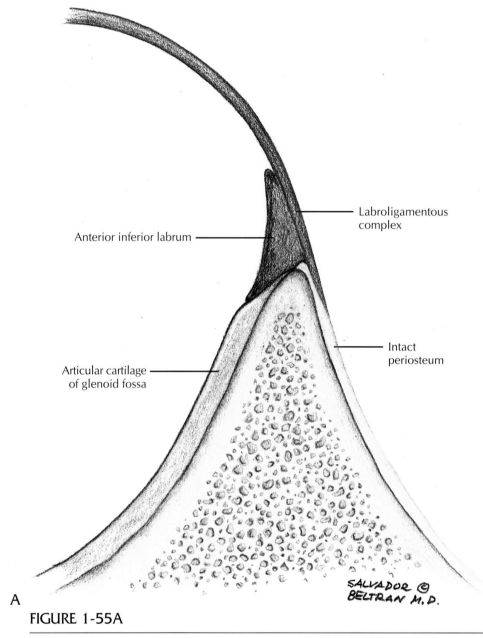

Labroligamentous
complex

Anterior inferior labrum

Intact
periosteum

Articular cartilage
of glenoid fossa

SALVADOR ©
BELTRAN M.D.

A

FIGURE 1-55A

(A) Normal anterior labrum and capsulolabral complex. For related MR, arthroscopy, and surgical anatomy image see Figure 1-77.

SHOULDER: PERTHES LESION, AXIAL VIEW

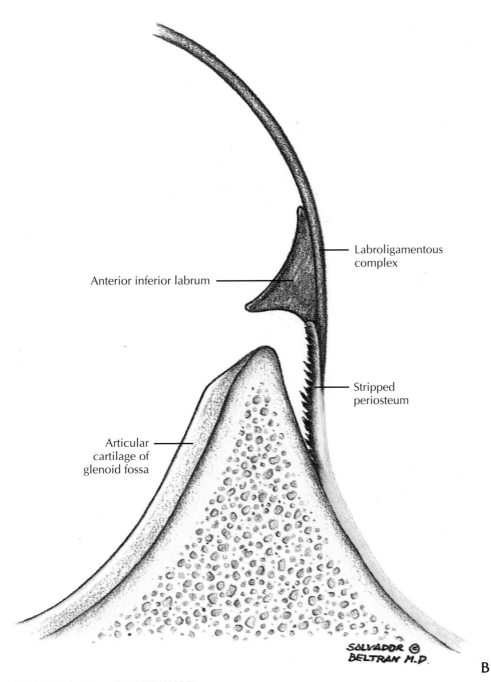

Labroligamentous
complex

Anterior inferior labrum

Stripped
periosteum

Articular
cartilage of
glenoid fossa

SALVADOR ©
BELTRAN M.D.

B

FIGURE 1-55B *CONTINUED*

(B) Perthes lesion with medially stripped but intact scapular periosteum. The Perthes lesion represents a labroligamentous avulsion. For related MR, arthroscopy, and surgical anatomy image see Figure 1-77.

SHOULDER: ALPSA LESION, AXIAL VIEW

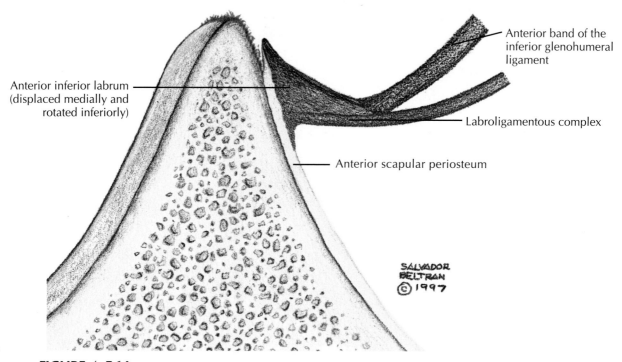

Anterior band of the
inferior glenohumeral
ligament

Anterior inferior labrum
(displaced medially and
rotated inferiorly)

Labroligamentous complex

Anterior scapular periosteum

A

FIGURE 1-56A

ALPSA lesion. Axial **(A)** and lateral **(B)** views of the anterior labroligamentous periosteal sleeve avulsion (ALPSA lesion), which represents an avulsion of the inferior glenohumeral ligament through its anterior band attachment to the anterior labrum. The ALPSA lesion differs from the Bankart lesion, in that the ALPSA lesion has an intact anterior scapular periosteum allowing the labroligamentous structures to displace medially and rotate inferiorly on the scapular neck. There may be synovial fibrous tissue deposition between the medial displaced inferior glenohumeral ligament labral complex and the glenoid margin in the chronic ALPSA lesion. For related MR, arthroscopy, and surgical anatomy image see Figure 1-87.

SHOULDER: ALPSA LESION, LATERAL VIEW

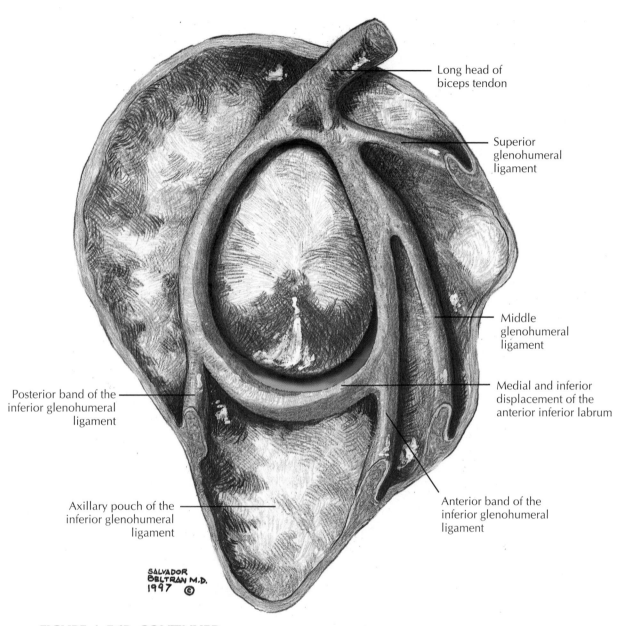

Long head of
biceps tendon

Superior
glenohumeral
ligament

Middle
glenohumeral
ligament

Medial and inferior
displacement of the
anterior inferior labrum

Posterior band of the
inferior glenohumeral
ligament

Anterior band of the
inferior glenohumeral
ligament

Axillary pouch of the
inferior glenohumeral
ligament

SALVADOR
BELTRAN M.D.
1997 ©

B

FIGURE 1-56B *CONTINUED*

For related MR, arthroscopy, and surgical anatomy image see Figure 1-87.

SHOULDER: GLAD LESION, AXIAL VIEW

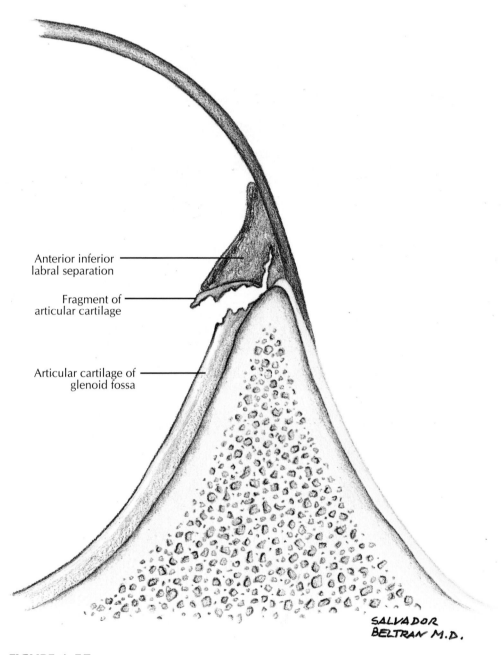

Anterior inferior
labral separation

Fragment of
articular cartilage

Articular cartilage of
glenoid fossa

SALVADOR
BELTRAN M.D.

FIGURE 1-57

GLAD lesion. Glenolabral articular disruption (GLAD lesion) is a superficial anterior inferior labral tear, associated with an anterior inferior glenoid articular cartilage injury.

SHOULDER: HAGL LESION, ANTERIOR VIEW

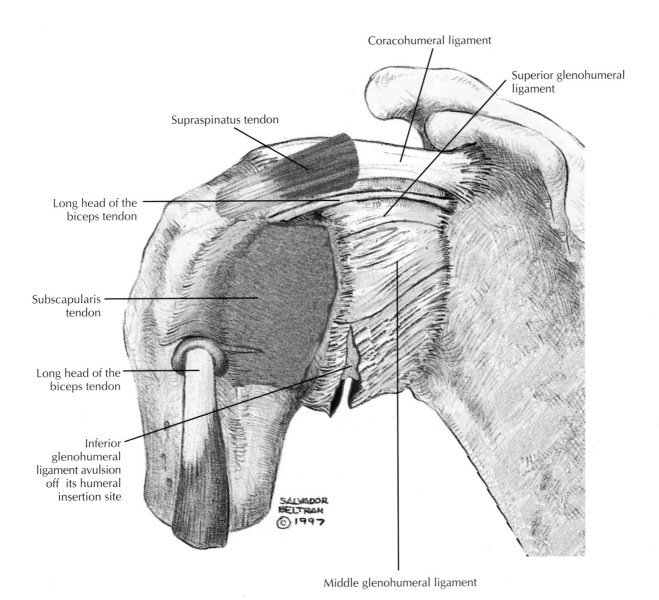

Coracohumeral ligament

Superior glenohumeral ligament

Supraspinatus tendon

Long head of the biceps tendon

Subscapularis tendon

Long head of the biceps tendon

Inferior glenohumeral ligament avulsion off its humeral insertion site

SALVADOR BELTRAN © 1997

Middle glenohumeral ligament

FIGURE 1-58

HAGL lesion. Humeral avulsion of the glenohumeral ligament (HAGL lesion) involves tearing of the anatomic humeral neck attachment of the inferior glenohumeral ligament. The axillary pouch may display a j-shaped configuration (from the coronal perspective) as the humeral attachment of the inferior glenohumeral ligament drops inferiorly. For related MR, arthroscopy, and surgical anatomy image see Figure 1-89.

SHOULDER: OSSEOUS BANKART LESION, LATERAL VIEW

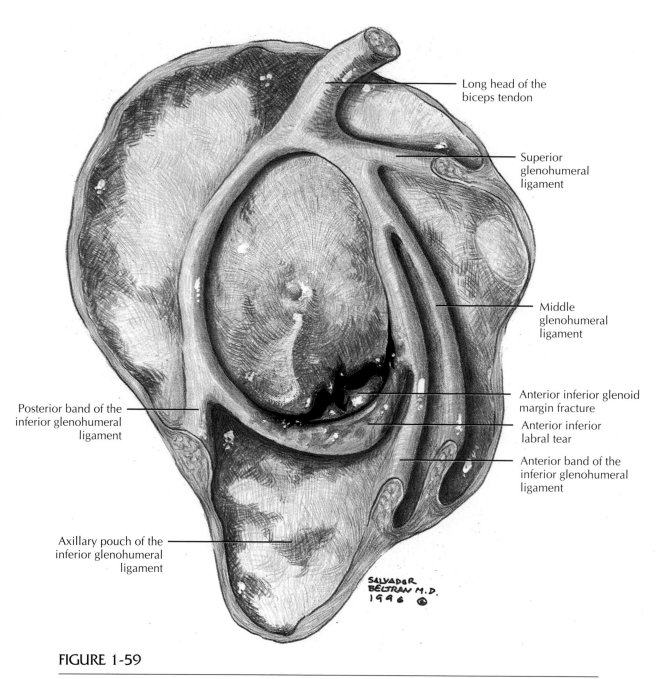

FIGURE 1-59

Osseous Bankart lesion with a fracture of the anteroinferior glenoid rim.

SHOULDER: EXTENSIVE ANTERIOR LABRAL TEAR, LATERAL VIEW

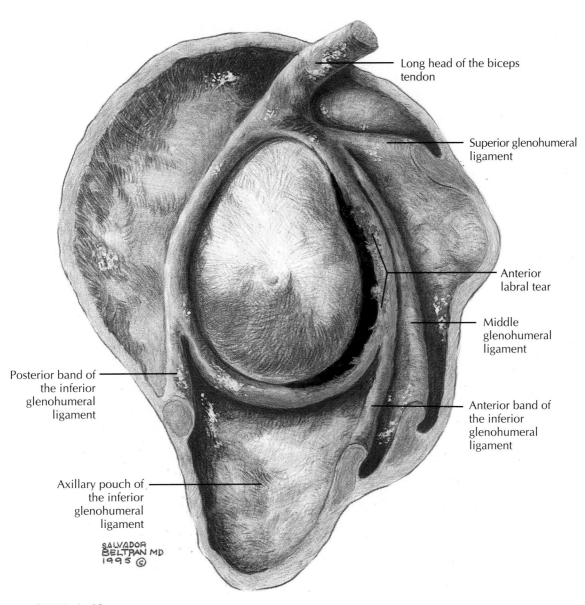

Long head of the biceps tendon

Superior glenohumeral ligament

Anterior labral tear

Middle glenohumeral ligament

Posterior band of the inferior glenohumeral ligament

Anterior band of the inferior glenohumeral ligament

Axillary pouch of the inferior glenohumeral ligament

SALVADOR
BELTRAN MD
1995 ©

FIGURE 1-60

An extensive anterior labral tear from the insertion of the middle glenohumeral ligament to the inferior glenoid rim. For related MR, arthroscopy, and surgical anatomy image see Figure 1-86.

SHOULDER: ANTEROSUPERIOR LABRAL TEAR, LATERAL VIEW

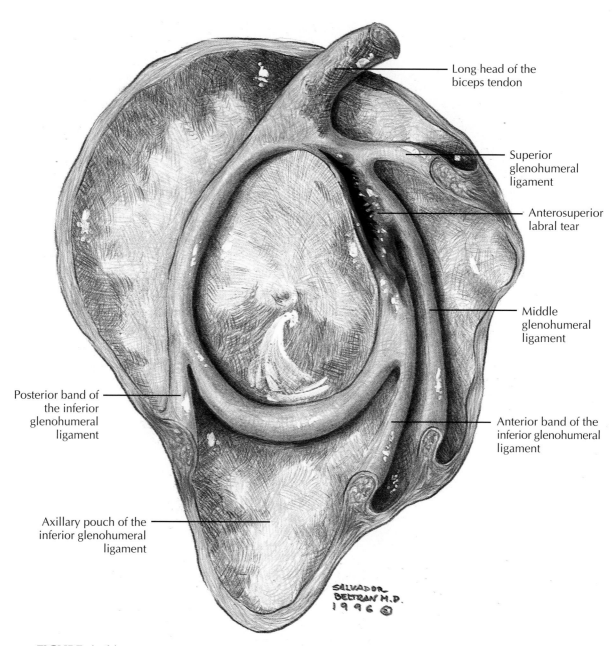

Long head of the biceps tendon

Superior glenohumeral ligament

Anterosuperior labral tear

Middle glenohumeral ligament

Anterior band of the inferior glenohumeral ligament

Posterior band of the inferior glenohumeral ligament

Axillary pouch of the inferior glenohumeral ligament

FIGURE 1-61

An anterosuperior labral tear at the insertion of the middle glenohumeral ligament. Anterosuperior labral tears may be associated with stretching or tearing of the middle glenohumeral ligament and present with microinstability. Superior extension to the biceps labral complex may further increase anterosuperior instability.

SHOULDER: POSTERIOR LABRAL TEAR, LATERAL VIEW

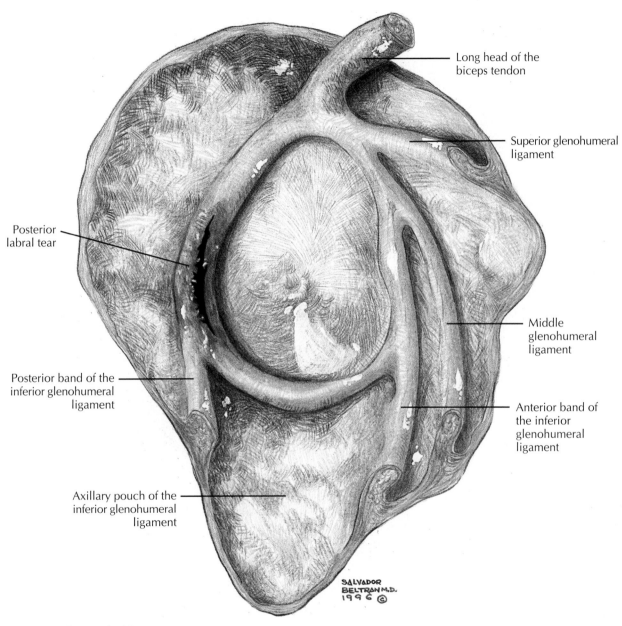

Long head of the biceps tendon

Superior glenohumeral ligament

Posterior labral tear

Middle glenohumeral ligament

Posterior band of the inferior glenohumeral ligament

Anterior band of the inferior glenohumeral ligament

Axillary pouch of the inferior glenohumeral ligament

SALVADOR BELTRAN M.D. 1996 ©

FIGURE 1-62

Posterior labral tear. A tear of the posterior labrum is illustrated in the nine o'clock position. In a reverse Bankart lesion, a posterior labral tear is associated with an anteromedial superior humeral head impaction (reverse Hill–Sachs lesion). For related MR, arthroscopy, and surgical anatomy image see Figure 1-88.

SHOULDER: TYPE I SLAP LESION, LATERAL VIEW

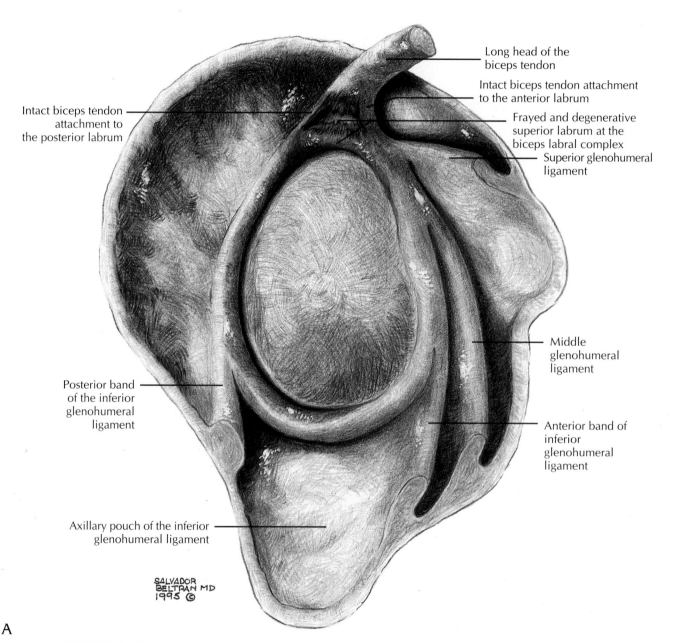

Long head of the biceps tendon

Intact biceps tendon attachment to the anterior labrum

Frayed and degenerative superior labrum at the biceps labral complex

Superior glenohumeral ligament

Intact biceps tendon attachment to the posterior labrum

Middle glenohumeral ligament

Anterior band of inferior glenohumeral ligament

Posterior band of the inferior glenohumeral ligament

Axillary pouch of the inferior glenohumeral ligament

SALVADOR BELTRAN MD 1995 ©

A

FIGURE 1-63A

SLAP (superior labrum from anterior to posterior) lesions. **(A)** Type I SLAP lesion with frayed and degenerative superior labrum.

SHOULDER: TYPE II SLAP LESION, LATERAL VIEW

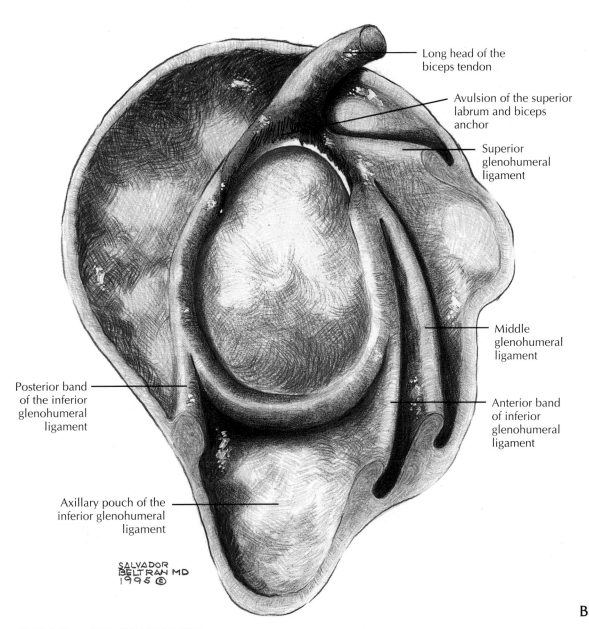

Long head of the
biceps tendon

Avulsion of the superior
labrum and biceps
anchor

Superior
glenohumeral
ligament

Middle
glenohumeral
ligament

Anterior band
of inferior
glenohumeral
ligament

Posterior band
of the inferior
glenohumeral
ligament

Axillary pouch of the
inferior glenohumeral
ligament

SALVADOR
BELTRAN MD
1995 ©

B

FIGURE 1-63B *CONTINUED*

(B) Type II SLAP lesion with avulsion of the superior labrum and biceps anchor. Note that the term "biceps anchor" is misleading. The long head of the biceps tendon has a primary attachment to the supraglenoid tubercle, which is not disrupted in the SLAP lesion. The biceps anchor, as referred to in a SLAP lesion, should be more properly thought of as a biceps expansion. For related MR, arthroscopy, and surgical anatomy images see Figures 1-82 and 1-83.

SHOULDER: TYPE III SLAP LESION, LATERAL VIEW

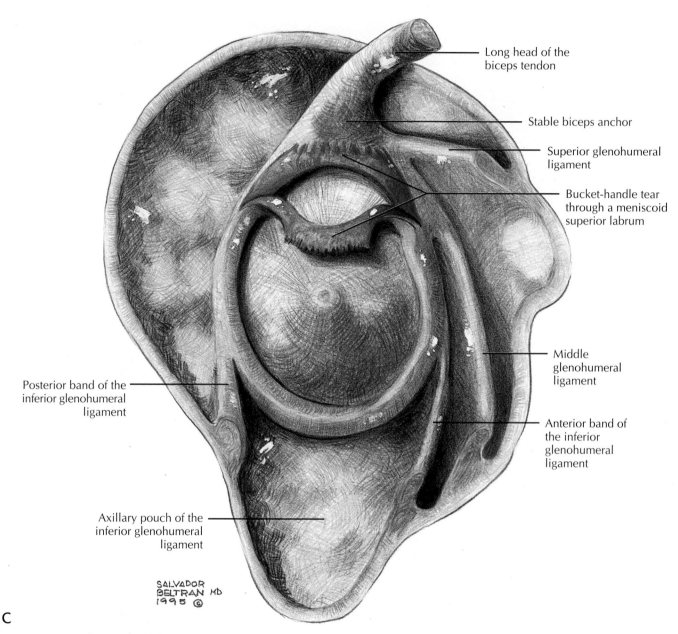

Long head of the
biceps tendon

Stable biceps anchor

Superior glenohumeral
ligament

Bucket-handle tear
through a meniscoid
superior labrum

Middle
glenohumeral
ligament

Anterior band of
the inferior
glenohumeral
ligament

Posterior band of the
inferior glenohumeral
ligament

Axillary pouch of the
inferior glenohumeral
ligament

SALVADOR
BELTRAN MD
1995 ©

C

FIGURE 1-63C *CONTINUED*

(C) Type III SLAP lesion with a bucket handle tear through a meniscoid superior labrum and intact biceps anchor.

SHOULDER: TYPE IV SLAP LESION, LATERAL VIEW

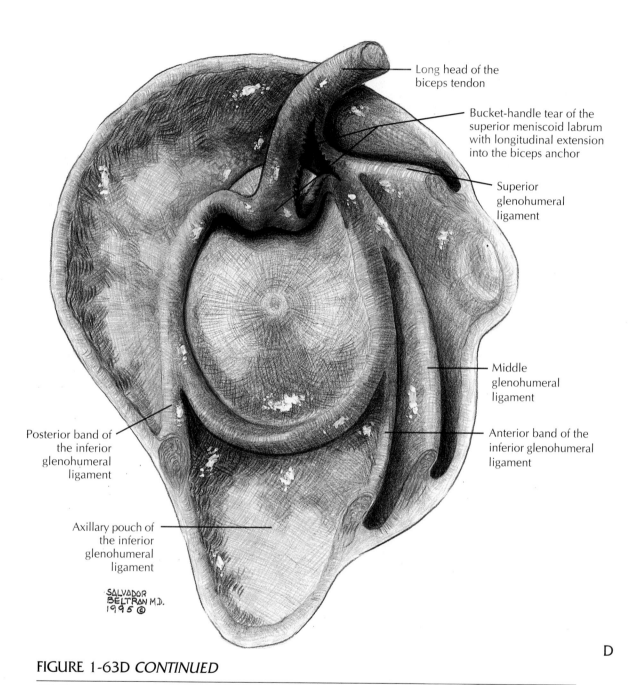

Long head of the biceps tendon

Bucket-handle tear of the superior meniscoid labrum with longitudinal extension into the biceps anchor

Superior glenohumeral ligament

Middle glenohumeral ligament

Anterior band of the inferior glenohumeral ligament

Posterior band of the inferior glenohumeral ligament

Axillary pouch of the inferior glenohumeral ligament

SALVADOR BELTRAN M.D. 1995 ©

D

FIGURE 1-63D *CONTINUED*

(D) Type IV SLAP lesion with a bucket handle tear of the superior meniscoid labrum and extension into the biceps tendon.

SHOULDER: TYPE V SLAP LESION, LATERAL VIEW

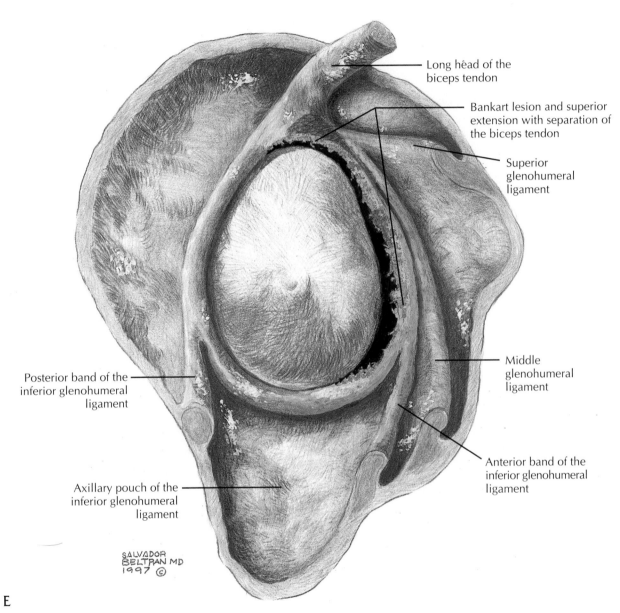

Long head of the
biceps tendon

Bankart lesion and superior
extension with separation of
the biceps tendon

Superior
glenohumeral
ligament

Middle
glenohumeral
ligament

Anterior band of the
inferior glenohumeral
ligament

Posterior band of the
inferior glenohumeral
ligament

Axillary pouch of the
inferior glenohumeral
ligament

SALVADOR
BELTRAN MD
1997 ©

E

FIGURE 1-63E *CONTINUED*

(E) Type V SLAP lesion with superior extension of an anteroinferior Bankart lesion to include the superior labrum and separation of the biceps tendon. **(F)** Type VI SLAP lesion with an anteroposterior labral flap tear and a biceps tendon separation superiorly. **(G)** Type VII SLAP lesion with anterior extension of a Type II SLAP lesion to include the middle glenohumeral ligament.

SHOULDER: TYPE VI AND VII SLAP LESIONS, LATERAL VIEW

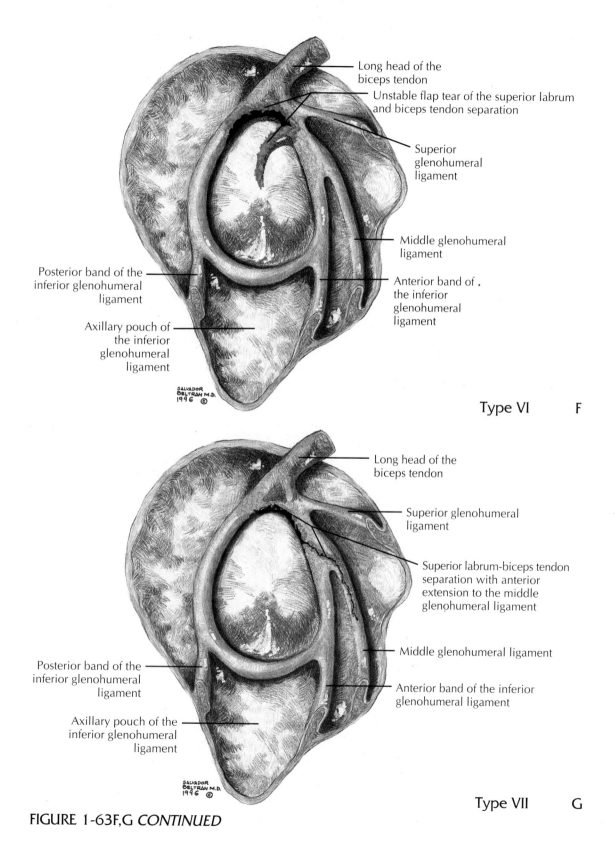

Long head of the biceps tendon

Unstable flap tear of the superior labrum and biceps tendon separation

Superior glenohumeral ligament

Middle glenohumeral ligament

Posterior band of the inferior glenohumeral ligament

Anterior band of the inferior glenohumeral ligament

Axillary pouch of the inferior glenohumeral ligament

SALVADOR
BELTRAN M.D.
1996 ©

Type VI   F

Long head of the biceps tendon

Superior glenohumeral ligament

Superior labrum-biceps tendon separation with anterior extension to the middle glenohumeral ligament

Middle glenohumeral ligament

Posterior band of the inferior glenohumeral ligament

Anterior band of the inferior glenohumeral ligament

Axillary pouch of the inferior glenohumeral ligament

SALVADOR
BELTRAN M.D.
1996 ©

Type VII   G

FIGURE 1-63F,G *CONTINUED*

SHOULDER: ROTATOR CUFF

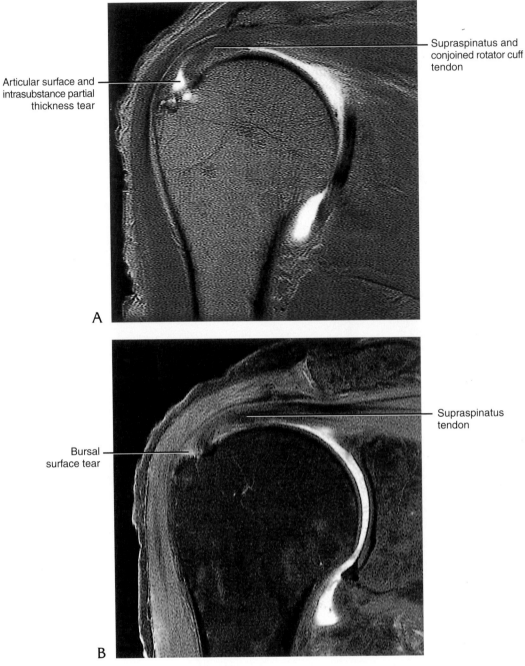

Supraspinatus and
conjoined rotator cuff
tendon

Articular surface and
intrasubstance partial
thickness tear

A

Bursal
surface tear

Supraspinatus
tendon

B

FIGURE 1-64A,B

Partial rotator cuff tear. **(A)** T1-weighted coronal oblique MR arthrogram with hyperintense intrasubstance and partial thickness articular surface tear of the supraspinatus tendon. **(B)** Fat-suppressed T2-weighted fast spin-echo coronal oblique MR arthrogram with partial thickness bursal surface tear. **(C** and **D)** Arthroscopic views of a partial thickness articular surface rotator cuff tear with calcification **(C)** and erosion of the coracoacromial ligament, which was associated with fraying of the bursal surface of the rotator cuff **(D)**. **(E)** Dissection with the cut coracoacromial ligament and rotator cuff tendons displayed. The humeral head is dislocated.

SHOULDER: ROTATOR CUFF

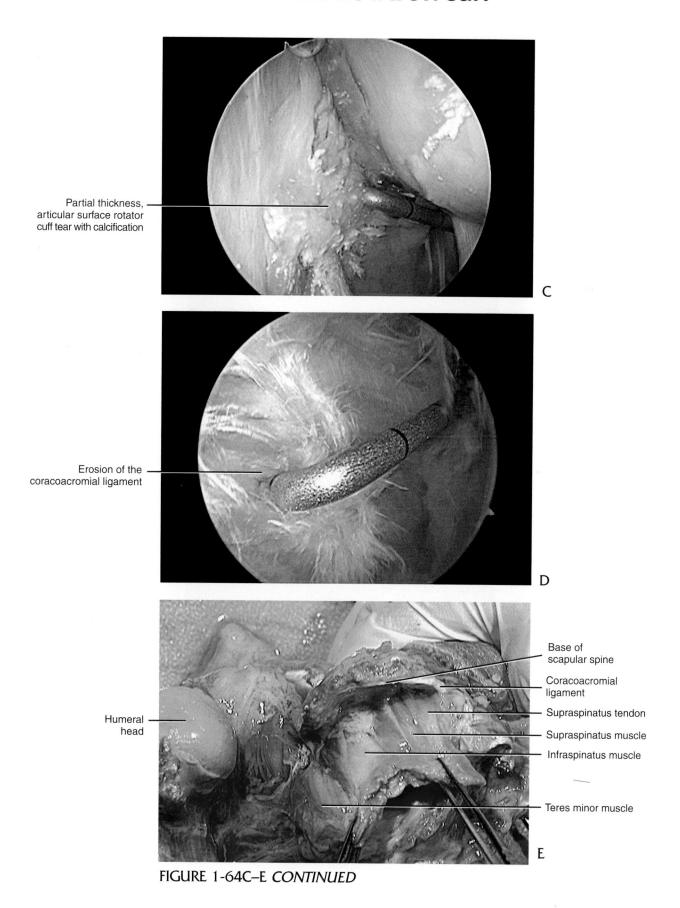

Partial thickness, articular surface rotator cuff tear with calcification

C

Erosion of the coracoacromial ligament

D

Humeral head

Base of scapular spine

Coracoacromial ligament

Supraspinatus tendon

Supraspinatus muscle

Infraspinatus muscle

Teres minor muscle

E

FIGURE 1-64C–E *CONTINUED*

SHOULDER: ROTATOR CUFF

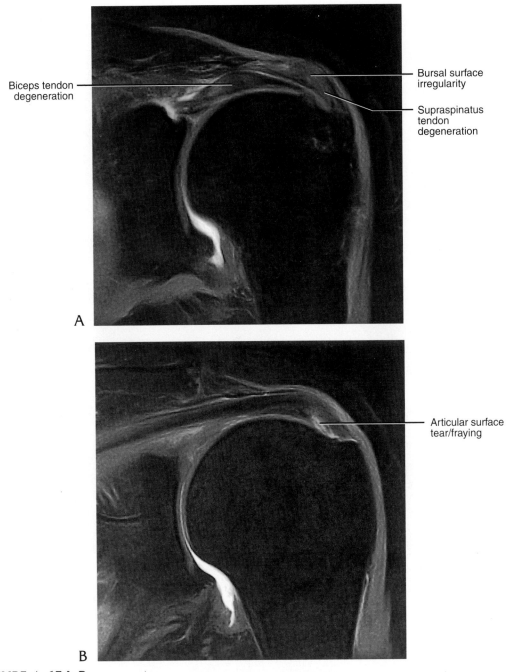

Biceps tendon degeneration

Bursal surface irregularity

Supraspinatus tendon degeneration

A

Articular surface tear/fraying

B

FIGURE 1-65A,B

Partial rotator cuff tear with tendinosis. **(A)** Fat-suppressed T1-weighted coronal oblique MR arthrogram with supraspinatus tendon thickening and bursal surface irregularity. **(B)** Partial thickness articular surface tear/fraying of the conjoined portion of the rotator cuff on a fat-suppressed coronal oblique MR arthrogram.

SHOULDER: ROTATOR CUFF

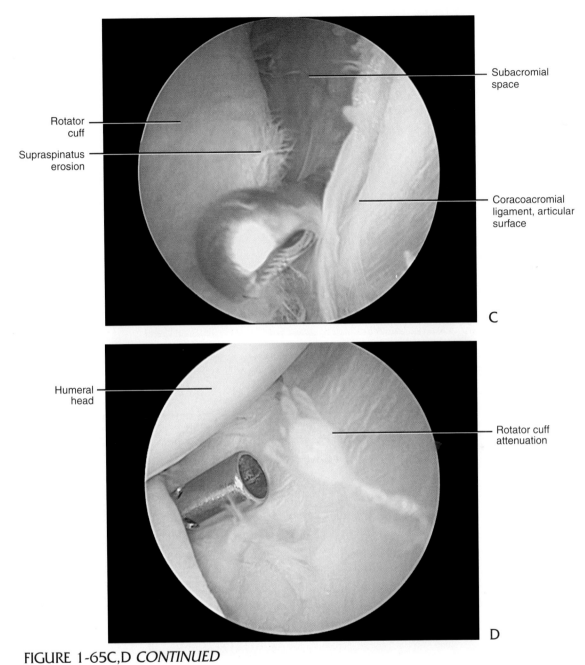

Subacromial space

Rotator cuff

Supraspinatus erosion

Coracoacromial ligament, articular surface

C

Humeral head

Rotator cuff attenuation

D

FIGURE 1-65C,D *CONTINUED*

(C) Arthroscopic view of supraspinatus bursal surface erosion and the coracoacromial ligament. (D) Arthroscopic view of articular surface partial thickness cuff tear.

SHOULDER: ROTATOR CUFF

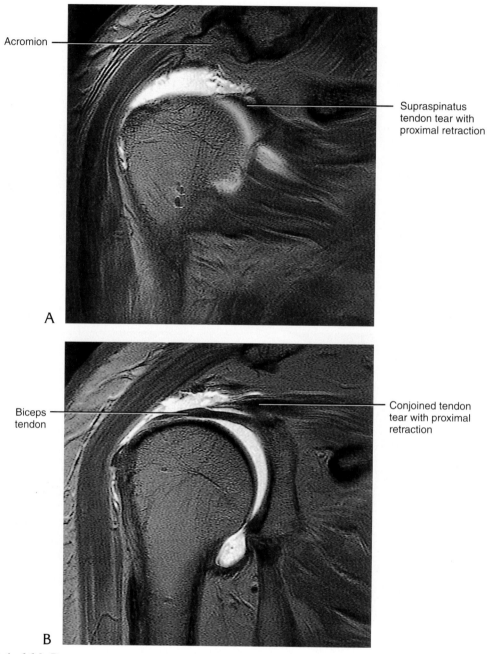

Acromion

Supraspinatus tendon tear with proximal retraction

A

Biceps tendon

Conjoined tendon tear with proximal retraction

B

FIGURE 1-66A,B

Complete rotator cuff tear. Cuff retraction to the level of the glenoid can be seen on anterior **(A)** and more posterior **(B)** T1-weighted coronal oblique MR arthrograms. The posterior margin of the cuff tear **(C)** and acromial erosion **(D)** are shown on corresponding arthroscopic views. **(E)** The corresponding gross specimen demonstrates the massive cuff tear exposing the intraarticular passage of the biceps tendon.

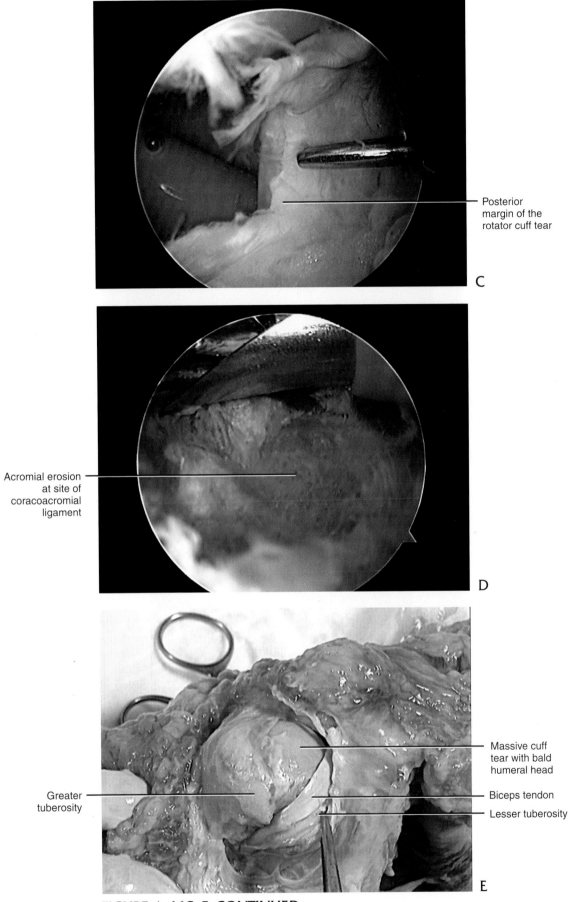

Posterior margin of the rotator cuff tear

C

Acromial erosion at site of coracoacromial ligament

D

Massive cuff tear with bald humeral head

Biceps tendon

Lesser tuberosity

Greater tuberosity

E

FIGURE 1-66C–E *CONTINUED*

SHOULDER: ROTATOR CUFF

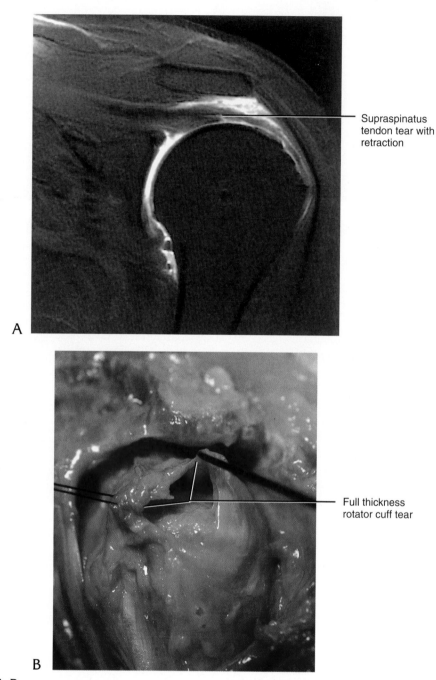

Supraspinatus
tendon tear with
retraction

Full thickness
rotator cuff tear

A

B

FIGURE 1-67A,B

(A) Supraspinatus tendon tear with partial retraction on a fat-suppressed T1-weighted coronal oblique MR arthrogram. **(B)** Corresponding cuff defect on gross specimen.

SHOULDER: ROTATOR CUFF

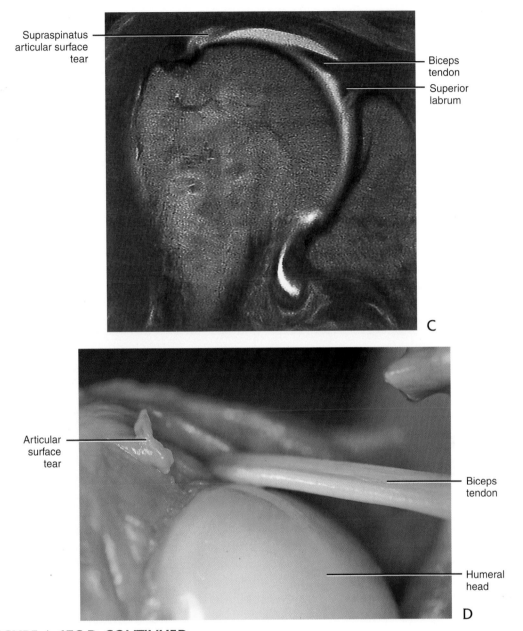

Supraspinatus articular surface tear

Biceps tendon

Superior labrum

C

Articular surface tear

Biceps tendon

Humeral head

D

FIGURE 1-67C,D *CONTINUED*

(C) Partial thickness articular surface tear on a T1-weighted coronal oblique MR arthrogram. **(D)** Articular surface irregularity on the undersurface of the cuff. The long head of the biceps tendon is intact.

SHOULDER: CORACOACROMIAL LIGAMENT

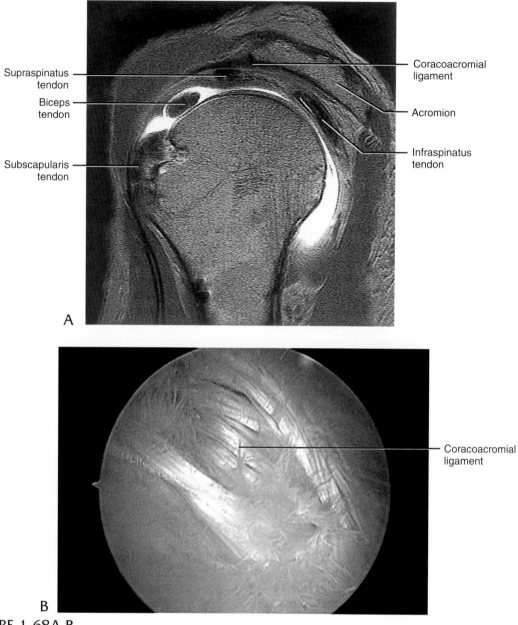

FIGURE 1-68A,B

(A) Normal attachment of the coracoacromial ligament to the inferior surface of the acromion on a T1-weighted sagittal oblique MR arthrogram. (B) Arthroscopic view from the subacromial space showing the fascicles of the coracoacromial ligament as they attach to the inferior aspect of the acromion. The coracoacromial ligament attaches to the anterior, lateral, and inferior surfaces of the acromion and originates as a triangular band of two fascicles from the lateral aspect of the coracoid. (C) The corresponding coracoacromial ligament has been cut, with the acromial attachment intact. There are erosive changes on the undersurface of the anterolateral acromial margin. (D) A separate gross specimen highlighting the anatomy of the coracohumeral and coracoacromial ligaments.

SHOULDER: CORACOACROMIAL LIGAMENT

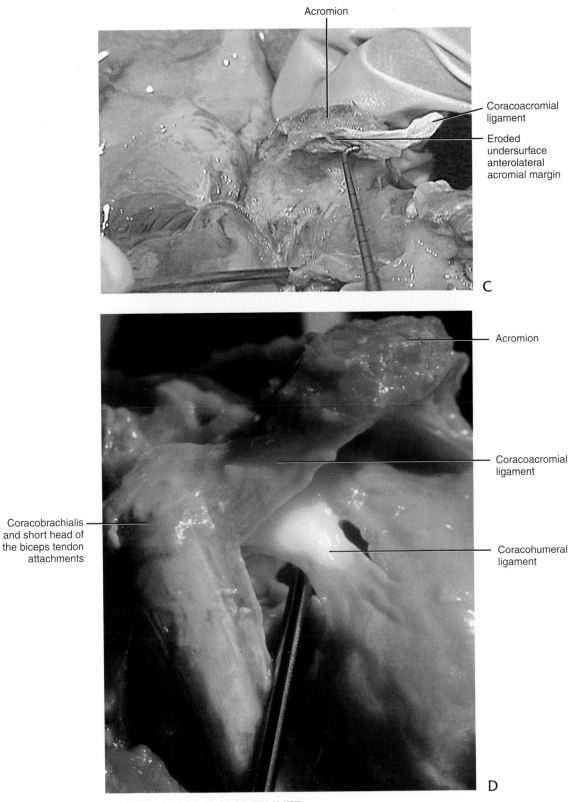

FIGURE 1-68C,D *CONTINUED*

SHOULDER: BICEPS TENDON

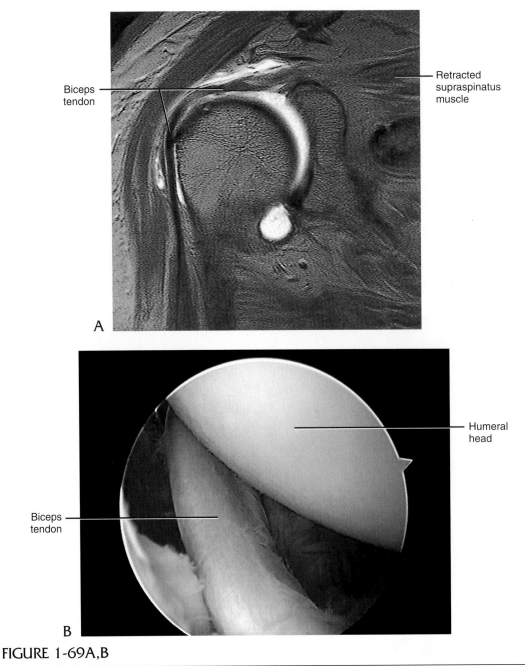

FIGURE 1-69A,B

(A) Long head of the biceps tendon with complete absence of overlying cuff tendons on a T1-weighted coronal oblique MR arthrogram. **(B)** Arthroscopic view of the biceps tendon entering the glenohumeral joint through a massive cuff tear.

SHOULDER: BICEPS TENDON

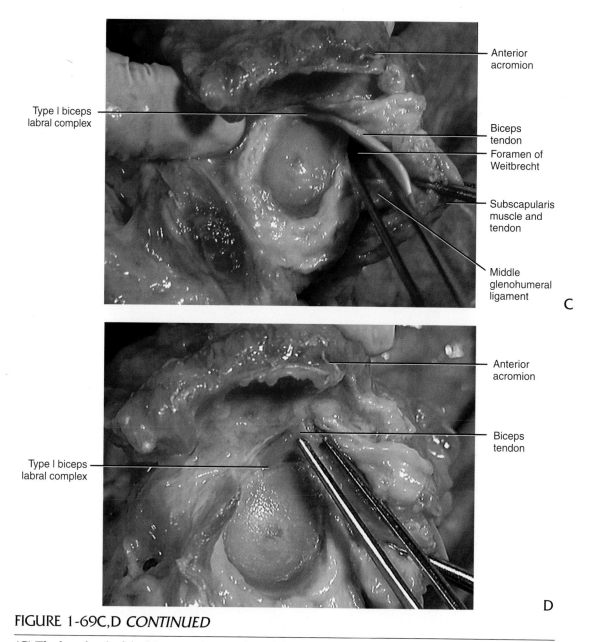

Anterior
acromion

Type I biceps
labral complex

Biceps
tendon

Foramen of
Weitbrecht

Subscapularis
muscle and
tendon

Middle
glenohumeral
ligament

C

Anterior
acromion

Biceps
tendon

Type I biceps
labral complex

D

FIGURE 1-69C,D *CONTINUED*

(C) The long head of the biceps tendon attaches to the supraglenoid tubercle and contributes to the biceps labral complex. **(D)** The cut long head of the biceps tendon is mobilized to show the superior pole of the glenoid.

SHOULDER: BICEPS TENDON

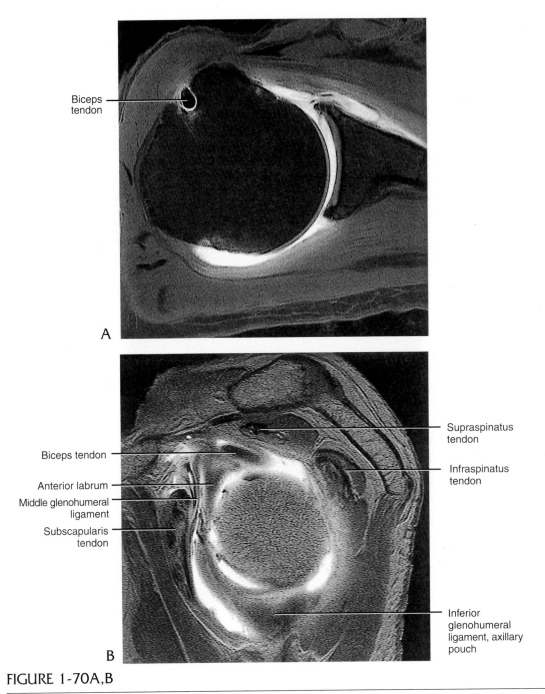

FIGURE 1-70A,B

The long head of the biceps tendon on a fat-suppressed T1-weighted axial MR arthrogram **(A)** and a T1-weighted sagittal oblique MR arthrogram **(B)**.

SHOULDER: BICEPS TENDON

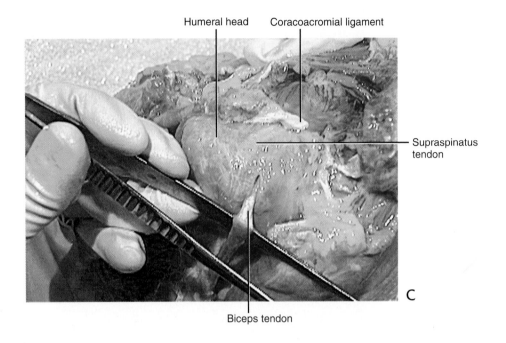

Humeral head   Coracoacromial ligament

Supraspinatus tendon

C

Biceps tendon

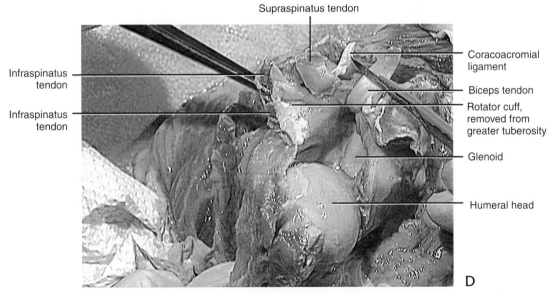

Supraspinatus tendon

Infraspinatus tendon

Infraspinatus tendon

Coracoacromial ligament

Biceps tendon

Rotator cuff, removed from greater tuberosity

Glenoid

Humeral head

D

FIGURE 1-70C,D *CONTINUED*

(C) The extraarticular portion of the long head of the biceps tendon in the bicipital groove in the hiatus between the subscapularis and supraspinatus tendons. **(D)** The relationship of the long head of the biceps tendon is shown relative to the rotator cuff and coracoacromial ligament. Fibers of the biceps contribute to the posterior and superior labrum. The long head of the biceps, with the biceps labral complex, centralizes and stabilizes the joint, as does the rotator cuff.

SHOULDER: BICEPS TENDON

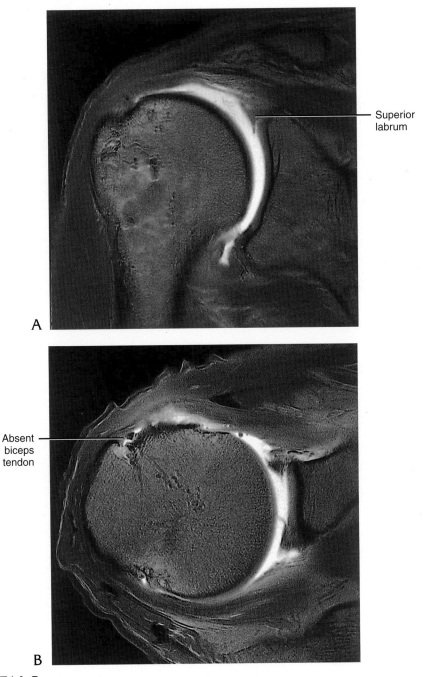

Superior labrum

Absent biceps tendon

A

B

FIGURE 1-71A,B

Absent biceps tendon on T1-weighted coronal oblique **(A)** and T1-weighted axial **(B)** MR arthrograms. The superior labrum is shown in part **A** without a biceps attachment.

SHOULDER: BICEPS TENDON

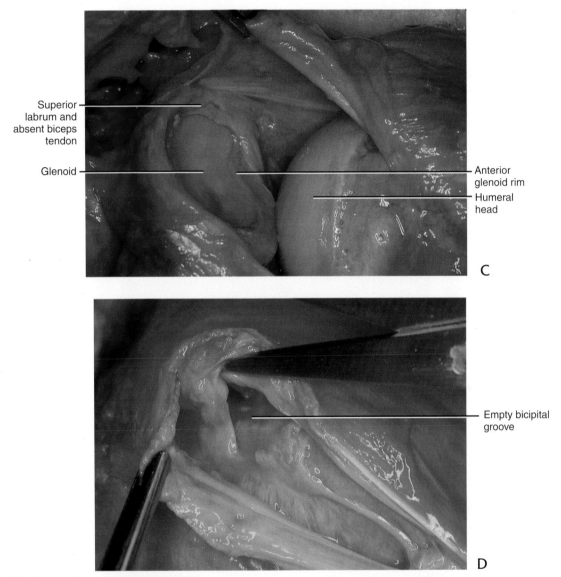

Superior labrum and absent biceps tendon

Glenoid

Anterior glenoid rim

Humeral head

C

Empty bicipital groove

D

FIGURE 1-71C,D *CONTINUED*

(**C** and **D**) Corresponding specimens displaying the intraarticular absence of the biceps tendon (**C**) and an empty bicipital groove (**D**).

SHOULDER: SUPERIOR GLENOHUMERAL LIGAMENT AND SUBSCAPULARIS TENDON

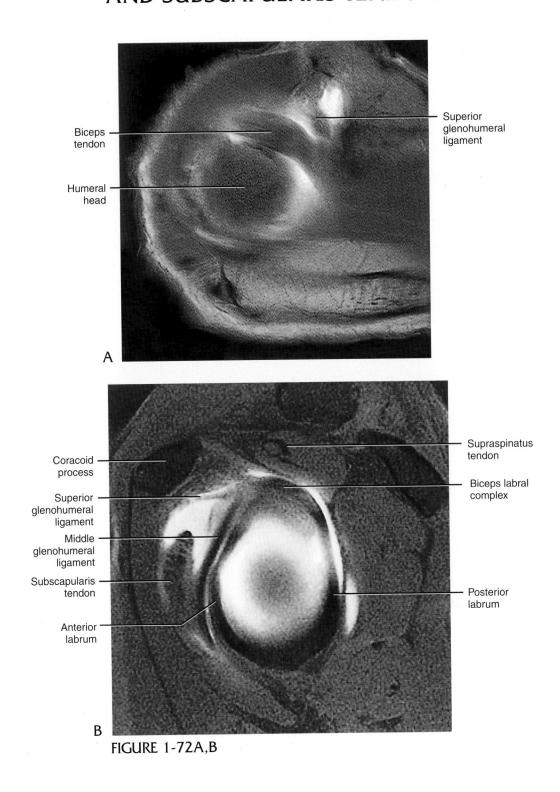

FIGURE 1-72A,B

SHOULDER: SUPERIOR GLENOHUMERAL LIGAMENT AND SUBSCAPULARIS TENDON

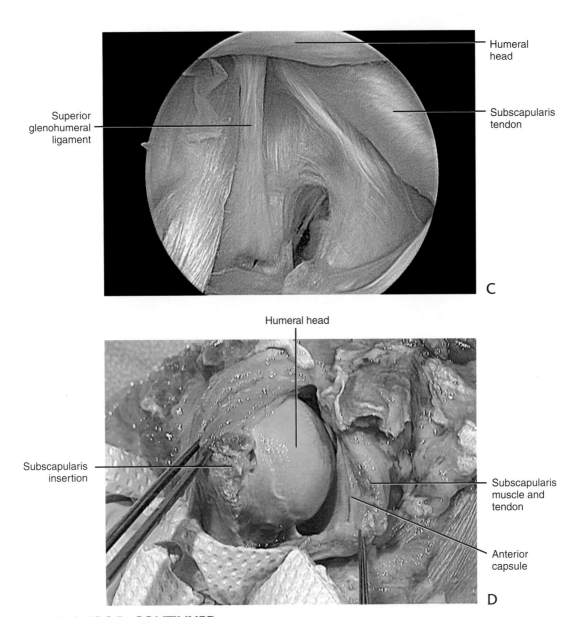

FIGURE 1-72C,D *CONTINUED*

(A) The long head of the biceps tendon and more medially located superior glenohumeral ligament are shown on a T1-weighted MR arthrogram through the superior aspect of the glenohumeral joint. **(B)** The superior glenohumeral ligament and biceps labral complex are demonstrated on a T1-weighted sagittal oblique MR arthrogram. The size of the superior glenohumeral ligament varies, ranging from a thin, thread-like thickening of the capsule to a more substantial ligament. The insertion of the superior glenohumeral ligament is superior to the lesser tuberosity in the region of the bicipital groove. The superior glenohumeral ligament has attachments to the middle glenohumeral ligament, biceps tendon, and labrum. **(C)** Posterior arthroscopic view showing the subscapularis tendon and the superior glenohumeral ligament. **(D)** Corresponding gross specimen with the subscapularis tendon lying on the anterior aspect of the anterior capsule. The superior portion of the subscapularis tendon is intraarticular (see part **C**). The subscapularis tendon insertion on the lesser tuberosity is also identified.

SHOULDER: ANTERIOR CAPSULE AND GLENOID

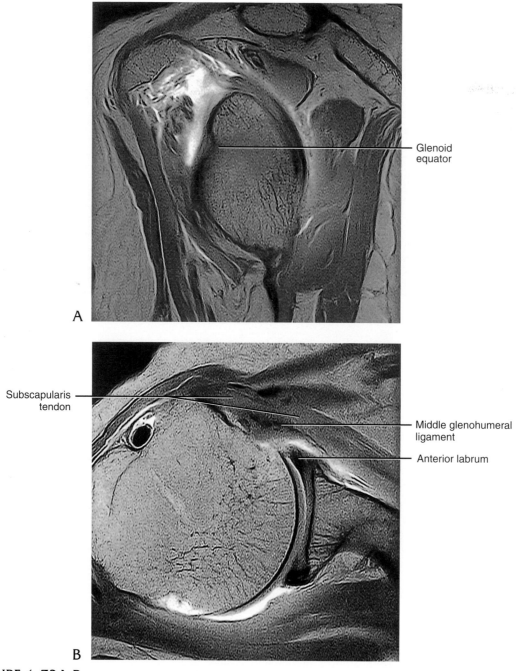

FIGURE 1-73A,B

(A) The equator of the glenoid corresponding to the epiphyseal line of the glenoid fossa is demonstrated on a T1-weighted sagittal oblique MR arthrogram. (B) The subscapularis tendon, the middle glenohumeral ligament, and the anterior labrum shown on a T1-weighted axial MR arthrogram at the level of the equator.

SHOULDER: ANTERIOR CAPSULE AND GLENOID

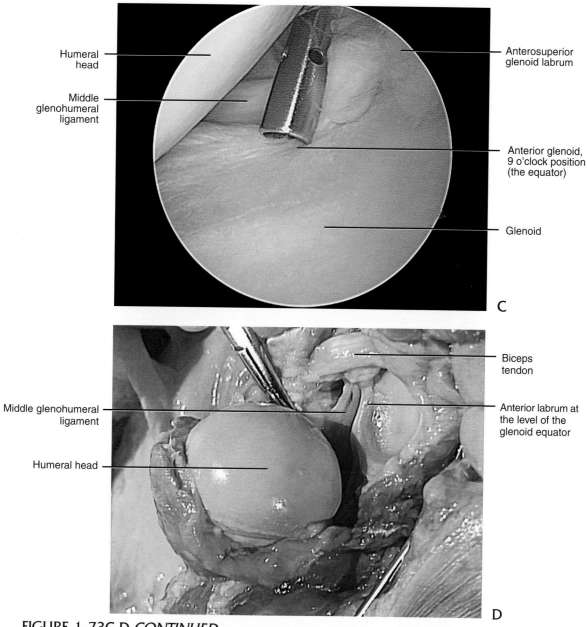

Humeral head

Middle glenohumeral ligament

Anterosuperior glenoid labrum

Anterior glenoid, 9 o'clock position (the equator)

Glenoid

C

Middle glenohumeral ligament

Humeral head

Biceps tendon

Anterior labrum at the level of the glenoid equator

D

FIGURE 1-73C,D *CONTINUED*

(C) Arthroscopic view of the anterior glenoid indentation at the nine o'clock position of the equator. **(D)** Corresponding gross specimen with the middle glenohumeral ligament and anterior labrum at the glenoid equator.

SHOULDER: MIDDLE GLENOHUMERAL LIGAMENT

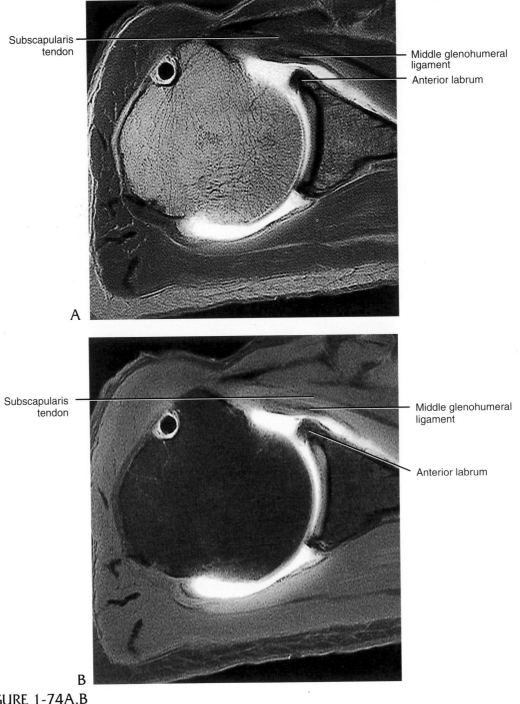

Subscapularis
tendon

Middle glenohumeral
ligament

Anterior labrum

A

Subscapularis
tendon

Middle glenohumeral
ligament

Anterior labrum

B

FIGURE 1-74A,B

Middle glenohumeral ligament (MGL). T1-weighted **(A)** and fat-suppressed T1-weighted **(B)** MR arthrograms showing the MGL between the subscapularis tendon and the anterior labrum. The MGL, which may present as thin ligamentous tissue or a more cordlike structure, has a role in the stability of the shoulder joint from 0° to 45° of abduction. It demonstrates a more vertical orientation with internal rotation and courses horizontally (elongates) with external rotation. The MGL is seen passing across the subscapularis tendon on corresponding arthroscopic **(C)** and gross **(D)** specimens.

SHOULDER: MIDDLE GLENOHUMERAL LIGAMENT

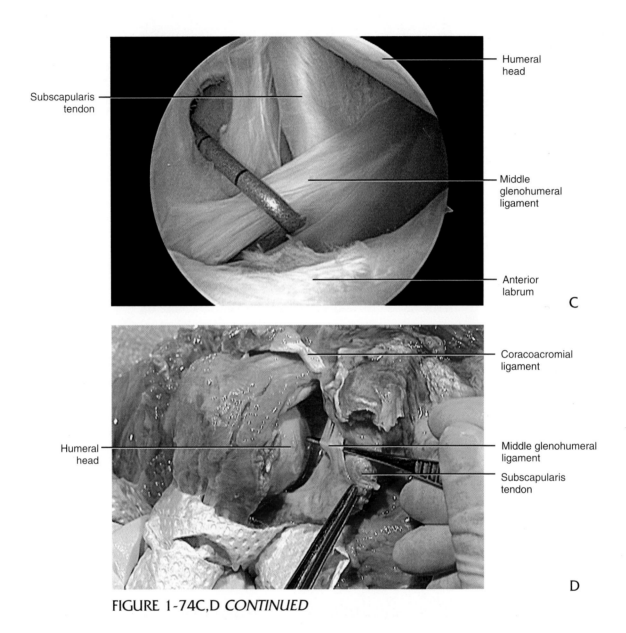

FIGURE 1-74C,D *CONTINUED*

SHOULDER: INFERIOR GLENOHUMERAL LIGAMENT

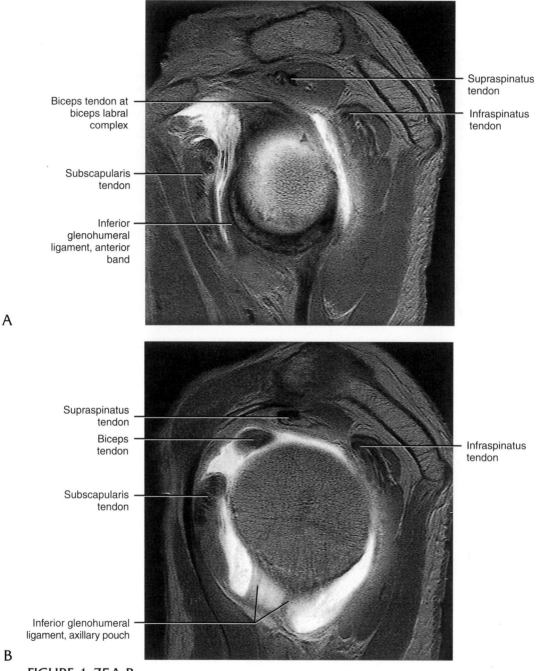

Supraspinatus
tendon

Biceps tendon at
biceps labral
complex

Subscapularis
tendon

Infraspinatus
tendon

Inferior
glenohumeral
ligament, anterior
band

A

Supraspinatus
tendon

Biceps
tendon

Subscapularis
tendon

Infraspinatus
tendon

Inferior glenohumeral
ligament, axillary pouch

B

FIGURE 1-75A,B

T1-weighted sagittal oblique MR arthrograms showing the anterior band **(A)** and the axillary pouch **(B)** of the inferior glenohumeral ligament. The inferior glenohumeral ligament is lax in the adducted position. As it tightens with increasing abduction, the anterior and posterior bands move superiorly with respect to the humeral head. At 90° of abduction, the inferior glenohumeral ligament is the primary restraint for anterior and posterior dislocations.

SHOULDER: INFERIOR GLENOHUMERAL LIGAMENT

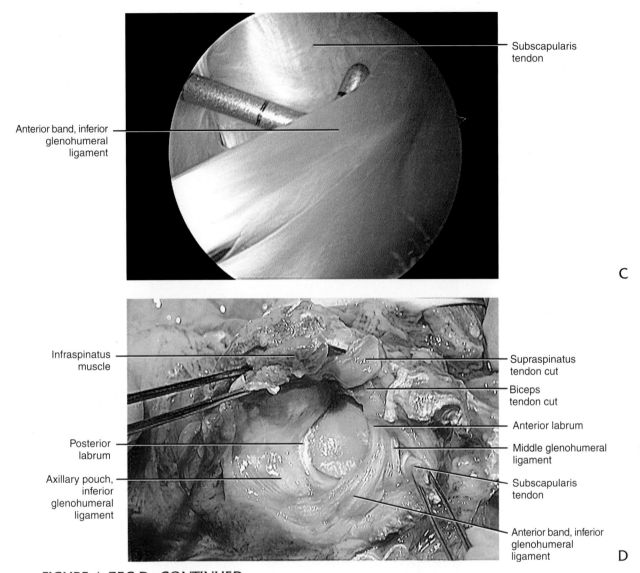

Subscapularis
tendon

Anterior band, inferior
glenohumeral
ligament

C

Infraspinatus
muscle

Supraspinatus
tendon cut

Biceps
tendon cut

Anterior labrum

Posterior
labrum

Middle glenohumeral
ligament

Axillary pouch,
inferior
glenohumeral
ligament

Subscapularis
tendon

Anterior band, inferior
glenohumeral
ligament

D

FIGURE 1-75C,D, *CONTINUED*

(C) An arthroscopic view showing the anterior band of the inferior glenohumeral ligament. The anterior band forms the anterior labrum at the medial attachment of the inferior glenohumeral ligament to the glenoid. The posterior band contributes to the formation of the posterior labrum. **(D)** The well-defined anterior band and axillary pouch are demonstrated on this corresponding gross specimen with the humeral head removed. The origin of the anterior band is located near the three o'clock position on the glenoid.

SHOULDER: INFERIOR GLENOHUMERAL LIGAMENT

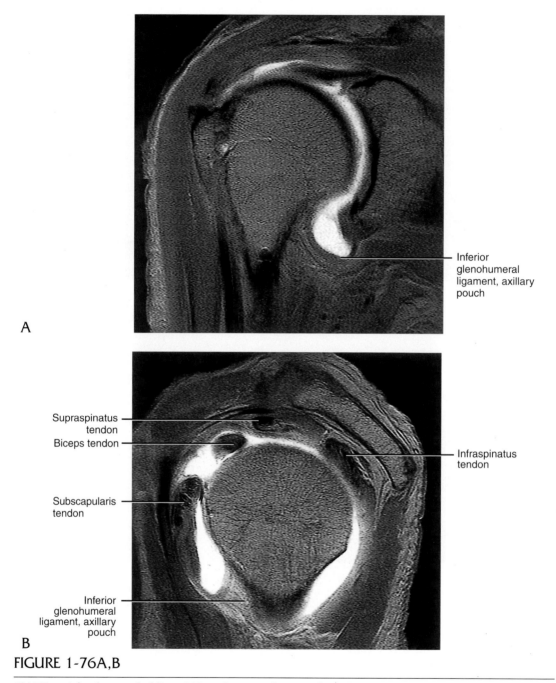

A

B

FIGURE 1-76A,B

(A) T1-weighted coronal oblique MR arthrogram showing the axillary pouch of the inferior glenohumeral ligament, which extends inferior to the glenohumeral joint as a redundancy of thickened capsular tissue. **(B)** T1-weighted sagittal oblique MR arthrogram showing the inferior glenohumeral ligament complex, which inserts onto the anatomic neck of the humerus either as a collar-like attachment or as a V-shaped attachment.

SHOULDER: INFERIOR GLENOHUMERAL LIGAMENT

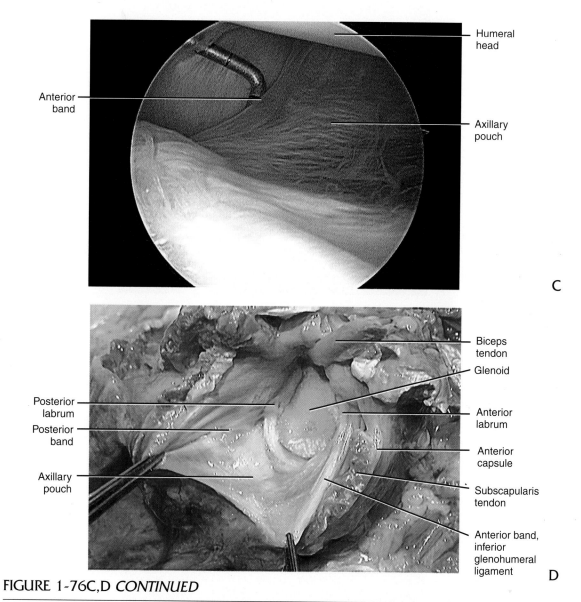

C

D

FIGURE 1-76C,D *CONTINUED*

(C and **D)** The inferior glenohumeral ligament complex shown on corresponding arthroscopic **(C)** and gross **(D)** views. Note that the posterior band of the inferior glenohumeral ligament is not as well-defined as the anterior band.

SHOULDER: ANTERIOR LABRUM

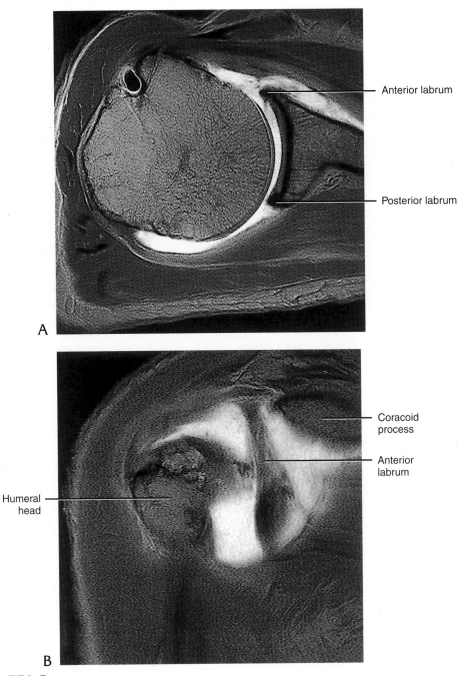

Anterior labrum

Posterior labrum

Coracoid process

Anterior labrum

Humeral head

B

FIGURE 1-77A,B

The glenoid labrum on T1-weighted axial **(A)** and coronal oblique **(B)** MR arthrograms. The labrum represents the fibrous attachment of the glenohumeral ligaments and capsule to the glenoid rim. Above the epiphyseal line (i.e., the junction of the upper and middle thirds of the glenoid body fossa), the attachment of the labrum is variable. Inferior to the epiphyseal line, the labrum is continuous with the glenoid articular cartilage and serves as the insertion site for the inferior glenohumeral ligament. Corresponding arthroscopic **(C)** and gross **(D)** views of the anterior labrum.

SHOULDER: ANTERIOR LABRUM

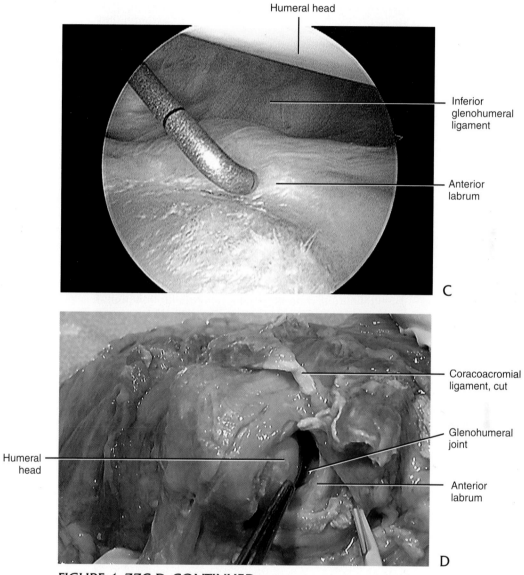

Humeral head

Inferior
glenohumeral
ligament

Anterior
labrum

C

Coracoacromial
ligament, cut

Glenohumeral
joint

Humeral
head

Anterior
labrum

D

FIGURE 1-77C,D *CONTINUED*

SHOULDER: BICEPS LABRAL COMPLEX

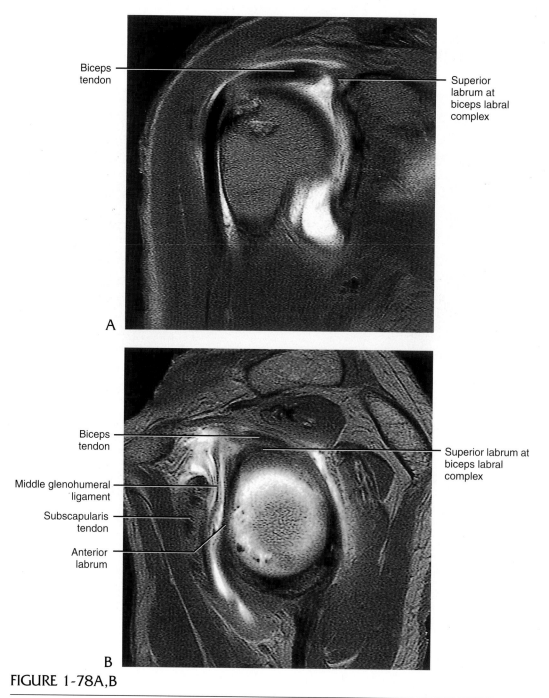

Biceps tendon

Superior labrum at biceps labral complex

Biceps tendon

Superior labrum at biceps labral complex

Middle glenohumeral ligament

Subscapularis tendon

Anterior labrum

FIGURE 1-78A,B

The biceps labral complex on T1-weighted coronal oblique (**A**) and sagittal oblique (**B**) MR arthrograms. The superior labrum functions in conjunction with the biceps tendon to form the biceps labral complex (BLC). The BLC corresponds to the labrum above the equator (epiphyseal line) and represents the upper one-third of the glenoid labrum. (**C** and **D**) Arthroscopic views of the BLC. (**E**) Corresponding dissection with the BLC shown at the level of the superior pole of the glenoid.

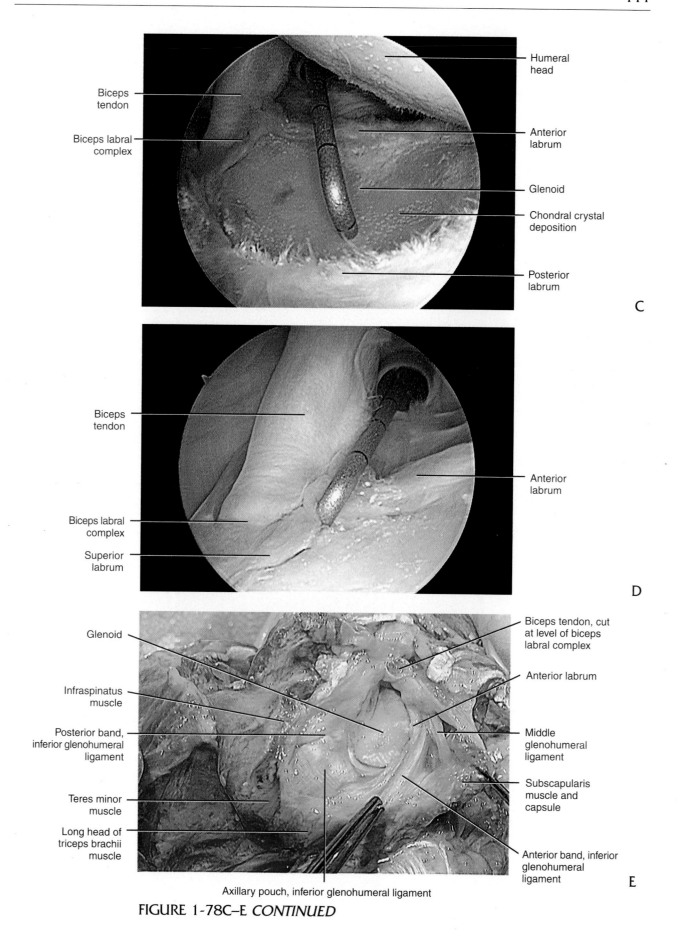

Biceps tendon

Biceps labral complex

Humeral head

Anterior labrum

Glenoid

Chondral crystal deposition

Posterior labrum

C

Biceps tendon

Biceps labral complex

Superior labrum

Anterior labrum

D

Glenoid

Infraspinatus muscle

Posterior band, inferior glenohumeral ligament

Teres minor muscle

Long head of triceps brachii muscle

Biceps tendon, cut at level of biceps labral complex

Anterior labrum

Middle glenohumeral ligament

Subscapularis muscle and capsule

Anterior band, inferior glenohumeral ligament

Axillary pouch, inferior glenohumeral ligament

E

FIGURE 1-78C–E CONTINUED

SHOULDER: BICEPS LABRAL COMPLEX, TYPE 1

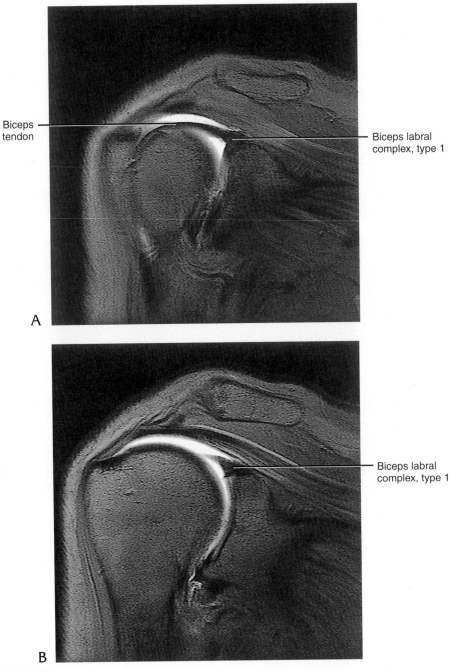

Biceps
tendon

Biceps labral
complex, type 1

A

Biceps labral
complex, type 1

B

FIGURE 1-79A,B

(**A** and **B**) Type 1 biceps labral complex on T1-weighted coronal oblique MR arthrogram. The image in part **A** is anterior to the image in part **B**. In a Type 1 attachment, the biceps labral complex is firmly attached to the superior pole of the glenoid.

SHOULDER: BICEPS LABRAL COMPLEX, TYPE 1

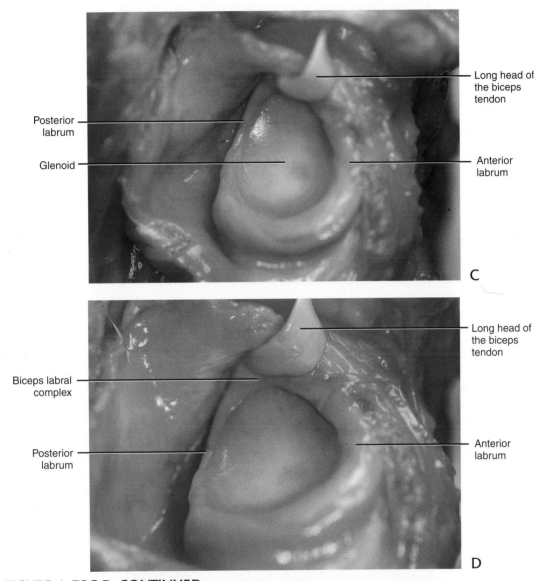

FIGURE 1-79C,D *CONTINUED*

(**C** and **D**) Corresponding gross specimens identifying the long head of the biceps tendon and the biceps labral complex. The superior labrum is adherent to the superior pole of the glenoid, and a sulcus does not exist between the superior labrum and the glenoid articular cartilage. In addition, there is no associated anterosuperior sublabral foramen in this type of biceps labral complex.

SHOULDER: BICEPS LABRAL COMPLEX, TYPE 2

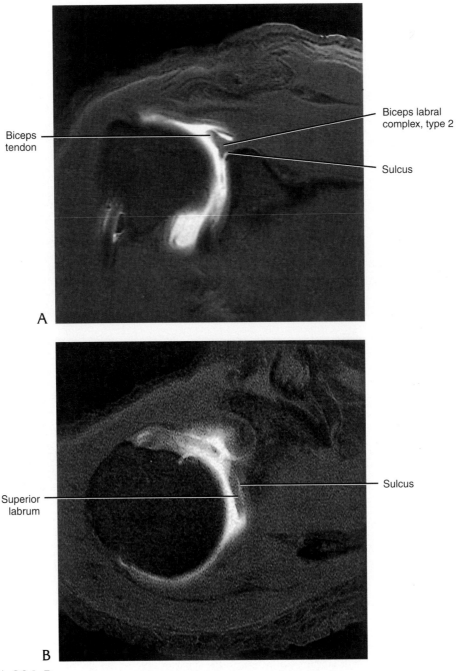

FIGURE 1-80A,B

Type 2 biceps labral complex with the biceps attached to the superior labrum lateral to the superior glenoid. The biceps tendon continues medially and attaches to the supraglenoid tubercle. **(A)** A fat-suppressed T1-weighted coronal oblique MR arthrogram showing the fluid-filled sulcus that formed at the superior pole of the glenoid. **(B)** A fat-suppressed T1-weighted axial image, obtained through the biceps labral sulcus, shows a layer of fluid interposed between the labrum and glenoid corresponding to the sulcus. This could be mistaken for a SLAP (superior labrum from anterior to posterior) lesion. The frayed superior labrum and sulcus are demonstrated on a corresponding fat-suppressed T1-weighted sagittal oblique MR arthrogram **(C)** and a lateral view of glenoid dissection **(D)**.

SHOULDER: BICEPS LABRAL COMPLEX, TYPE 2

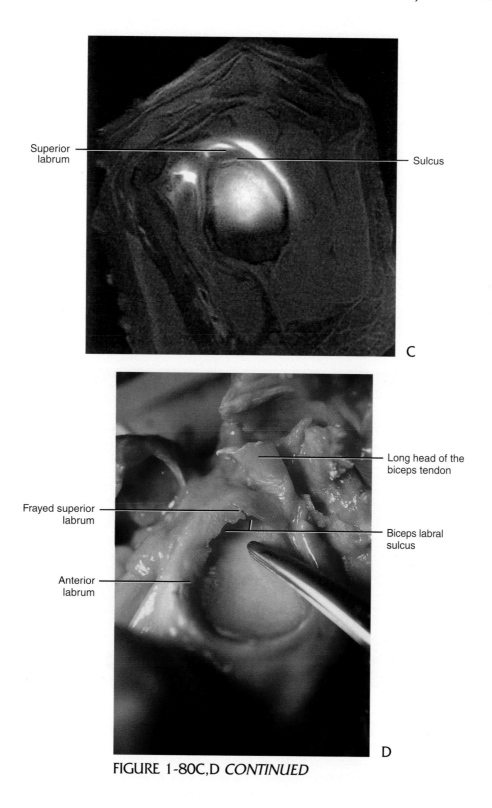

FIGURE 1-80C,D *CONTINUED*

SHOULDER: BICEPS LABRAL COMPLEX, TYPE 3

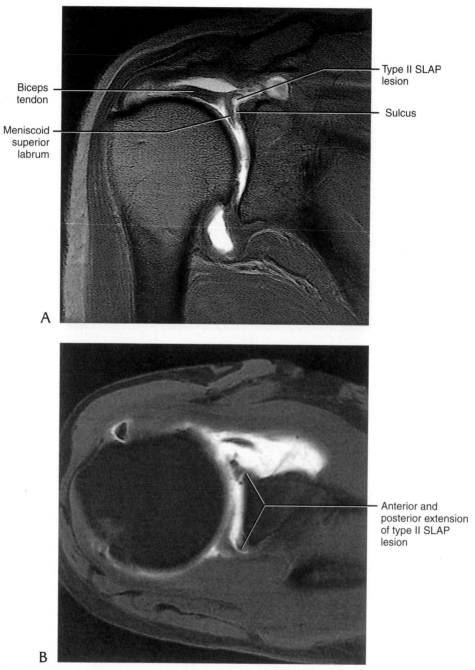

FIGURE 1-81A,B

(A) T1-weighted coronal oblique MR arthrogram illustrating a Type 3 biceps labral complex with a large sulcus extending underneath a meniscoid superior labrum. This meniscoid labrum has an associated Type II SLAP (superior labrum from anterior to posterior) lesion with detachment of the superior labrum and biceps tendon expansion (when present the finding of intralabral signal intensity can be used to differentiate a true SLAP lesion from a normal biceps labral sulcus). (B) Fat-suppressed T1-weighted axial MR arthrogram identifying the anterior to posterior extension of the Type II SLAP lesion. The Type II SLAP lesion and meniscoid labrum with posterior superior labral tear is shown on a T1-weighted sagittal MR arthrogram (C) and on a corresponding gross specimen (D).

SHOULDER: BICEPS LABRAL COMPLEX, TYPE 3

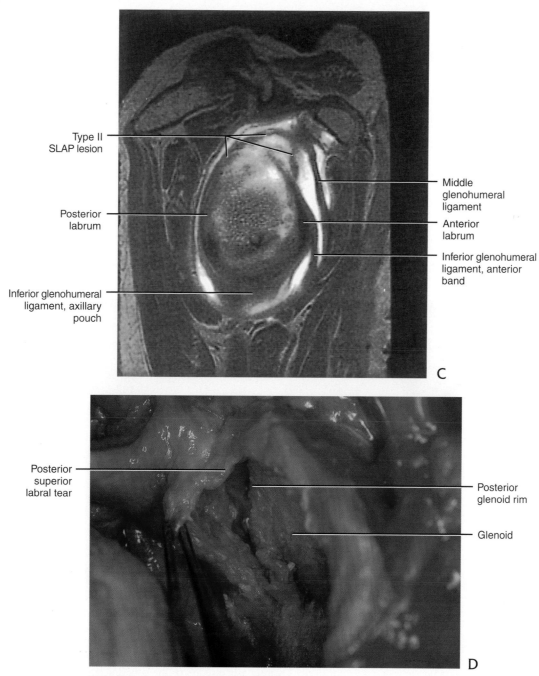

Type II
SLAP lesion

Posterior
labrum

Inferior glenohumeral
ligament, axillary
pouch

Middle
glenohumeral
ligament

Anterior
labrum

Inferior glenohumeral
ligament, anterior
band

C

Posterior
superior
labral tear

Posterior
glenoid rim

Glenoid

D

FIGURE 1-81C,D *CONTINUED*

SHOULDER: SLAP II LESION

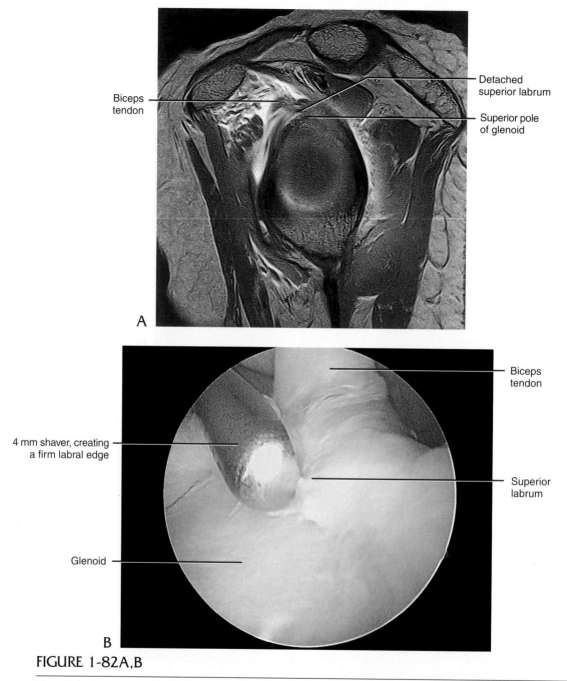

Biceps tendon

Detached superior labrum

Superior pole of glenoid

A

Biceps tendon

4 mm shaver, creating a firm labral edge

Superior labrum

Glenoid

B

FIGURE 1-82A,B

Type II SLAP (superior labrum from anterior to posterior) lesion. **(A)** T1–weighted sagittal MR arthrogram showing separation of the superior labrum and biceps anchor (expansion) from the superior pole of the glenoid. **(B)** Arthroscopic view of a 4.0 mm shaver creating a firm edge to the superior labrum at the site of detachment.

SHOULDER: SLAP II LESION

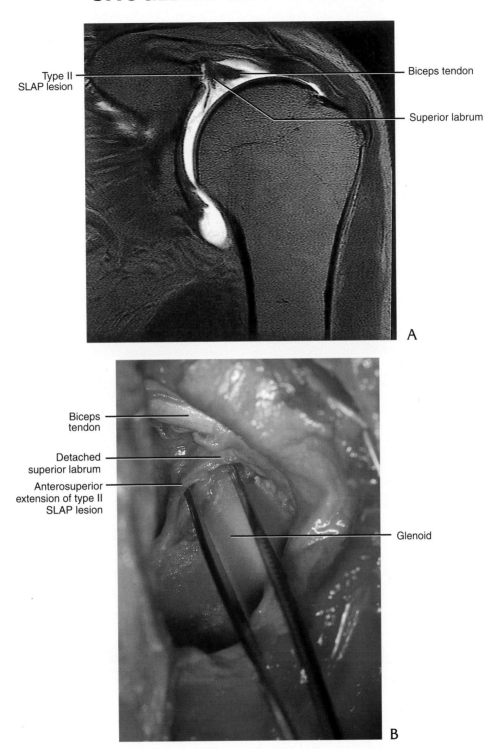

Type II
SLAP lesion

Biceps tendon

Superior labrum

A

Biceps
tendon

Detached
superior labrum

Anterosuperior
extension of type II
SLAP lesion

Glenoid

B

FIGURE 1-83A,B

Type II SLAP (superior labrum from anterior to posterior) lesion. A T1-weighted coronal oblique MR arthrogram **(A)** and a corresponding gross dissection **(B)** identifying superior labral and biceps tendon detachment. The term biceps expansion should be used to replace the torn biceps anchor since the origin of the biceps tendon from the supraglenoid tubercle is not involved. The biceps tendon has a separate expansion or attachment directly to the anterior and posterior glenoid labrum. Except for the frayed appearance of the superior labrum this SLAP lesion could be mistaken for a prominent biceps labral sulcus on the coronal oblique MR image.

SHOULDER: SUBLABRAL FORAMEN

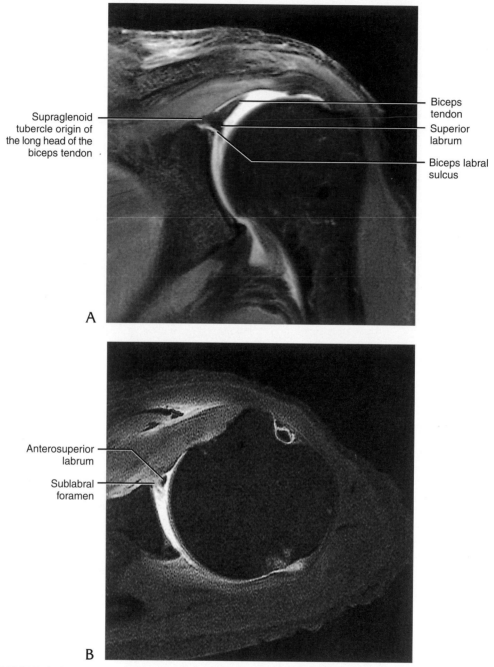

Supraglenoid
tubercle origin of
the long head of the
biceps tendon

Biceps
tendon

Superior
labrum

Biceps labral
sulcus

A

Anterosuperior
labrum

Sublabral
foramen

B

FIGURE 1-84A,B

Sublabral foramen. **(A)** The biceps labral sulcus between the superior labrum and the superior pole of the glenoid is not the sublabral foramen. **(B)** The sublabral foramen is shown with fluid undermining the anterosuperior labrum.

SHOULDER: SUBLABRAL FORAMEN

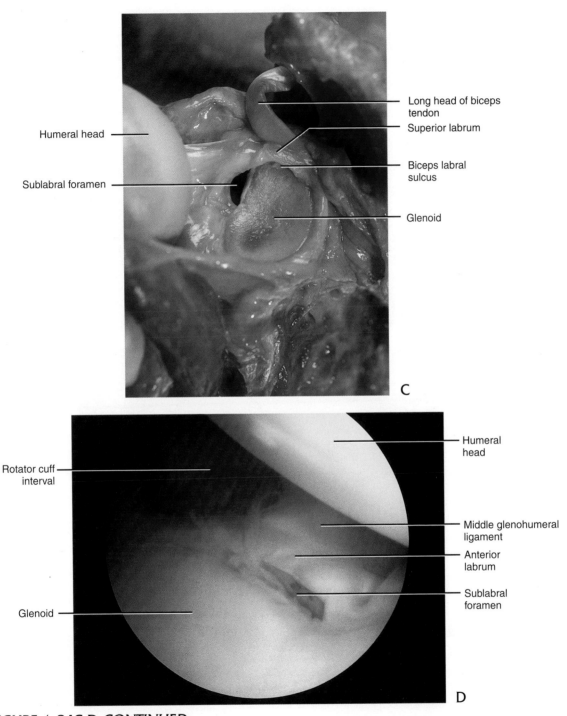

Long head of biceps tendon

Humeral head

Superior labrum

Biceps labral sulcus

Sublabral foramen

Glenoid

C

Rotator cuff interval

Humeral head

Middle glenohumeral ligament

Anterior labrum

Sublabral foramen

Glenoid

D

FIGURE 1-84C,D *CONTINUED*

(C) Corresponding gross specimen has both an anterosuperior sublabral foramen and a superior biceps labral sulcus. This is a common association in a meniscoid superior labrum. **(D)** An arthroscopic photograph of a separate specimen showing a sublabral foramen with an absent anterior labral attachment above the epiphyseal line of the glenoid.

SHOULDER: BUFORD COMPLEX

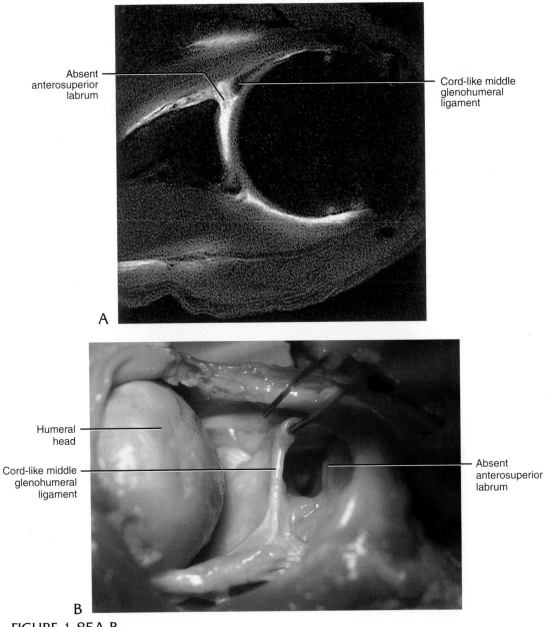

FIGURE 1-85A,B

Buford complex. **(A)** A fat-suppressed T1-weighted axial MR arthrogram showing a cord-like middle glenohumeral ligament with an absent anterosuperior labrum. The labrum below the level of the subscapularis (inferior labrum) is normal. **(B)** Corresponding gross specimen demonstrates the cord-like middle glenohumeral ligament, which attaches directly to the superior labrum.

SHOULDER: BUFORD COMPLEX

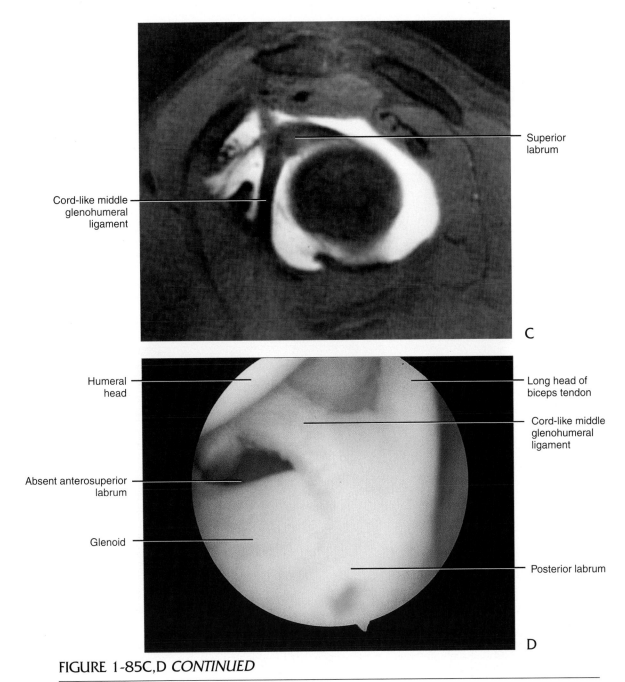

FIGURE 1-85C,D *CONTINUED*

(**C** and **D**) In a separate specimen, a cord-like middle glenohumeral ligament is shown as part of the Buford complex on a fat-suppressed T1-weighted sagittal image (**C**) and an arthroscopic view (**D**). The middle glenohumeral ligament can be seen to be directly attached to the superior labrum at the base of the biceps anchor.

SHOULDER: ANTERIOR LABRAL TEAR

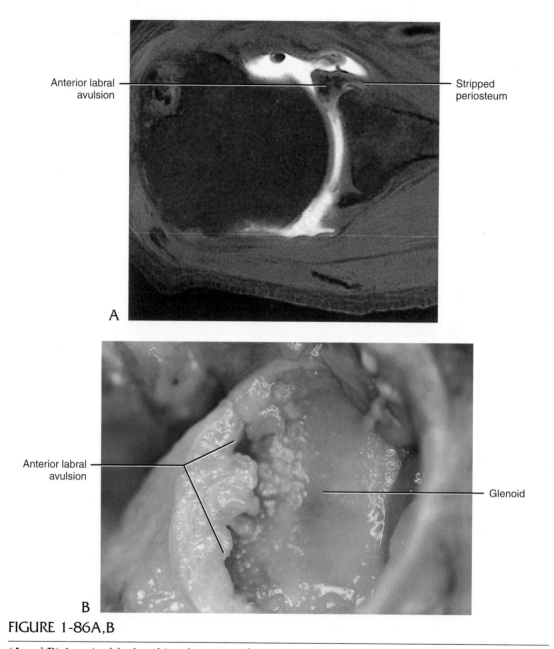

FIGURE 1-86A,B

(**A** and **B**) Anterior labral avulsion shown on a fat-suppressed T1-weighted MR arthrogram (**A**) and on the corresponding glenoid dissection (lateral view) (**B**).

SHOULDER: ANTERIOR LABRAL TEAR, THE ALPSA LESION

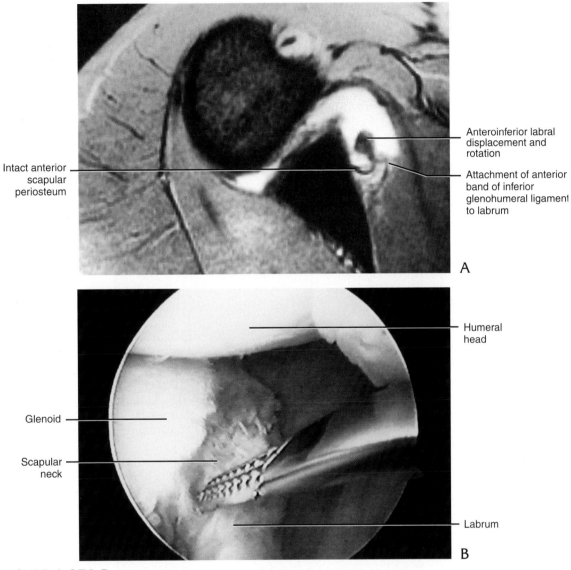

Intact anterior
scapular
periosteum

Anteroinferior labral
displacement and
rotation

Attachment of anterior
band of inferior
glenohumeral ligament
to labrum

A

Humeral
head

Glenoid

Scapular
neck

Labrum

B

FIGURE 1-87A,B

An ALPSA lesion (anterior labroligamentous periosteal sleeve avulsion) is demonstrated on a T2*-weighted axial MR image (**A**) and an arthroscopic view (**B**). The labrum is displayed medially along the anterior neck of the glenoid. The associated inferior rotation of the labrum produces a blunted morphology as appreciated on the axial MR image in part **A**.

SHOULDER: POSTERIOR CAPSULE TEAR

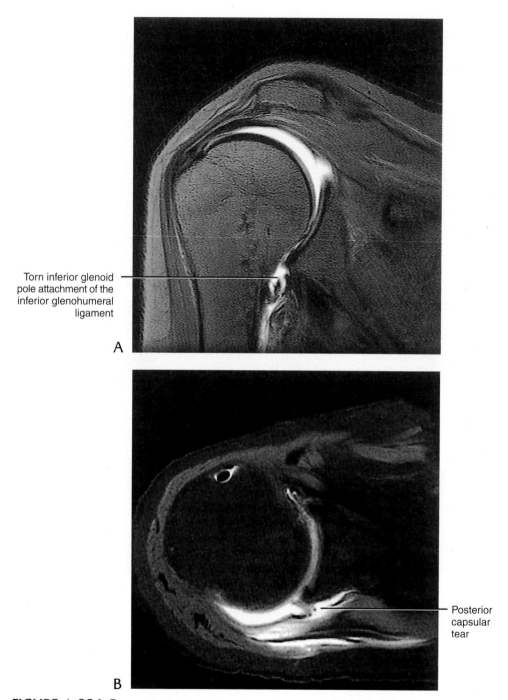

Torn inferior glenoid pole attachment of the inferior glenohumeral ligament

A

Posterior capsular tear

B

FIGURE 1-88A,B

A posterior capsule tear with an inferior glenohumeral ligament defect is shown on a T1-weighted posterior coronal oblique MR arthrogram **(A)**, a fat-suppressed T1-weighted axial MR arthrogram **(B)**, and an external rotation and abduction (ABER) MR arthrogram **(C)**. **(D)** The corresponding capsular defect is shown on the gross dissection.

SHOULDER: POSTERIOR CAPSULE TEAR

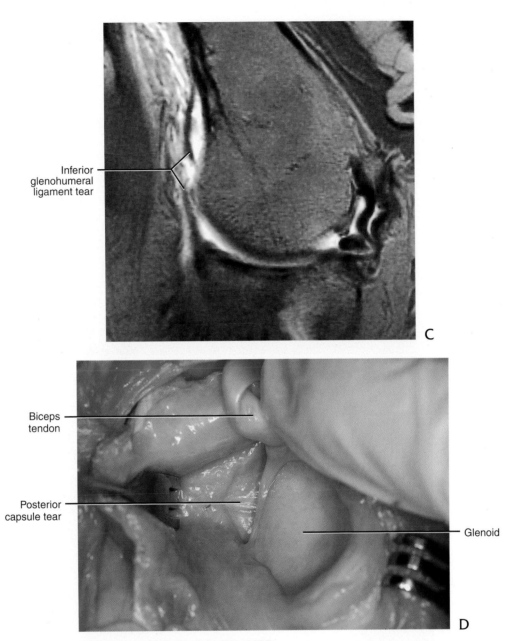

FIGURE 1-88C,D *CONTINUED*

SHOULDER: HAGL LESION

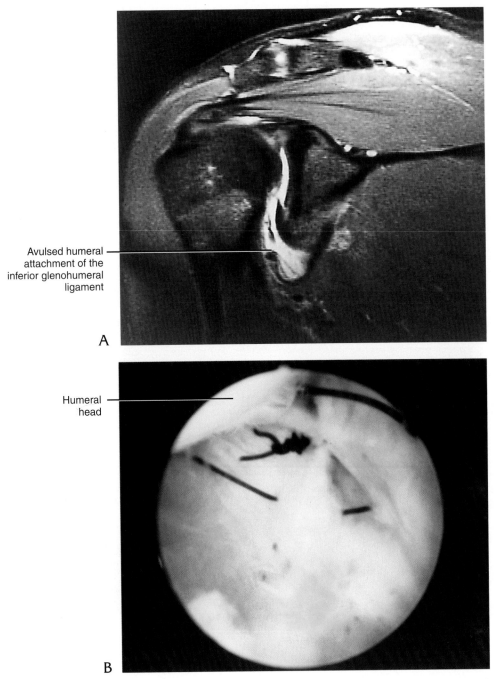

Avulsed humeral
attachment of the
inferior glenohumeral
ligament

A

Humeral
head

B

FIGURE 1-89A,B

Humeral avulsion of the glenohumeral ligament (HAGL lesion). **(A)** A fat-suppressed T2-weighted fast spin-echo coronal oblique MR arthrogram showing tearing of the humeral attachment of the inferior gleno-humeral ligament. **(B)** The corresponding arthroscopic view showing suturing with coaptation of the de-tached portion of the inferior glenohumeral ligament.

SHOULDER: HAGL LESION

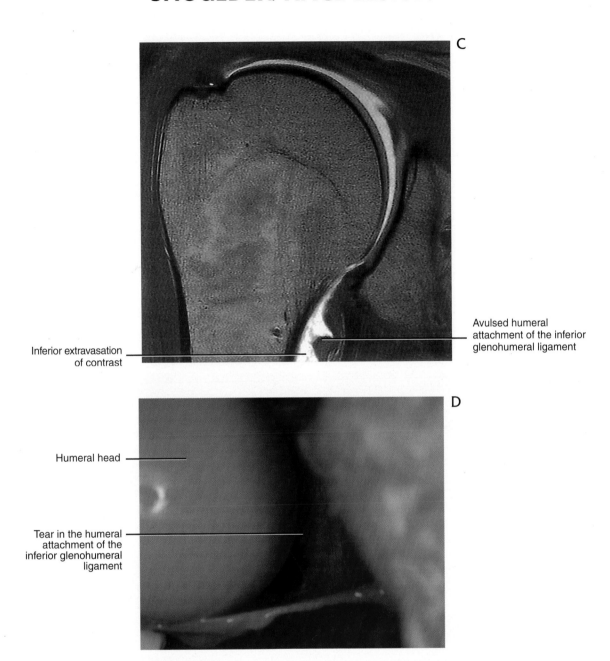

C

Avulsed humeral
attachment of the inferior
glenohumeral ligament

Inferior extravasation
of contrast

D

Humeral head

Tear in the humeral
attachment of the
inferior glenohumeral
ligament

FIGURE 1-89C,D *CONTINUED*

(**C** and **D**) In a separate case, the T1-weighted coronal oblique MR arthrogram (**C**) and gross specimen (**D**) demonstrate the defect in the humeral attachment of the inferior glenohumeral ligament. The HAGL lesion may exist in patients with anterior instability with or without an associated anterior labral tear.

SHOULDER: OSTEOARTHRITIS

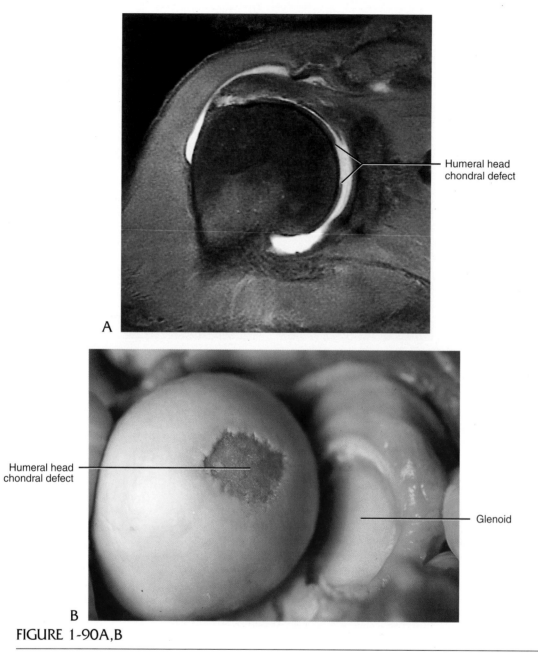

FIGURE 1-90A,B

Articular cartilage loss of the humeral head in osteoarthritis. **(A)** Fat-suppressed T1-weighted coronal oblique MR arthrogram. **(B)** Gross dissection of the disarticulated humeral head.

SHOULDER: AVASCULAR NECROSIS

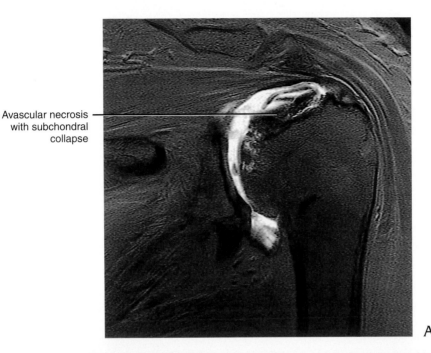

Avascular necrosis
with subchondral
collapse

A

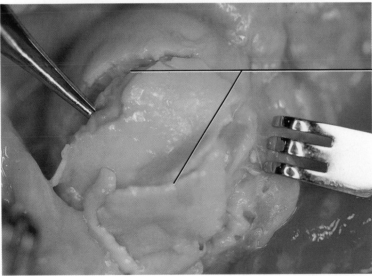

Subchondral collapse in
avascular necrosis of the
humeral head

B

FIGURE 1-91A,B

(**A** and **B**) A fat-suppressed T1-weighted coronal oblique MR arthrogram (**A**) and a humeral head superior view (**B**) demonstrate extensive subchondral collapse producing flattening of the humeral head in avascular necrosis.

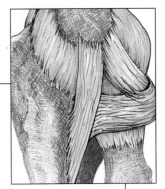

CHAPTER 2

THE ELBOW

David W. Stoller
Salvador Beltran
Mathias Masem
Louis Keppler
Russell C. Fritz

ELBOW ARTHROSCOPY AND DISSECTION
MR NORMAL ANATOMY

COLOR ANATOMIC ILLUSTRATIONS
MR, ARTHROSCOPY, AND SURGICAL CORRELATION

——— ELBOW ARTHROSCOPY ———

ARTHROSCOPY OF THE ELBOW with the patient in the prone position permits improved arthroscopic manipulation and flexion and extension of the elbow. The lateral epicondyle, the olecranon, and the radial head form a triangle on the lateral aspect of the elbow. The soft spot in the center of this anconeus triangle is the landmark for injection to distend the capsule prior to establishing the arthroscopic portals. When the elbow joint is distended and positioned in 90° of flexion, the neurovascular structures are displaced anteriorly making anterior portal placement safer.

The common portals used for elbow arthroscopy include the antero-medial portal (the primary diagnostic portal) and the posterolateral, antero-lateral, and straight posterior portals. A proximal lateral portal can be used in place of the anterolateral approach, which is more hazardous with respect to radial nerve injury. The proximal medial or anteromedial portal allows visu-alization of the humeroulnar joint, the radiocapitellar joint, the coronoid fossa, and the medial and lateral gutters. The posterolateral portal facilitates visualization of the olecranon and the olecranon fossa.

The trochlea is devoid of articular cartilage in the centrally located bare areas of the trochlear notch, between the proximal and distal articular facets. Loose bodies, usually the result of osteochondritis, may be identified arthroscopically in the lateral and posterior compartments. Posterior im-pingement in athletes who use a throwing motion may cause posteromedial olecranon osteophytes with associated chondromalacia of the trochlea.

Arthroscopy can be used to evaluate medial and posterolateral instability of the elbow. Since only a portion of the anterior and posterior bundles of the medial collateral ligament (MCL) can be seen during arthroscopy, a complete tear of the anterior bundle may be missed. Synovitis of the elbow may be associated with thickened synovial bands, synovial chondromatosis, and inflammatory (rheumatoid) arthritis. Anterior lesions of the elbow joint include hypertrophy of the coronoid process and coronoid fractures. Since there is no capsular attachment to the coronoid process, a fracture of the tip of the coronoid is associated with either elbow subluxation or dislocation and is not an avulsion injury. Posttraumatic arthrofibrosis may develop as a result of elbow dislocation or fracture of the radial head. Degenerative arthritis is usually related to a traumatic episode or to a chronic repetitive injury. In the athlete who uses a throwing motion, osteochondritis dissecans of the capitellum occurs with valgus movement, resulting in compression of the radial capitellar articulation.

SURGICAL DISSECTION OF THE ELBOW

The triceps mechanism converges and inserts onto the olecranon. The interposition of fat between the distal fascicles of the triceps tendon may produce heterogeneity of signal intensity on corresponding axial, sagittal, and posterior coronal T1-weighted images. In full elbow extension, increased laxity of the triceps may be seen as a normal finding, without any loss of tendon continuity. In triceps tendon injury, tendinosis usually precedes rupture. Triceps tendon rupture typically occurs adjacent to the olecranon and may follow or accompany olecranon bursitis. The ulnar nerve courses within the cubital tunnel, posterior to the medial epicondyle. It is bordered by a posteromedial epicondylar groove, the medial trochlear edge, and the ulnar collateral ligament. The flexor carpi ulnaris aponeurosis (the arcuate ligament) and the cubital tunnel retinaculum (Osborne's band) contribute to the formation of the roof of the cubital tunnel. The flexor carpi ulnaris aponeurosis forms the roof of the cubital tunnel just distal to the medial epicondyle and the cubital tunnel retinaculum. The cubital tunnel retinaculum extends from the medial epicondyle to the olecranon. Anatomic variations of the cubital tunnel retinaculum may contribute to the development of ulnar neuropathy. The cubital tunnel retinaculum may be absent in as many as 10% of cases, allowing anterior dislocation of the nerve over the medial epicondyle during flexion and friction neuritis. In approximately 11% of the population the cubital tunnel retinaculum is replaced by an anomalous muscle, the anconeus epitrochlearis, resulting in static compression of the ulnar nerve. Thickening of the MCL and medial bony spurring may undermine the floor of the cubital tunnel, which is formed by the capsule of the elbow and posterior and transverse portions of the MCL. If cubital tunnel syndrome is secondary to an accessory anconeus epitrochlearis muscle, then myotomy or excision of the muscle can be performed in place of an ulnar nerve transposition or medial epicondylectomy.

Distal to the cubital tunnel, the ulnar nerve courses through the humeral and ulnar heads of the flexor carpi ulnaris. The ulnar nerve sends muscular branches to the ulnar side of the flexor carpi ulnaris muscle and the flexor digitorum profundus. The flexor carpi radialis, the palmaris longus, the flexor digitorum superficialis, and the flexor carpi ulnaris have a common tendon origin from the medial epicondyle. The pronator teres muscle has a larger humeral head origin and a smaller deep ulnar head origin. The common flexor tendon origin of the flexor carpi radialis is deep to the pronator teres. The palmaris longus origin from the common flexor tendon is deep to the flexor carpi radialis. The origin of the humeral ulnar head of the flexor digitorum superficialis is at the common flexor tendon. The origin of the flexor carpi ulnaris, at the common extensor tendon, is medial to the origin of the pronator teres, the flexor carpi radialis, the palmaris longus, and the flexor digitorum superficialis.

Medial epicondylitis is secondary to tendinosis of the common flexor tendon. It may progress to complete tendon avulsion and is often associated with ulnar neuritis. In a valgus stress injury, medial tension overload may present as an extraarticular injury, such as MCL sprain, flexor pronator muscle strain, medial epicondylitis, ulnar traction spurs, and ulnar neuritis. Valgus stress may also produce lateral compression overload with intraarticular injury, bone contusions, and osteochondritis dissecans of the capitellum or radial head. In a submuscular transposition, the ulnar nerve is placed anteriorly underneath the common flexor tendon. The MCL complex is deep to the common flexor tendon and is the primary medial stabilizer of the elbow. The anterior bundle of the MCL is the key static stabilizing ligament to valgus stress, whereas the common flexor tendon functions as a dynamic stabilizer. The anterior bundle consists of deep and superficial capsular layers. The transverse bundle lacks a humeral attachment and is not important in maintaining elbow stability. Throwers may develop undersurface partial tears or midsubstance ruptures of the MCL, which require reconstruction.

The common extensor tendon is composed of the extensor carpi radialis brevis, the extensor digitorum, the extensor digiti minimi, and the extensor carpi ulnaris. The extensor carpi radialis brevis has the most lateral extensor tendon origin from the epicondyle and is deep to the extensor carpi radialis longus. The extensor carpi ulnaris is the most medial of the common extensor tendon origins. The origin of the extensor digitorum is from the distal anterior aspect of the lateral epicondyle. Lateral epicondylitis is secondary to tendinosis of the common extensor tendon and primarily involves the extensor carpi radialis brevis tendon. Macroscopic tears of the common extensor tendon occur in 35% of surgical cases. Associated lateral collateral ligament complex injuries may result in posterolateral rotatory instability. The lateral collateral ligament complex consists of the radial collateral ligament proper, the lateral ulnar collateral ligament (LUCL), and the annular ligament. An accessory lateral collateral ligament, variably present, extends from the annular ligament to insert onto the ulna. The LUCL represents the primary restraint to varus stress and when incompetent is associated with posterolateral rotatory instability and a pivot shift phenomenon.

In distal biceps impingement syndrome, biceps tendinosis develops from mechanical impingement and a poor distal tendon blood supply. Tendinosis typically precedes rupture, which usually occurs adjacent to the radial tuberosity. The lacertus fibrosus often tears in association with biceps rupture. Partial tears of the biceps tendon and cubital bursitis are less common findings.

ELBOW: CORONAL

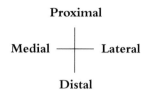

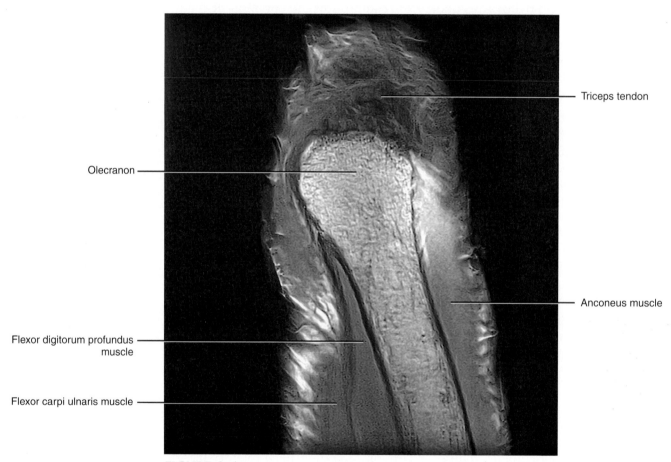

Triceps tendon

Olecranon

Anconeus muscle

Flexor digitorum profundus muscle

Flexor carpi ulnaris muscle

FIGURE 2-1

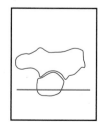

ELBOW: CORONAL

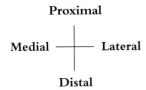

Proximal

Medial ——— Lateral

Distal

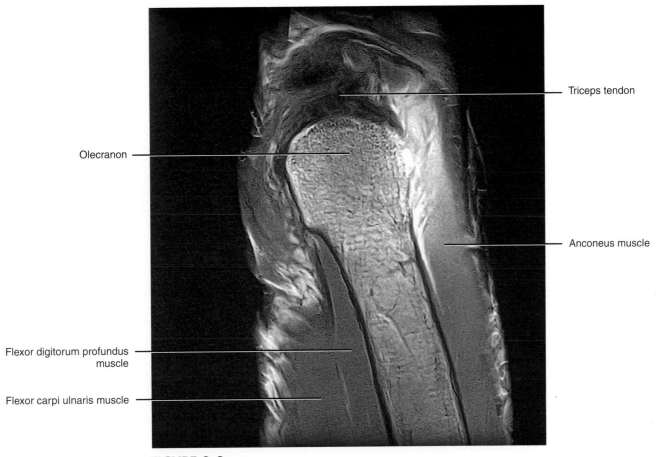

Triceps tendon

Olecranon

Anconeus muscle

Flexor digitorum profundus
muscle

Flexor carpi ulnaris muscle

FIGURE 2-2

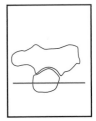

ELBOW: CORONAL

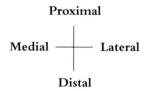

Proximal

Medial ——|—— Lateral

Distal

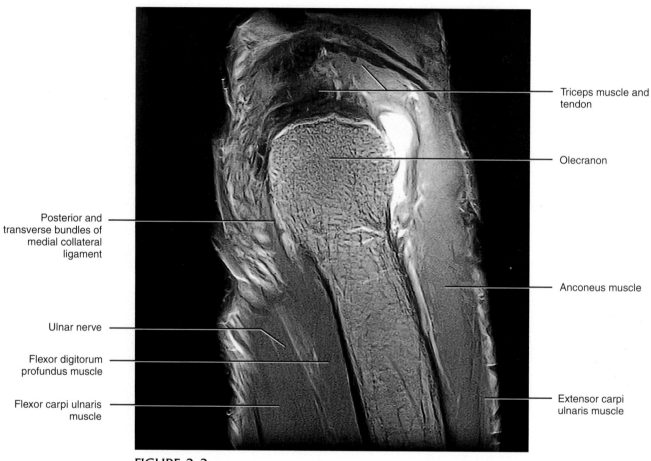

Triceps muscle and tendon

Olecranon

Posterior and transverse bundles of medial collateral ligament

Anconeus muscle

Ulnar nerve

Flexor digitorum profundus muscle

Flexor carpi ulnaris muscle

Extensor carpi ulnaris muscle

FIGURE 2-3

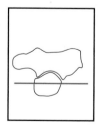

ELBOW: CORONAL

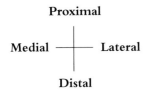

Proximal

Medial ——|—— Lateral

Distal

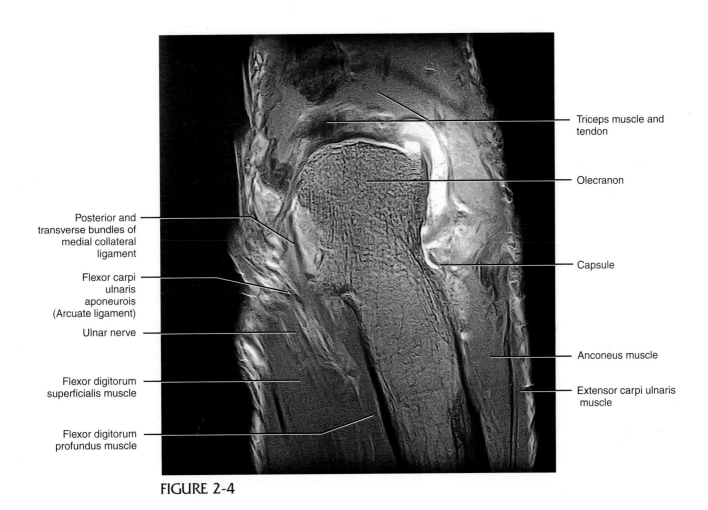

Triceps muscle and tendon

Olecranon

Capsule

Anconeus muscle

Extensor carpi ulnaris muscle

Posterior and transverse bundles of medial collateral ligament

Flexor carpi ulnaris aponeurois (Arcuate ligament)

Ulnar nerve

Flexor digitorum superficialis muscle

Flexor digitorum profundus muscle

FIGURE 2-4

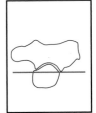

ELBOW: CORONAL

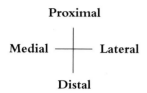

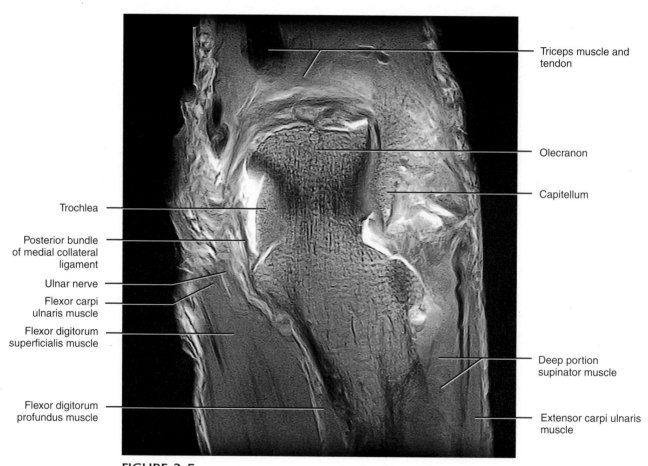

FIGURE 2-5

Triceps muscle and tendon

Olecranon

Capitellum

Trochlea

Posterior bundle of medial collateral ligament

Ulnar nerve

Flexor carpi ulnaris muscle

Flexor digitorum superficialis muscle

Deep portion supinator muscle

Flexor digitorum profundus muscle

Extensor carpi ulnaris muscle

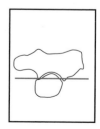

ELBOW: CORONAL

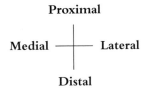

Proximal

Medial ─┼─ Lateral

Distal

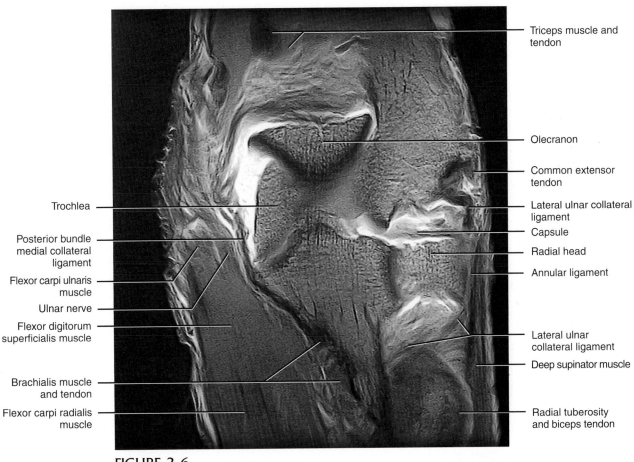

Triceps muscle and tendon

Olecranon

Common extensor tendon

Trochlea

Lateral ulnar collateral ligament

Capsule

Posterior bundle medial collateral ligament

Radial head

Flexor carpi ulnaris muscle

Annular ligament

Ulnar nerve

Flexor digitorum superficialis muscle

Lateral ulnar collateral ligament

Deep supinator muscle

Brachialis muscle and tendon

Flexor carpi radialis muscle

Radial tuberosity and biceps tendon

FIGURE 2-6

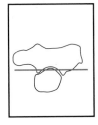

ELBOW: CORONAL

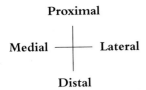

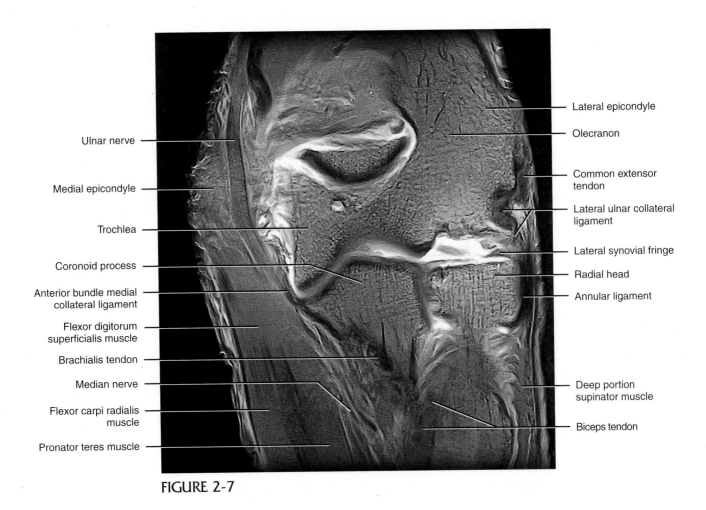

Ulnar nerve

Medial epicondyle

Trochlea

Coronoid process

Anterior bundle medial collateral ligament

Flexor digitorum superficialis muscle

Brachialis tendon

Median nerve

Flexor carpi radialis muscle

Pronator teres muscle

Lateral epicondyle

Olecranon

Common extensor tendon

Lateral ulnar collateral ligament

Lateral synovial fringe

Radial head

Annular ligament

Deep portion supinator muscle

Biceps tendon

FIGURE 2-7

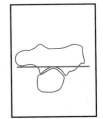

ELBOW: CORONAL

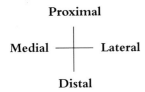

Proximal

Medial — Lateral

Distal

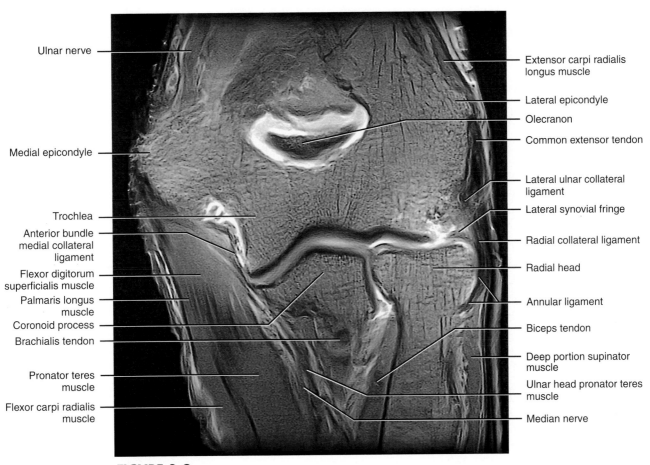

Ulnar nerve

Medial epicondyle

Trochlea

Anterior bundle
medial collateral
ligament

Flexor digitorum
superficialis muscle

Palmaris longus
muscle

Coronoid process

Brachialis tendon

Pronator teres
muscle

Flexor carpi radialis
muscle

Extensor carpi radialis
longus muscle

Lateral epicondyle

Olecranon

Common extensor tendon

Lateral ulnar collateral
ligament

Lateral synovial fringe

Radial collateral ligament

Radial head

Annular ligament

Biceps tendon

Deep portion supinator
muscle

Ulnar head pronator teres
muscle

Median nerve

FIGURE 2-8

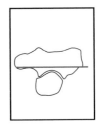

ELBOW: CORONAL

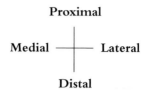

Proximal

Medial ———|——— Lateral

Distal

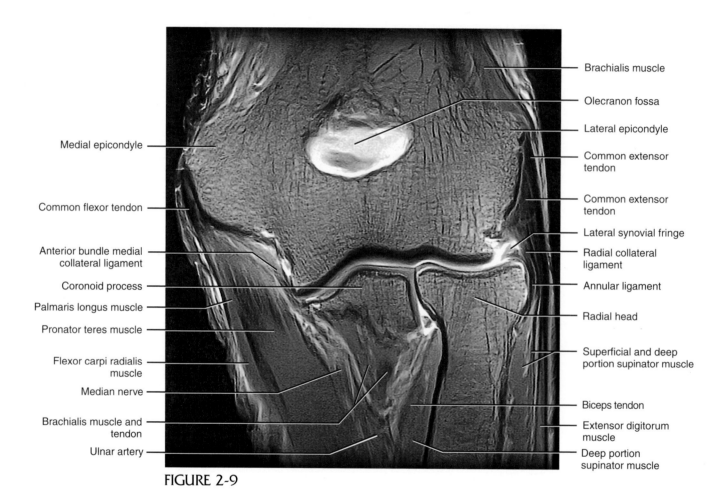

Medial epicondyle

Common flexor tendon

Anterior bundle medial collateral ligament

Coronoid process

Palmaris longus muscle

Pronator teres muscle

Flexor carpi radialis muscle

Median nerve

Brachialis muscle and tendon

Ulnar artery

Brachialis muscle

Olecranon fossa

Lateral epicondyle

Common extensor tendon

Common extensor tendon

Lateral synovial fringe

Radial collateral ligament

Annular ligament

Radial head

Superficial and deep portion supinator muscle

Biceps tendon

Extensor digitorum muscle

Deep portion supinator muscle

FIGURE 2-9

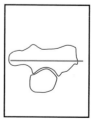

ELBOW: CORONAL

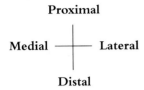

Proximal
Medial — Lateral
Distal

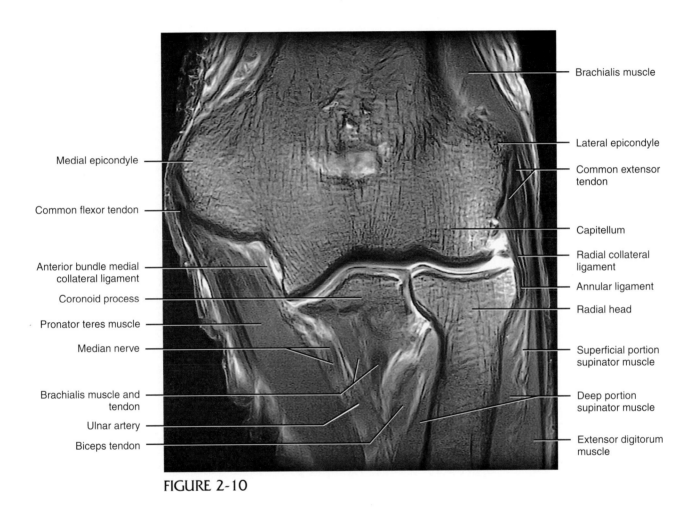

Brachialis muscle

Medial epicondyle

Common flexor tendon

Anterior bundle medial
collateral ligament

Coronoid process

Pronator teres muscle

Median nerve

Brachialis muscle and
tendon

Ulnar artery

Biceps tendon

Lateral epicondyle

Common extensor
tendon

Capitellum

Radial collateral
ligament

Annular ligament

Radial head

Superficial portion
supinator muscle

Deep portion
supinator muscle

Extensor digitorum
muscle

FIGURE 2-10

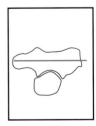

ELBOW: CORONAL

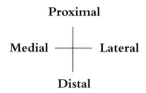

Proximal

Medial ——|—— Lateral

Distal

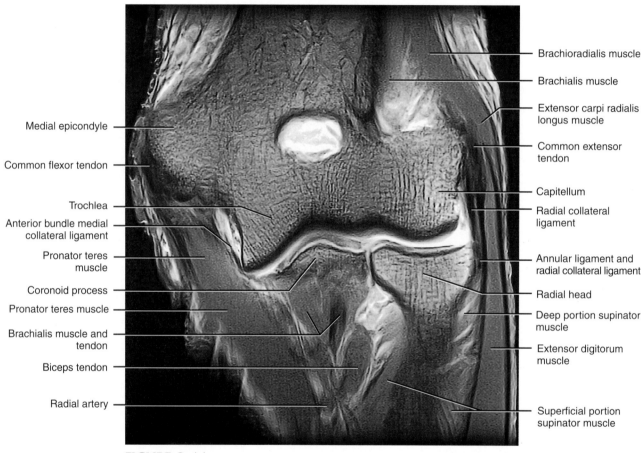

Medial epicondyle

Common flexor tendon

Trochlea

Anterior bundle medial
collateral ligament

Pronator teres
muscle

Coronoid process

Pronator teres muscle

Brachialis muscle and
tendon

Biceps tendon

Radial artery

Brachioradialis muscle

Brachialis muscle

Extensor carpi radialis
longus muscle

Common extensor
tendon

Capitellum

Radial collateral
ligament

Annular ligament and
radial collateral ligament

Radial head

Deep portion supinator
muscle

Extensor digitorum
muscle

Superficial portion
supinator muscle

FIGURE 2-11

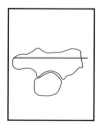

ELBOW: CORONAL

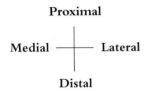

Proximal

Medial — Lateral

Distal

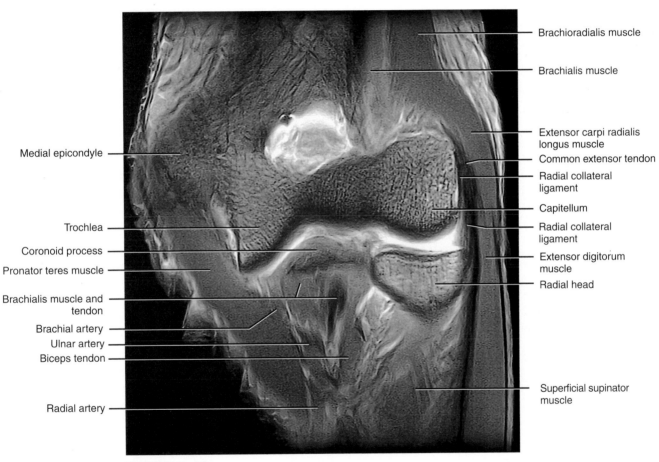

Brachioradialis muscle

Brachialis muscle

Extensor carpi radialis longus muscle

Common extensor tendon

Radial collateral ligament

Capitellum

Radial collateral ligament

Extensor digitorum muscle

Radial head

Superficial supinator muscle

Medial epicondyle

Trochlea

Coronoid process

Pronator teres muscle

Brachialis muscle and tendon

Brachial artery

Ulnar artery

Biceps tendon

Radial artery

FIGURE 2-12

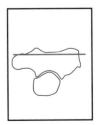

ELBOW: CORONAL

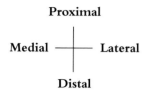

Proximal

Medial ——|—— Lateral

Distal

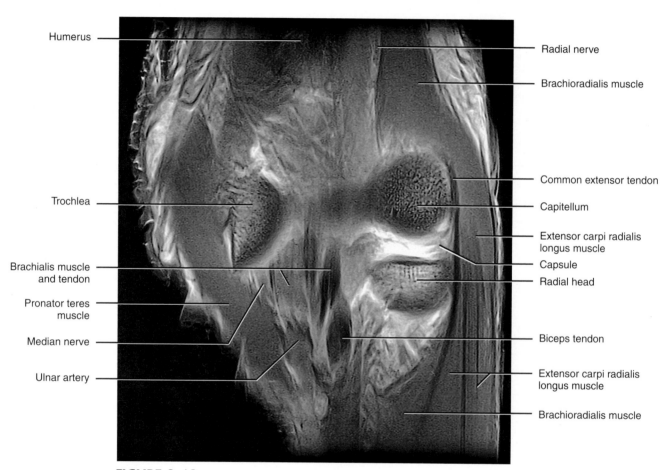

Humerus

Radial nerve

Brachioradialis muscle

Trochlea

Common extensor tendon

Capitellum

Extensor carpi radialis
longus muscle

Brachialis muscle
and tendon

Capsule

Radial head

Pronator teres
muscle

Median nerve

Biceps tendon

Ulnar artery

Extensor carpi radialis
longus muscle

Brachioradialis muscle

FIGURE 2-13

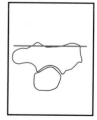

ELBOW: CORONAL

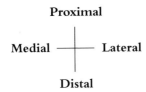

Proximal

Medial — Lateral

Distal

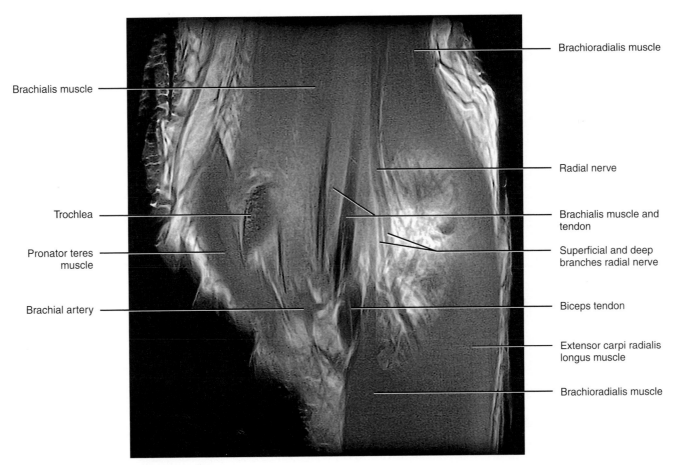

Brachialis muscle

Brachioradialis muscle

Trochlea

Radial nerve

Pronator teres muscle

Brachialis muscle and tendon

Brachial artery

Superficial and deep branches radial nerve

Biceps tendon

Extensor carpi radialis longus muscle

Brachioradialis muscle

FIGURE 2-14

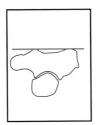

ELBOW: CORONAL

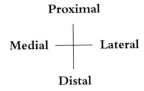

Proximal

Medial ——|—— Lateral

Distal

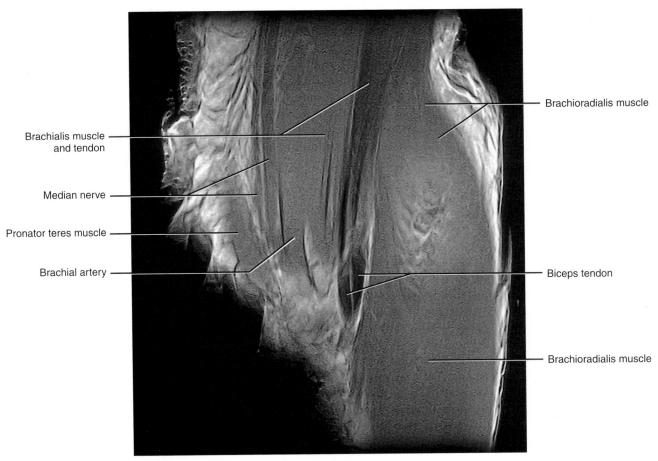

Brachialis muscle
and tendon

Median nerve

Pronator teres muscle

Brachial artery

Brachioradialis muscle

Biceps tendon

Brachioradialis muscle

FIGURE 2-15

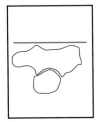

ELBOW: CORONAL

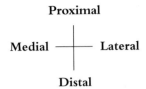

Proximal

Medial —|— **Lateral**

Distal

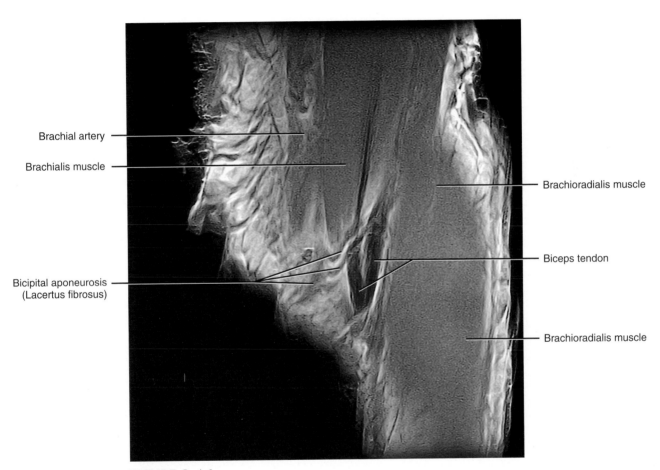

Brachial artery

Brachialis muscle

Bicipital aponeurosis
(Lacertus fibrosus)

Brachioradialis muscle

Biceps tendon

Brachioradialis muscle

FIGURE 2-16

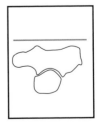

ELBOW: AXIAL

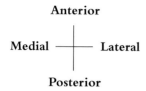

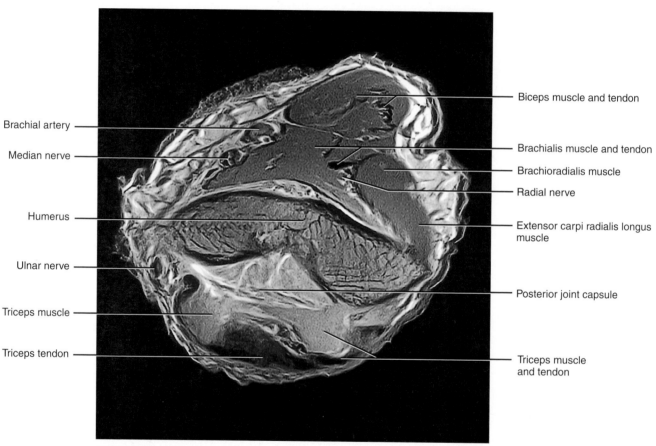

Brachial artery

Median nerve

Humerus

Ulnar nerve

Triceps muscle

Triceps tendon

Biceps muscle and tendon

Brachialis muscle and tendon

Brachioradialis muscle

Radial nerve

Extensor carpi radialis longus muscle

Posterior joint capsule

Triceps muscle and tendon

FIGURE 2-17

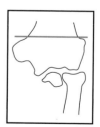

ELBOW: AXIAL

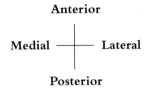

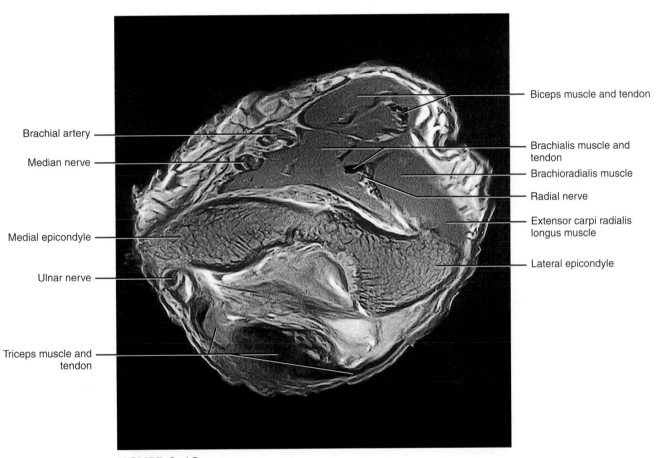

Brachial artery

Median nerve

Medial epicondyle

Ulnar nerve

Triceps muscle and tendon

Biceps muscle and tendon

Brachialis muscle and tendon

Brachioradialis muscle

Radial nerve

Extensor carpi radialis longus muscle

Lateral epicondyle

FIGURE 2-18

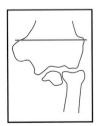

ELBOW: AXIAL

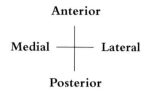

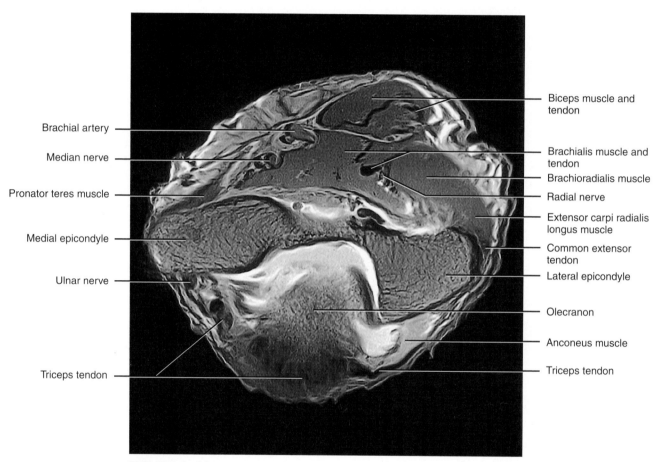

FIGURE 2-19

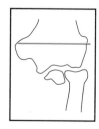

ELBOW: AXIAL

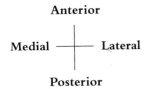

Anterior

Medial ——┼—— Lateral

Posterior

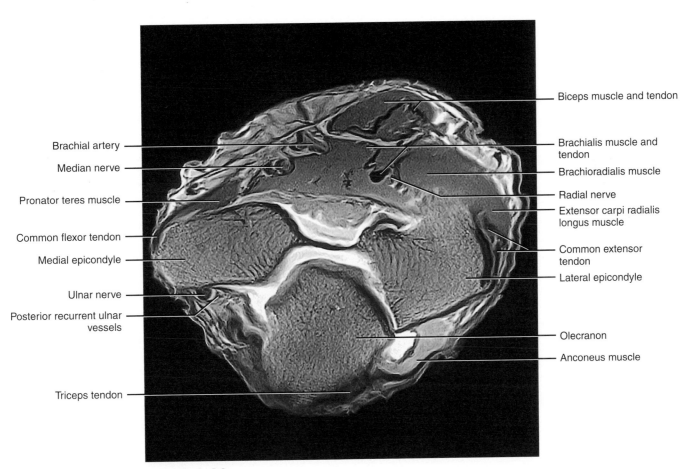

Biceps muscle and tendon

Brachial artery

Median nerve

Pronator teres muscle

Common flexor tendon

Medial epicondyle

Ulnar nerve

Posterior recurrent ulnar vessels

Triceps tendon

Brachialis muscle and tendon

Brachioradialis muscle

Radial nerve

Extensor carpi radialis longus muscle

Common extensor tendon

Lateral epicondyle

Olecranon

Anconeus muscle

FIGURE 2-20

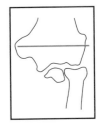

ELBOW: AXIAL

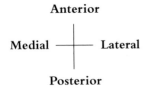

Anterior

Medial —— Lateral

Posterior

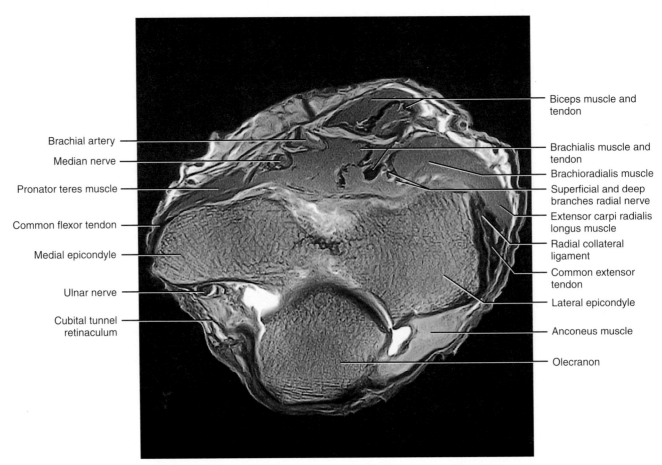

Brachial artery

Median nerve

Pronator teres muscle

Common flexor tendon

Medial epicondyle

Ulnar nerve

Cubital tunnel retinaculum

Biceps muscle and tendon

Brachialis muscle and tendon

Brachioradialis muscle

Superficial and deep branches radial nerve

Extensor carpi radialis longus muscle

Radial collateral ligament

Common extensor tendon

Lateral epicondyle

Anconeus muscle

Olecranon

FIGURE 2-21

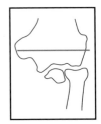

ELBOW: AXIAL

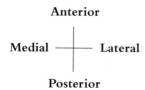

Anterior

Medial —|— **Lateral**

Posterior

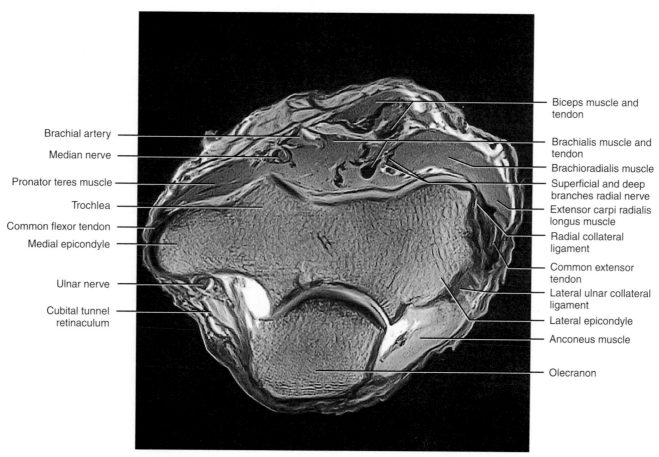

Brachial artery

Median nerve

Pronator teres muscle

Trochlea

Common flexor tendon

Medial epicondyle

Ulnar nerve

Cubital tunnel retinaculum

Biceps muscle and tendon

Brachialis muscle and tendon

Brachioradialis muscle

Superficial and deep branches radial nerve

Extensor carpi radialis longus muscle

Radial collateral ligament

Common extensor tendon

Lateral ulnar collateral ligament

Lateral epicondyle

Anconeus muscle

Olecranon

FIGURE 2-22

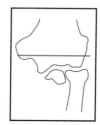

ELBOW: AXIAL

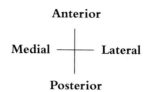

Anterior

Medial —— Lateral

Posterior

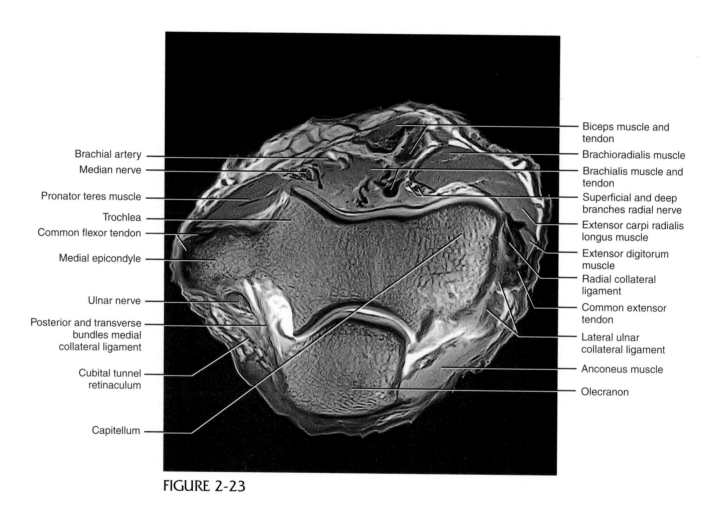

Brachial artery

Median nerve

Pronator teres muscle

Trochlea

Common flexor tendon

Medial epicondyle

Ulnar nerve

Posterior and transverse bundles medial collateral ligament

Cubital tunnel retinaculum

Capitellum

Biceps muscle and tendon

Brachioradialis muscle

Brachialis muscle and tendon

Superficial and deep branches radial nerve

Extensor carpi radialis longus muscle

Extensor digitorum muscle

Radial collateral ligament

Common extensor tendon

Lateral ulnar collateral ligament

Anconeus muscle

Olecranon

FIGURE 2-23

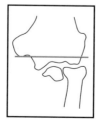

ELBOW: AXIAL

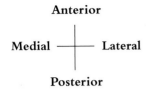

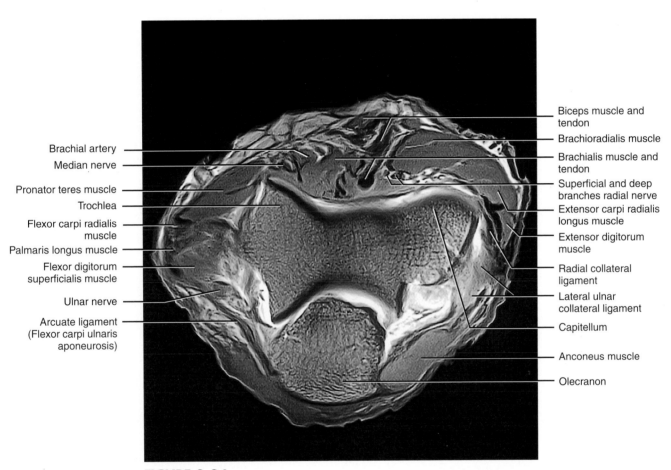

Biceps muscle and tendon

Brachioradialis muscle

Brachialis muscle and tendon

Superficial and deep branches radial nerve

Extensor carpi radialis longus muscle

Extensor digitorum muscle

Radial collateral ligament

Lateral ulnar collateral ligament

Capitellum

Anconeus muscle

Olecranon

Brachial artery

Median nerve

Pronator teres muscle

Trochlea

Flexor carpi radialis muscle

Palmaris longus muscle

Flexor digitorum superficialis muscle

Ulnar nerve

Arcuate ligament (Flexor carpi ulnaris aponeurosis)

FIGURE 2-24

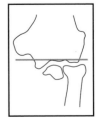

ELBOW: AXIAL

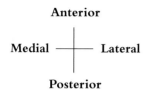

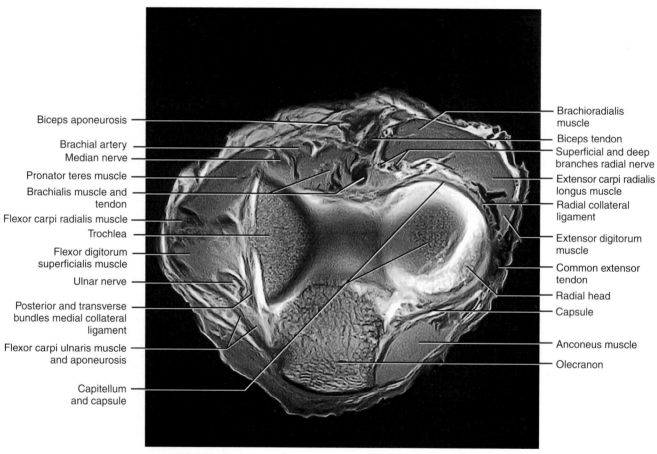

Biceps aponeurosis

Brachial artery
Median nerve

Pronator teres muscle

Brachialis muscle and
tendon

Flexor carpi radialis muscle

Trochlea

Flexor digitorum
superficialis muscle

Ulnar nerve

Posterior and transverse
bundles medial collateral
ligament

Flexor carpi ulnaris muscle
and aponeurosis

Capitellum
and capsule

Brachioradialis
muscle

Biceps tendon

Superficial and deep
branches radial nerve

Extensor carpi radialis
longus muscle

Radial collateral
ligament

Extensor digitorum
muscle

Common extensor
tendon

Radial head

Capsule

Anconeus muscle

Olecranon

FIGURE 2-25

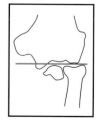

ELBOW: AXIAL

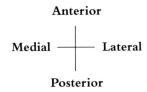

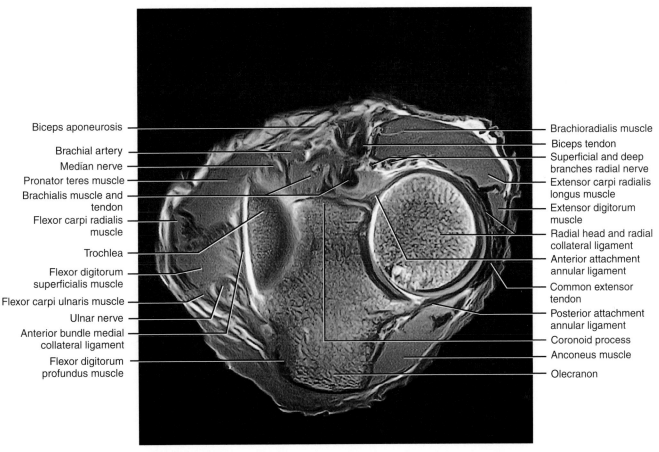

Biceps aponeurosis

Brachial artery

Median nerve

Pronator teres muscle

Brachialis muscle and tendon

Flexor carpi radialis muscle

Trochlea

Flexor digitorum superficialis muscle

Flexor carpi ulnaris muscle

Ulnar nerve

Anterior bundle medial collateral ligament

Flexor digitorum profundus muscle

Brachioradialis muscle

Biceps tendon

Superficial and deep branches radial nerve

Extensor carpi radialis longus muscle

Extensor digitorum muscle

Radial head and radial collateral ligament

Anterior attachment annular ligament

Common extensor tendon

Posterior attachment annular ligament

Coronoid process

Anconeus muscle

Olecranon

FIGURE 2-26

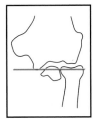

ELBOW: AXIAL

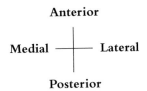

Anterior

Medial —|— Lateral

Posterior

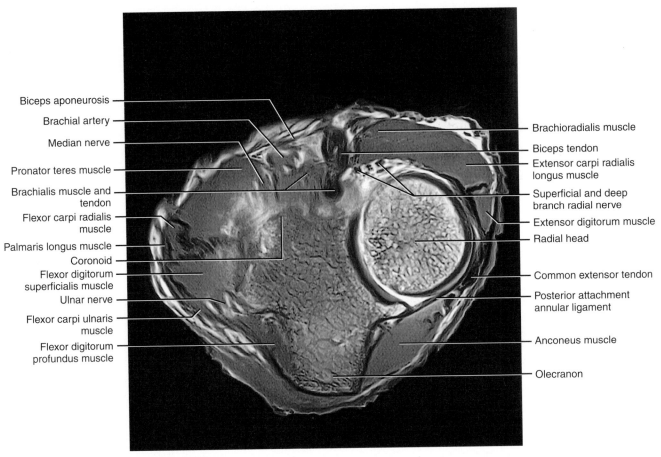

Biceps aponeurosis

Brachial artery

Median nerve

Pronator teres muscle

Brachialis muscle and tendon

Flexor carpi radialis muscle

Palmaris longus muscle

Coronoid

Flexor digitorum superficialis muscle

Ulnar nerve

Flexor carpi ulnaris muscle

Flexor digitorum profundus muscle

Brachioradialis muscle

Biceps tendon

Extensor carpi radialis longus muscle

Superficial and deep branch radial nerve

Extensor digitorum muscle

Radial head

Common extensor tendon

Posterior attachment annular ligament

Anconeus muscle

Olecranon

FIGURE 2-27

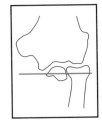

ELBOW: AXIAL

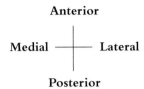

Anterior

Medial — Lateral

Posterior

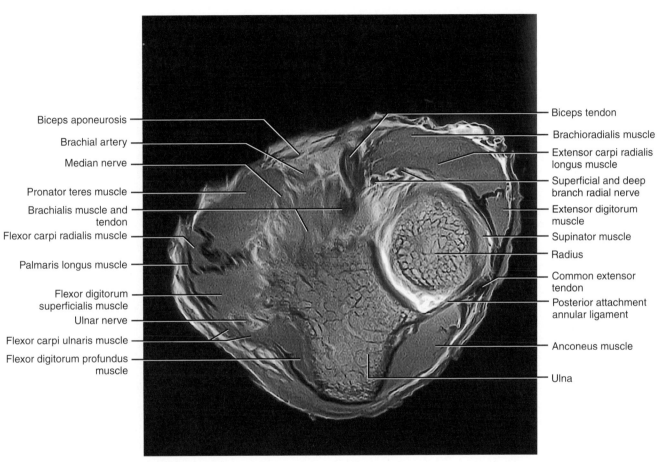

Biceps aponeurosis

Brachial artery

Median nerve

Pronator teres muscle

Brachialis muscle and tendon

Flexor carpi radialis muscle

Palmaris longus muscle

Flexor digitorum superficialis muscle

Ulnar nerve

Flexor carpi ulnaris muscle

Flexor digitorum profundus muscle

Biceps tendon

Brachioradialis muscle

Extensor carpi radialis longus muscle

Superficial and deep branch radial nerve

Extensor digitorum muscle

Supinator muscle

Radius

Common extensor tendon

Posterior attachment annular ligament

Anconeus muscle

Ulna

FIGURE 2-28

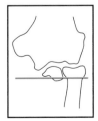

ELBOW: AXIAL

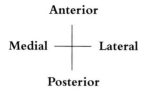

Anterior

Medial ——|—— Lateral

Posterior

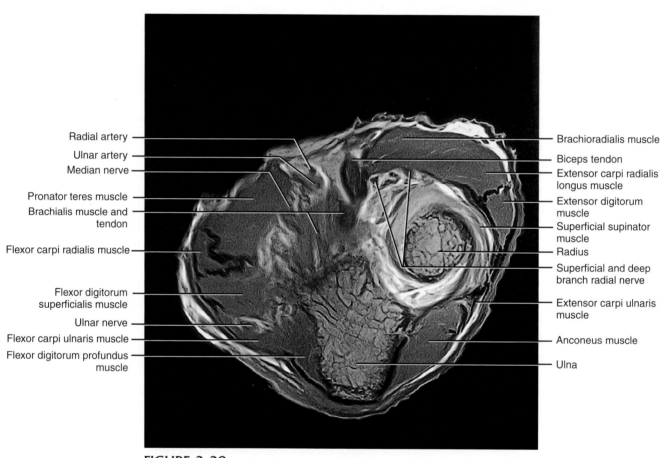

Radial artery —

Ulnar artery —

Median nerve —

Pronator teres muscle —

Brachialis muscle and tendon —

Flexor carpi radialis muscle —

Flexor digitorum superficialis muscle —

Ulnar nerve —

Flexor carpi ulnaris muscle —

Flexor digitorum profundus muscle —

— Brachioradialis muscle

— Biceps tendon

— Extensor carpi radialis longus muscle

— Extensor digitorum muscle

— Superficial supinator muscle

— Radius

— Superficial and deep branch radial nerve

— Extensor carpi ulnaris muscle

— Anconeus muscle

— Ulna

FIGURE 2-29

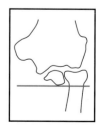

ELBOW: AXIAL

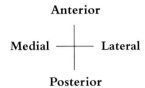

Anterior

Medial —|— Lateral

Posterior

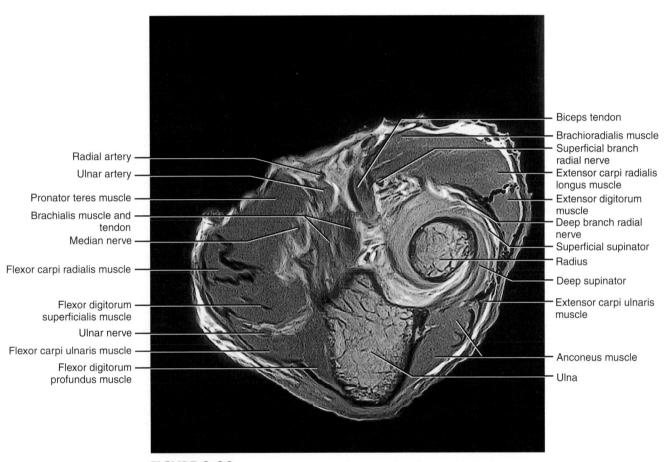

Radial artery

Ulnar artery

Pronator teres muscle

Brachialis muscle and tendon

Median nerve

Flexor carpi radialis muscle

Flexor digitorum superficialis muscle

Ulnar nerve

Flexor carpi ulnaris muscle

Flexor digitorum profundus muscle

Biceps tendon

Brachioradialis muscle

Superficial branch radial nerve

Extensor carpi radialis longus muscle

Extensor digitorum muscle

Deep branch radial nerve

Superficial supinator

Radius

Deep supinator

Extensor carpi ulnaris muscle

Anconeus muscle

Ulna

FIGURE 2-30

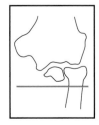

ELBOW: AXIAL

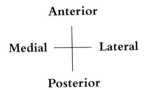

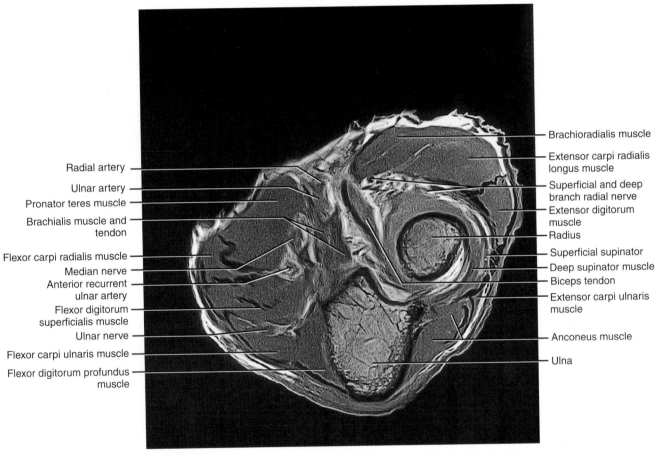

Radial artery

Ulnar artery

Pronator teres muscle

Brachialis muscle and
tendon

Flexor carpi radialis muscle

Median nerve

Anterior recurrent
ulnar artery

Flexor digitorum
superficialis muscle

Ulnar nerve

Flexor carpi ulnaris muscle

Flexor digitorum profundus
muscle

Brachioradialis muscle

Extensor carpi radialis
longus muscle

Superficial and deep
branch radial nerve

Extensor digitorum
muscle

Radius

Superficial supinator

Deep supinator muscle

Biceps tendon

Extensor carpi ulnaris
muscle

Anconeus muscle

Ulna

FIGURE 2-31

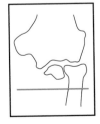

ELBOW: AXIAL

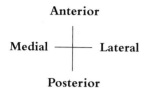

Anterior

Medial ─┼─ Lateral

Posterior

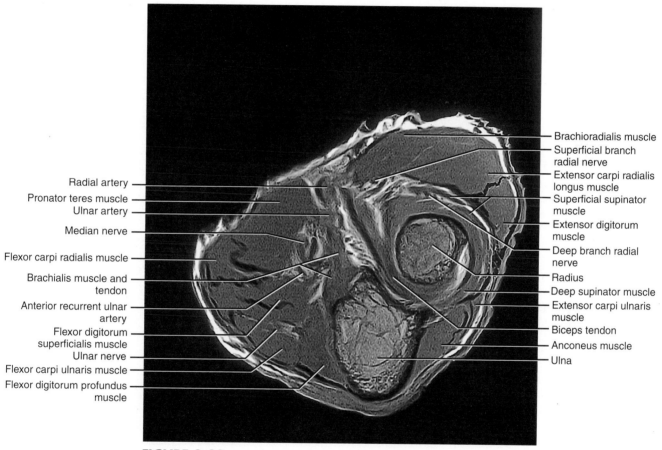

Radial artery

Pronator teres muscle

Ulnar artery

Median nerve

Flexor carpi radialis muscle

Brachialis muscle and tendon

Anterior recurrent ulnar artery

Flexor digitorum superficialis muscle

Ulnar nerve

Flexor carpi ulnaris muscle

Flexor digitorum profundus muscle

Brachioradialis muscle

Superficial branch radial nerve

Extensor carpi radialis longus muscle

Superficial supinator muscle

Extensor digitorum muscle

Deep branch radial nerve

Radius

Deep supinator muscle

Extensor carpi ulnaris muscle

Biceps tendon

Anconeus muscle

Ulna

FIGURE 2-32

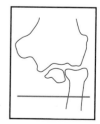

ELBOW: AXIAL

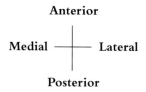

Anterior

Medial ——|—— Lateral

Posterior

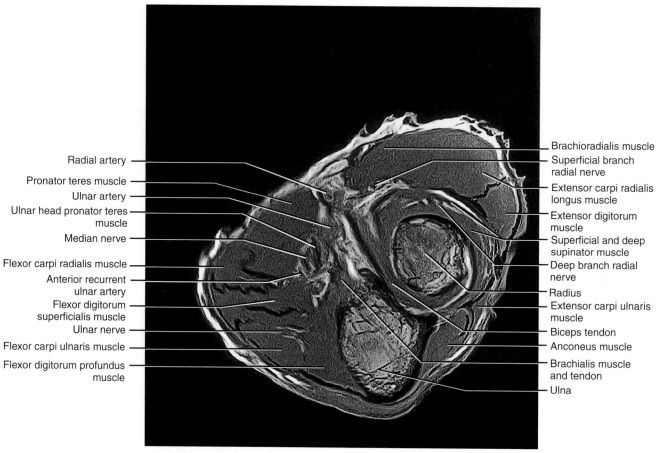

Radial artery

Pronator teres muscle

Ulnar artery

Ulnar head pronator teres muscle

Median nerve

Flexor carpi radialis muscle

Anterior recurrent ulnar artery

Flexor digitorum superficialis muscle

Ulnar nerve

Flexor carpi ulnaris muscle

Flexor digitorum profundus muscle

Brachioradialis muscle

Superficial branch radial nerve

Extensor carpi radialis longus muscle

Extensor digitorum muscle

Superficial and deep supinator muscle

Deep branch radial nerve

Radius

Extensor carpi ulnaris muscle

Biceps tendon

Anconeus muscle

Brachialis muscle and tendon

Ulna

FIGURE 2-33

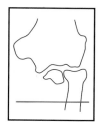

ELBOW: AXIAL

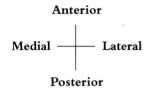

Anterior

Medial ——— Lateral

Posterior

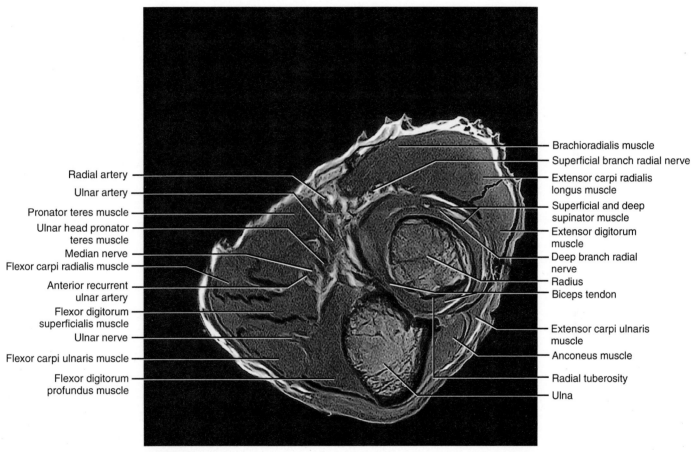

Radial artery

Ulnar artery

Pronator teres muscle

Ulnar head pronator
teres muscle

Median nerve

Flexor carpi radialis muscle

Anterior recurrent
ulnar artery

Flexor digitorum
superficialis muscle

Ulnar nerve

Flexor carpi ulnaris muscle

Flexor digitorum
profundus muscle

Brachioradialis muscle

Superficial branch radial nerve

Extensor carpi radialis
longus muscle

Superficial and deep
supinator muscle

Extensor digitorum
muscle

Deep branch radial
nerve

Radius

Biceps tendon

Extensor carpi ulnaris
muscle

Anconeus muscle

Radial tuberosity

Ulna

FIGURE 2-34

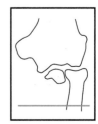

ELBOW: SAGITTAL

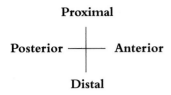

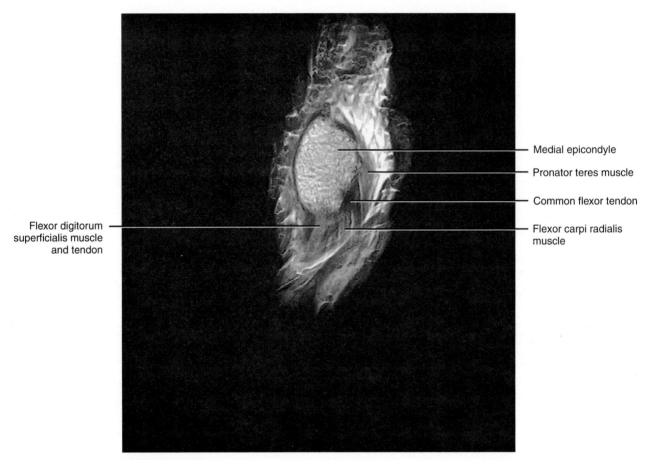

Medial epicondyle

Pronator teres muscle

Common flexor tendon

Flexor carpi radialis muscle

Flexor digitorum superficialis muscle and tendon

FIGURE 2-35

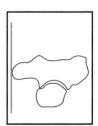

ELBOW: SAGITTAL

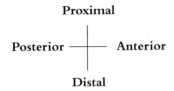

Proximal

Posterior ─┼─ Anterior

Distal

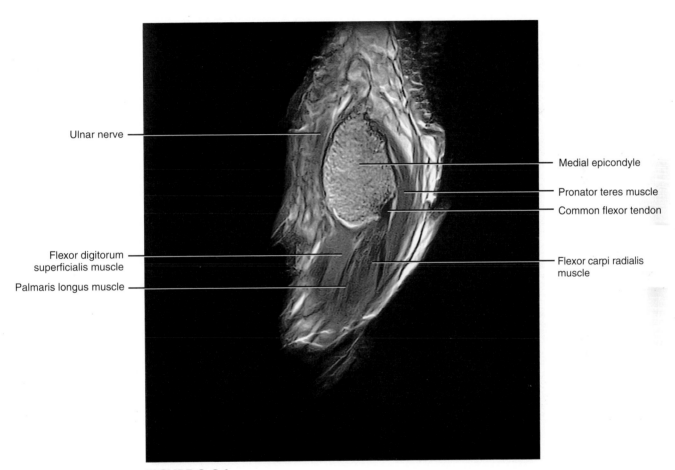

Ulnar nerve

Medial epicondyle

Pronator teres muscle

Common flexor tendon

Flexor digitorum superficialis muscle

Flexor carpi radialis muscle

Palmaris longus muscle

FIGURE 2-36

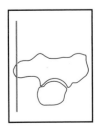

ELBOW: SAGITTAL

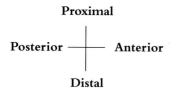

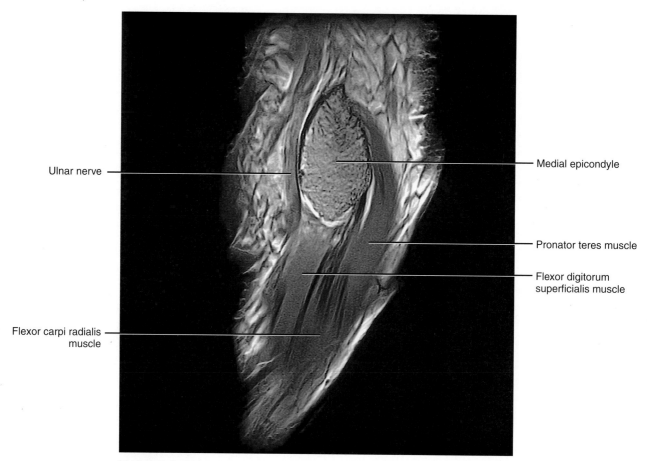

Ulnar nerve

Flexor carpi radialis muscle

Medial epicondyle

Pronator teres muscle

Flexor digitorum superficialis muscle

FIGURE 2-37

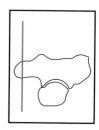

ELBOW: SAGITTAL

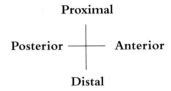

Proximal

Posterior ——|—— Anterior

Distal

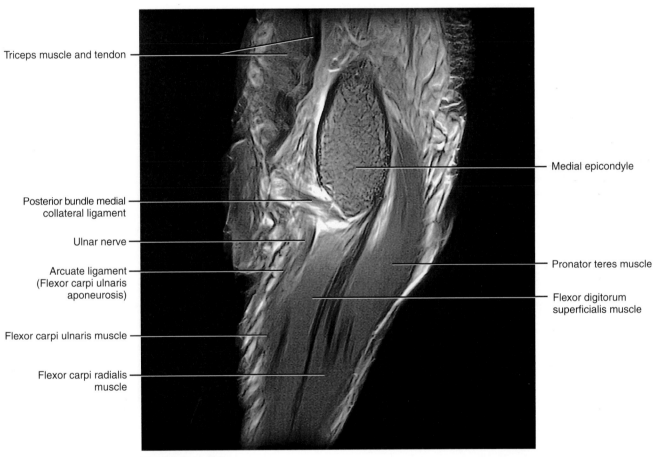

Triceps muscle and tendon

Medial epicondyle

Posterior bundle medial
collateral ligament

Ulnar nerve

Arcuate ligament
(Flexor carpi ulnaris
aponeurosis)

Pronator teres muscle

Flexor digitorum
superficialis muscle

Flexor carpi ulnaris muscle

Flexor carpi radialis
muscle

FIGURE 2-38

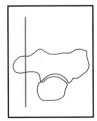

ELBOW: SAGITTAL

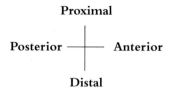

Triceps muscle

Medial epicondyle

Posterior bundle
medial collateral
ligament

Transverse bundle
medial collateral
ligament

Ulnar nerve

Flexor carpi
ulnaris muscle

Anterior bundle medial
collateral ligament

Pronator teres muscle

Flexor digitorum
superficialis muscle

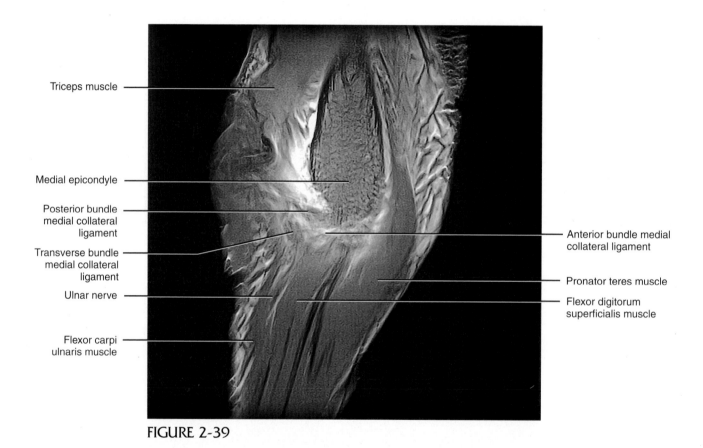

FIGURE 2-39

ELBOW: SAGITTAL

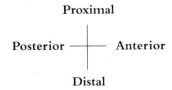

Proximal

Posterior ──┼── Anterior

Distal

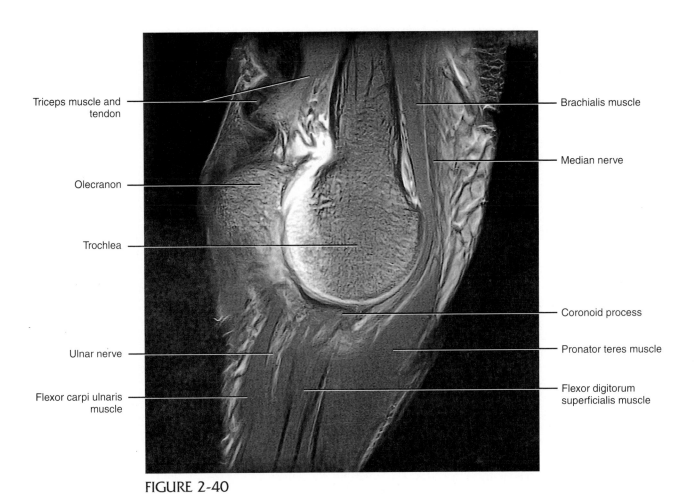

Triceps muscle and tendon

Olecranon

Trochlea

Ulnar nerve

Flexor carpi ulnaris muscle

Brachialis muscle

Median nerve

Coronoid process

Pronator teres muscle

Flexor digitorum superficialis muscle

FIGURE 2-40

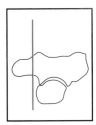

ELBOW: SAGITTAL

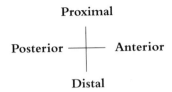

Proximal

Posterior —— Anterior

Distal

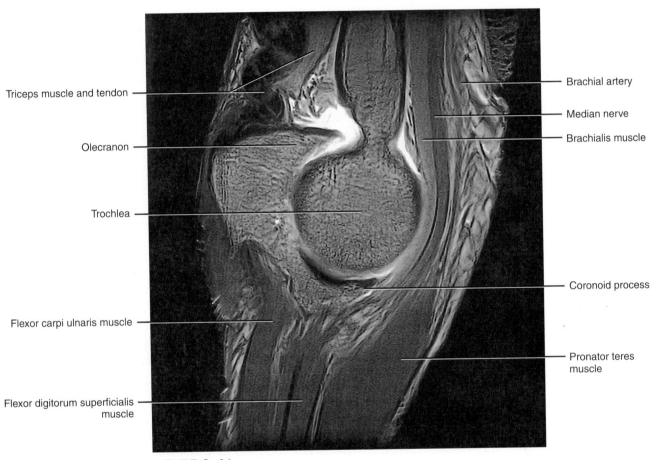

Triceps muscle and tendon

Brachial artery

Median nerve

Brachialis muscle

Olecranon

Trochlea

Coronoid process

Flexor carpi ulnaris muscle

Pronator teres muscle

Flexor digitorum superficialis muscle

FIGURE 2-41

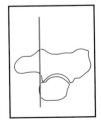

ELBOW: SAGITTAL

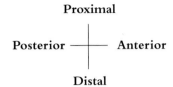

Proximal

Posterior ——+—— Anterior

Distal

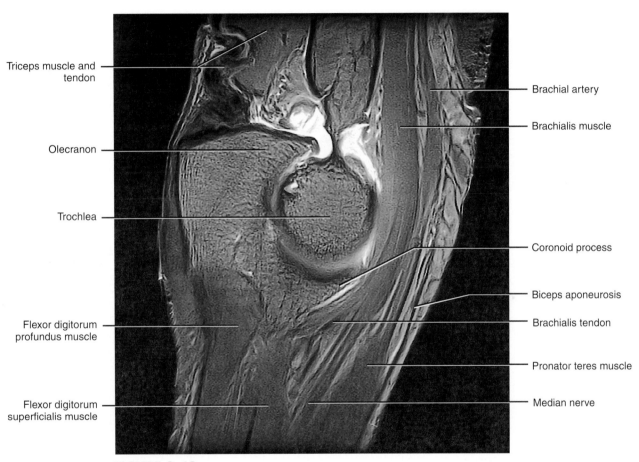

Triceps muscle and tendon

Olecranon

Trochlea

Flexor digitorum profundus muscle

Flexor digitorum superficialis muscle

Brachial artery

Brachialis muscle

Coronoid process

Biceps aponeurosis

Brachialis tendon

Pronator teres muscle

Median nerve

FIGURE 2-42

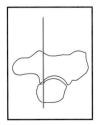

ELBOW: SAGITTAL

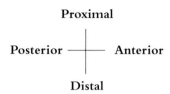

Proximal

Posterior —— Anterior

Distal

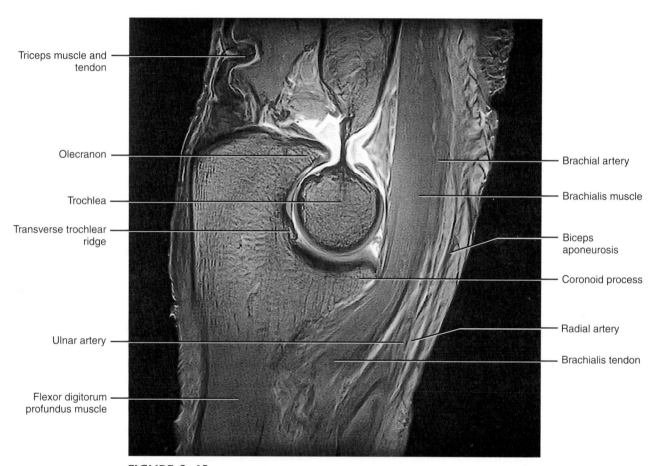

Triceps muscle and tendon

Olecranon

Trochlea

Transverse trochlear ridge

Ulnar artery

Flexor digitorum profundus muscle

Brachial artery

Brachialis muscle

Biceps aponeurosis

Coronoid process

Radial artery

Brachialis tendon

FIGURE 2-43

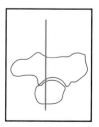

ELBOW: SAGITTAL

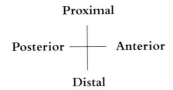

Proximal

Posterior ——|—— Anterior

Distal

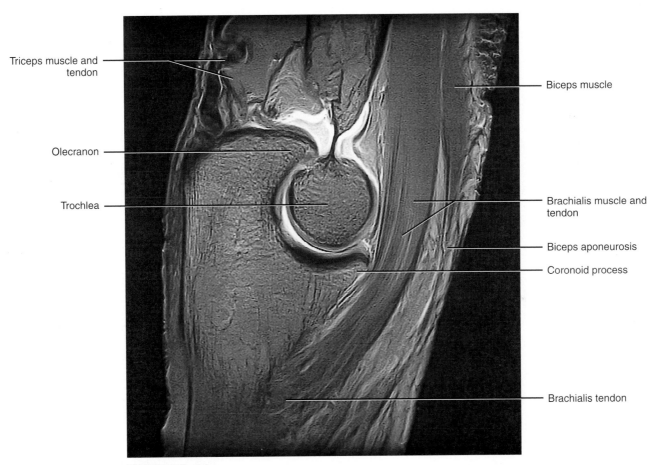

Triceps muscle and tendon

Biceps muscle

Olecranon

Trochlea

Brachialis muscle and tendon

Biceps aponeurosis

Coronoid process

Brachialis tendon

FIGURE 2-44

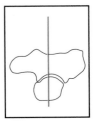

ELBOW: SAGITTAL

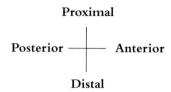

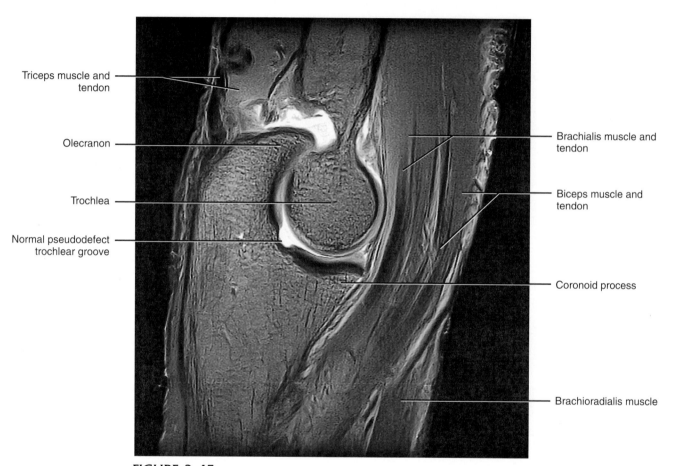

Triceps muscle and tendon

Olecranon

Trochlea

Normal pseudodefect trochlear groove

Brachialis muscle and tendon

Biceps muscle and tendon

Coronoid process

Brachioradialis muscle

FIGURE 2-45

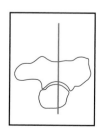

ELBOW: SAGITTAL

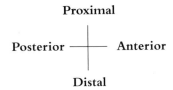

Proximal

Posterior —|— Anterior

Distal

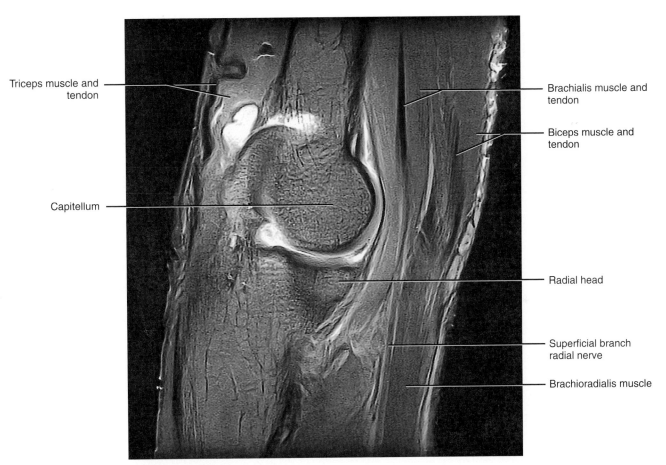

Triceps muscle and tendon

Capitellum

Brachialis muscle and tendon

Biceps muscle and tendon

Radial head

Superficial branch radial nerve

Brachioradialis muscle

FIGURE 2-46

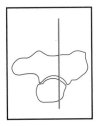

ELBOW: SAGITTAL

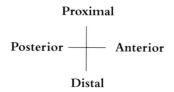

Proximal

Posterior —— Anterior

Distal

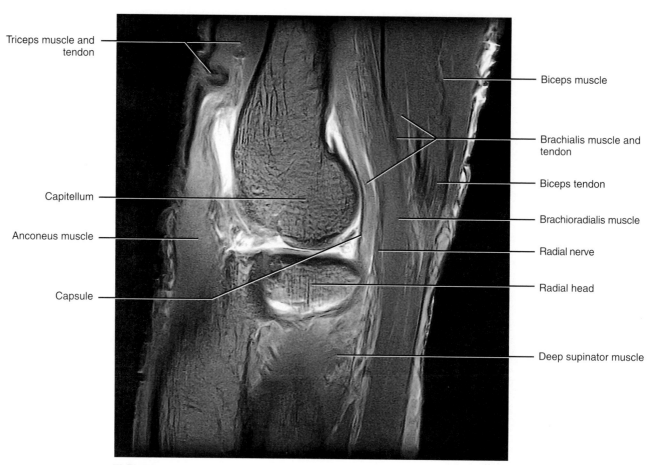

Triceps muscle and tendon

Biceps muscle

Brachialis muscle and tendon

Biceps tendon

Capitellum

Brachioradialis muscle

Anconeus muscle

Radial nerve

Radial head

Capsule

Deep supinator muscle

FIGURE 2-47

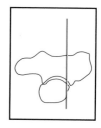

ELBOW: SAGITTAL

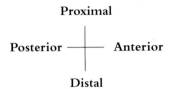

Proximal

Posterior ——+—— Anterior

Distal

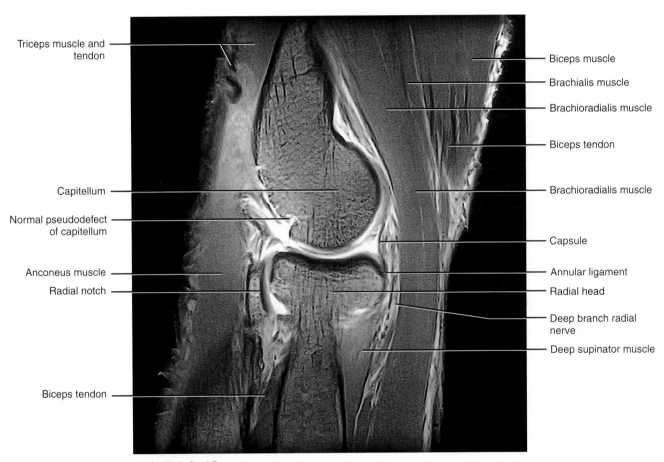

Triceps muscle and tendon

Capitellum

Normal pseudodefect of capitellum

Anconeus muscle

Radial notch

Biceps tendon

Biceps muscle

Brachialis muscle

Brachioradialis muscle

Biceps tendon

Brachioradialis muscle

Capsule

Annular ligament

Radial head

Deep branch radial nerve

Deep supinator muscle

FIGURE 2-48

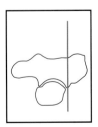

ELBOW: SAGITTAL

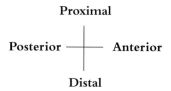

Proximal

Posterior ──┼── Anterior

Distal

Extensor carpi
radialis longus
muscle

Brachioradialis
muscle

Capitellum

Anconeus muscle

Biceps tendon

Radial tuberosity

Biceps muscle and
tendon

Brachialis muscle

Brachioradialis muscle

Capsule

Annular ligament

Radial head

Deep supinator muscle

Superficial supinator
muscle

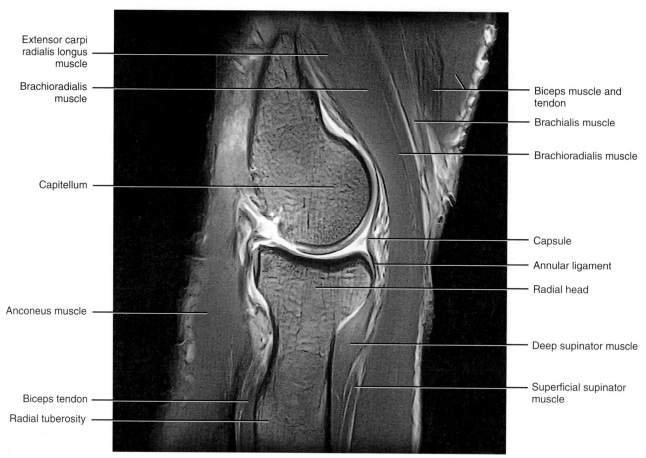

FIGURE 2-49

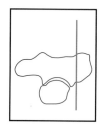

ELBOW: SAGITTAL

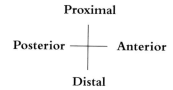

Proximal

Posterior ─── Anterior

Distal

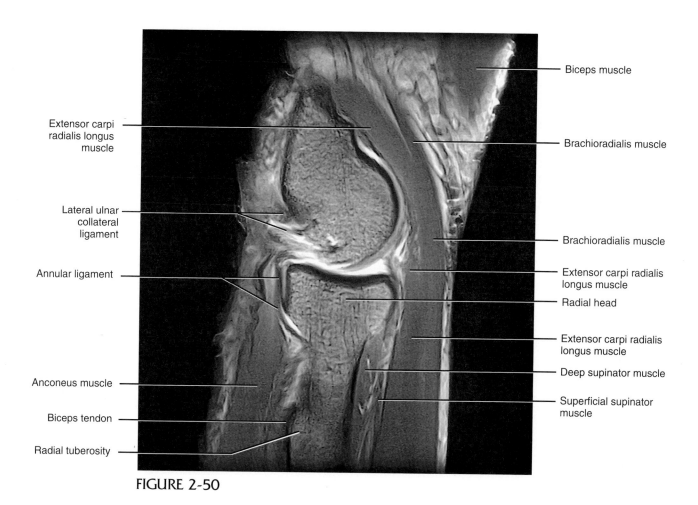

Extensor carpi radialis longus muscle

Lateral ulnar collateral ligament

Annular ligament

Anconeus muscle

Biceps tendon

Radial tuberosity

Biceps muscle

Brachioradialis muscle

Brachioradialis muscle

Extensor carpi radialis longus muscle

Radial head

Extensor carpi radialis longus muscle

Deep supinator muscle

Superficial supinator muscle

FIGURE 2-50

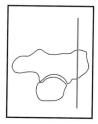

ELBOW: SAGITTAL

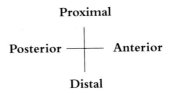

Proximal

Posterior — | — Anterior

Distal

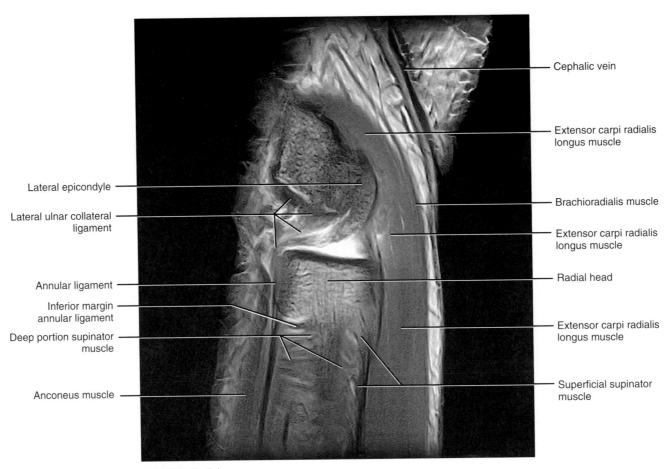

Lateral epicondyle

Lateral ulnar collateral ligament

Annular ligament

Inferior margin annular ligament

Deep portion supinator muscle

Anconeus muscle

Cephalic vein

Extensor carpi radialis longus muscle

Brachioradialis muscle

Extensor carpi radialis longus muscle

Radial head

Extensor carpi radialis longus muscle

Superficial supinator muscle

FIGURE 2-51

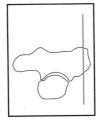

ELBOW: SAGITTAL

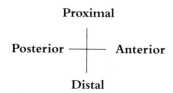

Proximal

Posterior ——|—— Anterior

Distal

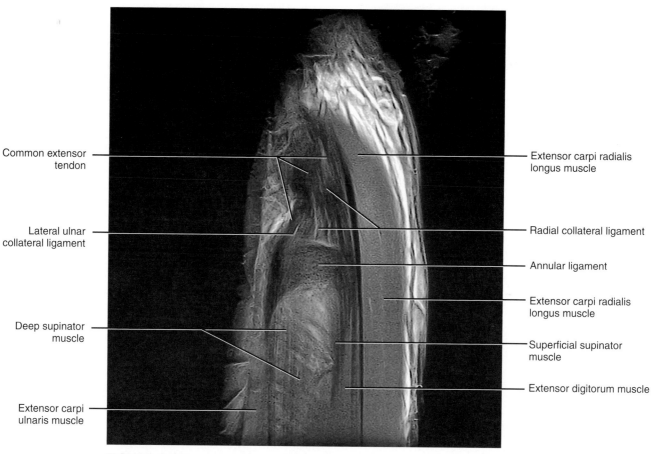

Common extensor tendon

Lateral ulnar collateral ligament

Deep supinator muscle

Extensor carpi ulnaris muscle

Extensor carpi radialis longus muscle

Radial collateral ligament

Annular ligament

Extensor carpi radialis longus muscle

Superficial supinator muscle

Extensor digitorum muscle

FIGURE 2-52

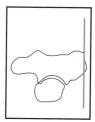

ELBOW: ARTICULAR ANATOMY

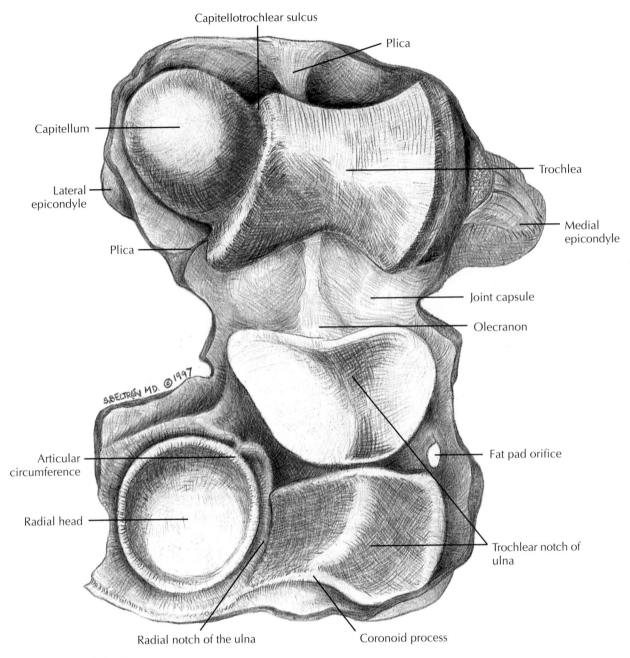

FIGURE 2-53

Interior exposure of the elbow joint shows the articular surfaces of the capitellum, trochlea, radial head, radial notch, and the trochlear notch. A bare area that is normally devoid of articular cartilage extends transversely across the midportion of the trochlear notch. For related MR, arthroscopy, and surgical anatomy images see Figures 2-68 through 2-70.

ELBOW: COLLATERAL LIGAMENTS, ANTERIOR VIEW

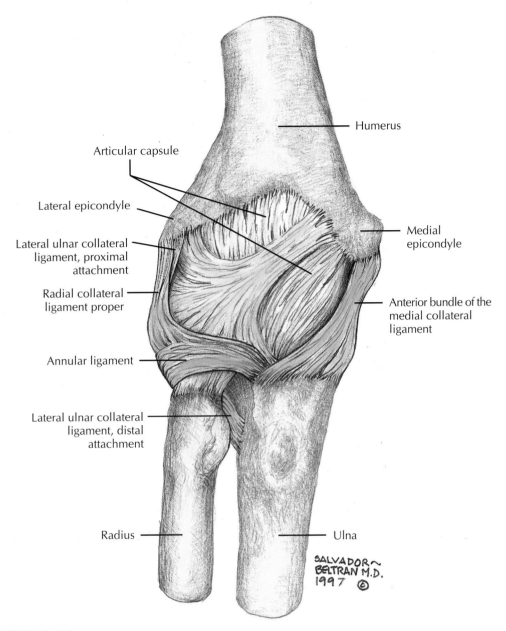

Humerus

Articular capsule

Lateral epicondyle

Lateral ulnar collateral
ligament, proximal
attachment

Radial collateral
ligament proper

Medial
epicondyle

Anterior bundle of the
medial collateral
ligament

Annular ligament

Lateral ulnar collateral
ligament, distal
attachment

Radius

Ulna

SALVADOR
BELTRAN M.D.
1997 ©

FIGURE 2-54

Collateral ligaments. The medial collateral ligament complex consists of anterior and posterior bundles as
well as an oblique band that is also known and more commonly referred to as the transverse ligament or
bundle. The lateral ligament complex consists of the radial collateral ligament, the annular ligament, a variably present accessory lateral collateral ligament, and the lateral ulnar collateral ligament. For related MR,
arthroscopy, and surgical anatomy images see Figures 2-62 through 2-65.

ELBOW: LATERAL LIGAMENT COMPLEX, LATERAL VIEW

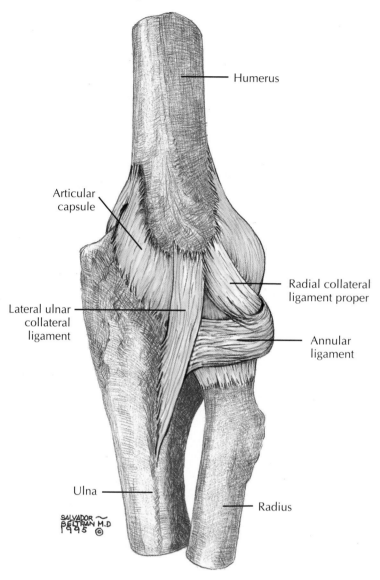

FIGURE 2-55

Lateral ligament complex—the radial collateral ligament, the annular ligament, and the lateral ulnar collateral ligament (LUCL). The radial collateral ligament proper arises from the lateral epicondyle anteriorly and blends with the fibers of the annular ligament, which surrounds the radial head. The LUCL arises from the lateral epicondyle and extends along the posterior aspect of the radius to insert on the tubercle of the supinator crest of the ulna. The LUCL is the primary restraint to varus and posterolateral rotatory stress. For related MR, arthroscopy, and surgical anatomy images see Figures 2-64 and 2-65.

ELBOW: MEDIAL COLLATERAL LIGAMENT COMPLEX, MEDIAL VIEW

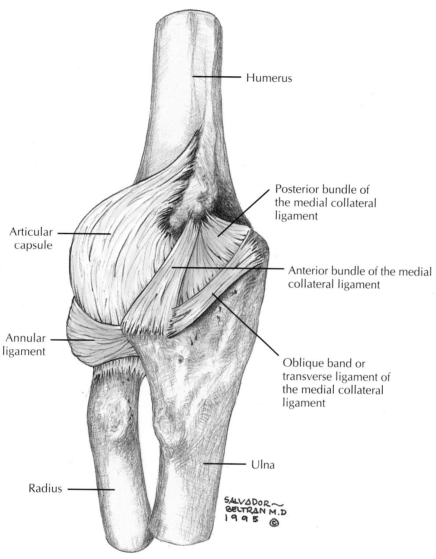

Humerus

Posterior bundle of the medial collateral ligament

Articular capsule

Anterior bundle of the medial collateral ligament

Annular ligament

Oblique band or transverse ligament of the medial collateral ligament

Ulna

Radius

SALVADOR~ BELTRAN M.D 1995 ©

FIGURE 2-56

Medial collateral ligament complex—the anterior and posterior bundles and transverse ligament (oblique band). The posterior bundle and the transverse ligament lie at the deep margin of the ulnar nerve and make up the floor of the cubital tunnel. The functionally important anterior bundle of the medial collateral ligament extends from the inferior aspect of the medial epicondyle to the medial aspect of the coronoid process. The anterior bundle provides the primary constraint to valgus stress and commonly is damaged in athletes who frequently use a throwing motion. For related MR, arthroscopy, and surgical anatomy images see Figures 2-62 and 2-63.

ELBOW: EXTENSORS OF THE HAND AND WRIST, LATERAL VIEW

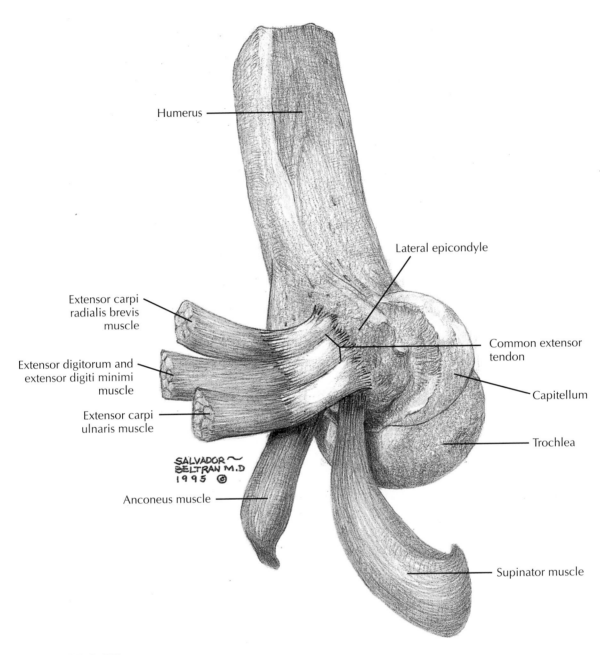

FIGURE 2-57

The extensor carpi radialis brevis, the extensor digitorum, the extensor digiti minimi, and the extensor carpi ulnaris arise from the lateral epicondyle as the common extensor tendon. The anconeus and supinator muscles are also shown. The anconeus arises from the posterior aspect of the lateral epicondyle and inserts more distally on the olecranon. The anconeus provides dynamic support to the lateral collateral ligament in resisting varus stress. For related MR, arthroscopy, and surgical anatomy image see Figure 2-67.

ELBOW: FLEXORS OF THE WRIST AND HAND, MEDIAL VIEW

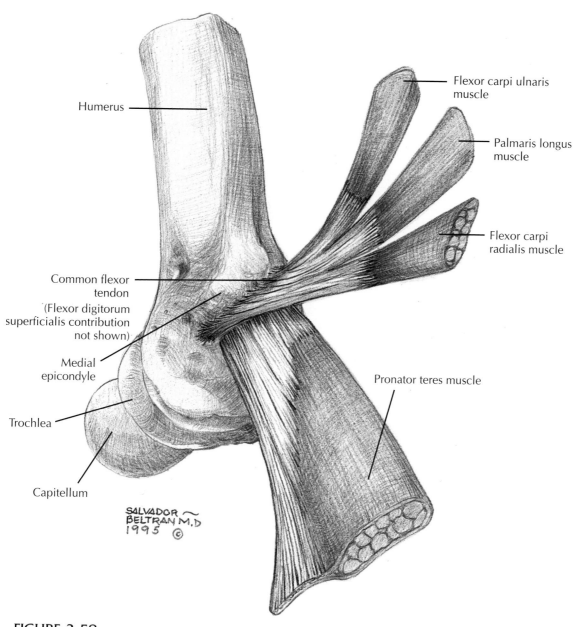

Flexor carpi ulnaris
muscle

Palmaris longus
muscle

Flexor carpi
radialis muscle

Humerus

Common flexor
tendon
(Flexor digitorum
superficialis contribution
not shown)

Medial
epicondyle

Pronator teres muscle

Trochlea

Capitellum

SALVADOR
BELTRAN M.D
1995 ©

FIGURE 2-58

The medial compartment structures include the pronator teres and the flexors of the hand and wrist, which arise from the medial epicondyle as the common flexor tendon. The common flexor tendon provides dynamic support to the medial collateral ligament complex in resisting valgus stress. For related MR, arthroscopy, and surgical anatomy image see Figure 2-66.

ELBOW: MUSCLES OF THE FOREARM, ANTERIOR VIEW

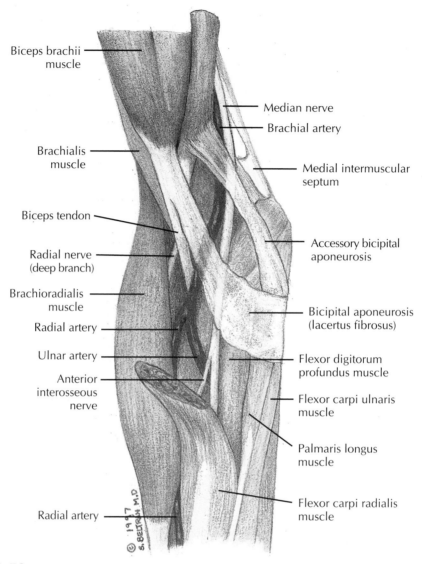

Biceps brachii
muscle

Brachialis
muscle

Biceps tendon

Radial nerve
(deep branch)

Brachioradialis
muscle

Radial artery

Ulnar artery

Anterior
interosseous
nerve

Radial artery

Median nerve

Brachial artery

Medial intermuscular
septum

Accessory bicipital
aponeurosis

Bicipital aponeurosis
(lacertus fibrosus)

Flexor digitorum
profundus muscle

Flexor carpi ulnaris
muscle

Palmaris longus
muscle

Flexor carpi radialis
muscle

© 1997
S. BELTRAN M.D.

FIGURE 2-59

The muscles of the elbow are divided into anterior, posterior, medial, and lateral compartments. The anterior compartment contains the biceps and brachialis muscles. The posterior compartment contains the triceps and anconeus muscles. The medial compartment contains the pronator teres and the flexors of the hand and wrist, which originate on the medial epicondyle. The lateral compartment contains the supinator, the brachioradialis, the extensor radialis longus, and the extensors of the hand and wrist, which originate on the lateral epicondyle. For related MR, arthroscopy, and surgical anatomy images see Figures 2-61 and 2-71.

ELBOW: ULNAR NERVE

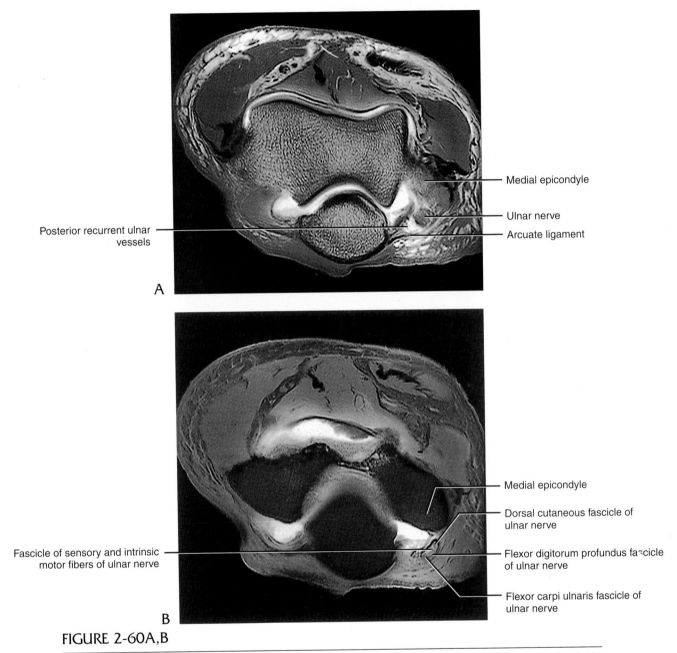

Medial epicondyle

Ulnar nerve

Arcuate ligament

Posterior recurrent ulnar vessels

A

Medial epicondyle

Dorsal cutaneous fascicle of ulnar nerve

Flexor digitorum profundus fascicle of ulnar nerve

Flexor carpi ulnaris fascicle of ulnar nerve

Fascicle of sensory and intrinsic motor fibers of ulnar nerve

B

FIGURE 2-60A,B

The ulnar nerve within the cubital tunnel is posterior to the medial epicondyle on axial T1-weighted **(A)** and fat-suppressed T2-weighted **(B)** MR arthrograms. The T1-weighted image is at the level of the capitellum and trochlea, whereas the fat-suppressed T2-weighted image is at the level of the olecranon and coronoid fossa. The ulnar nerve is medial to the posterior recurrent ulnar vessels. The arcuate ligament (flexor carpi ulnaris aponeurosis) and the cubital tunnel retinaculum (Osborne's band) form the roof of the cubital tunnel. The cubital tunnel is also defined anteriorly by the medial epicondyle, and laterally by the ulno-humeral ligament. The fat-suppressed MR image demonstrates intraneural topography of the ulnar nerve.

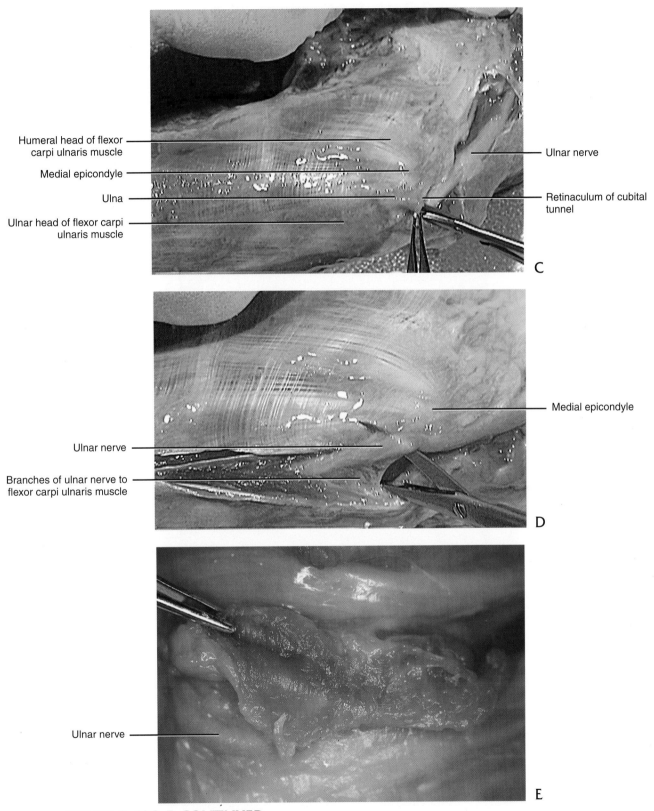

Humeral head of flexor carpi ulnaris muscle

Medial epicondyle

Ulna

Ulnar head of flexor carpi ulnaris muscle

Ulnar nerve

Retinaculum of cubital tunnel

C

Ulnar nerve

Branches of ulnar nerve to flexor carpi ulnaris muscle

Medial epicondyle

D

Ulnar nerve

E

FIGURE 2-60C–E *CONTINUED*

(**C** and **D**) Corresponding dissections. (**C**) The posteromedial course of the ulnar nerve at the level of the distal humerus. The retinaculum of the cubital tunnel is mobilized posterior to the medial epicondyle. (**D**) The ulnar nerve sends branches to the flexor carpi ulnaris muscle. The medial half of the flexor digitorum profundus muscles is also supplied by the ulnar nerve. (**E**) In a separate specimen, the anconeus epitrochlearis muscle occupies the cubital tunnel and is posteromedial to the ulnar nerve. This small accessory muscle may produce a compression neuropathy of the ulnar nerve by decreasing the volume of the cubital tunnel.

ELBOW: RADIAL NERVE

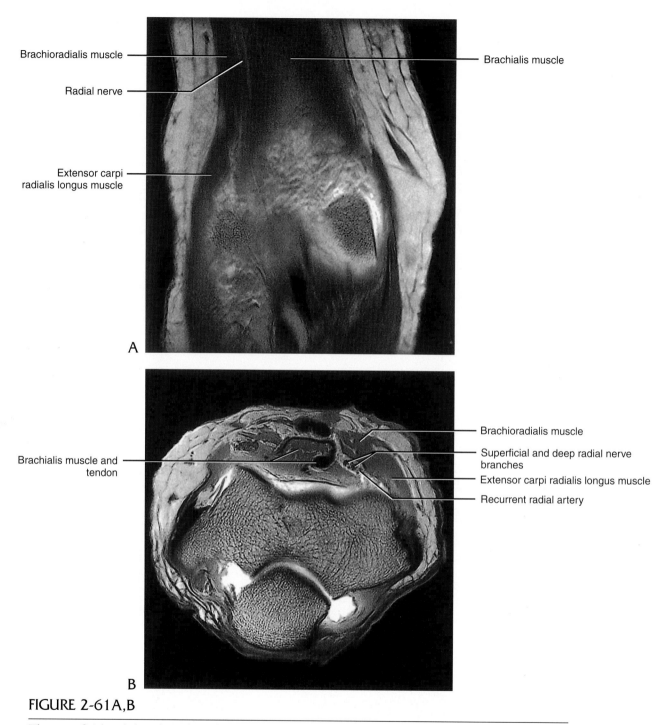

FIGURE 2-61A,B

The superficial and deep branches of the radial nerve are surrounded by fat and are located between the brachialis, brachioradialis, and extensor carpi radialis longus muscles. (A) T1-weighted coronal MR arthrogram. (B) T1-weighted axial MR arthrogram. The superficial branch courses distally, deep to the brachioradialis muscle.

ELBOW: RADIAL NERVE

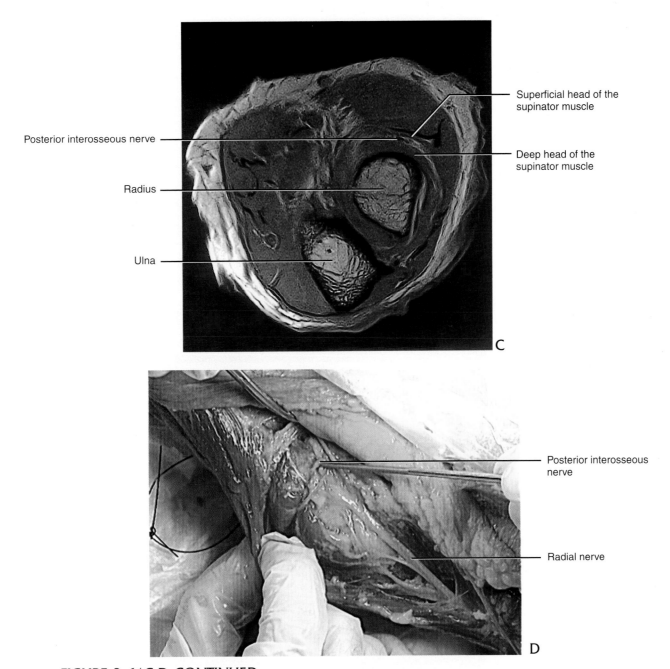

Superficial head of the supinator muscle

Posterior interosseous nerve

Deep head of the supinator muscle

Radius

Ulna

C

Posterior interosseous nerve

Radial nerve

D

FIGURE 2-61C,D *CONTINUED*

(C) T1-weighted axial image showing the deep branch coursing between the superficial and deep portions of the supinator muscle before continuing as the posterior interosseous nerve. The fibrous arcade of Frohse, at the proximal border of the superficial head of the supinator muscle, is frequently the cause of posterior interosseous neuropathy. Additional compression may be related to the fibrous edge of the extensor carpi radialis brevis muscle, the radial recurrent vessels of Henry (vascular leash of Henry), and fibrous bands. In radial tunnel syndrome, posterior interosseous nerve compression is not as severe and does not cause muscle paralysis. **(D)** Corresponding dissection of the radial nerve and posterior interosseous branch.

ELBOW: MEDIAL COLLATERAL LIGAMENT

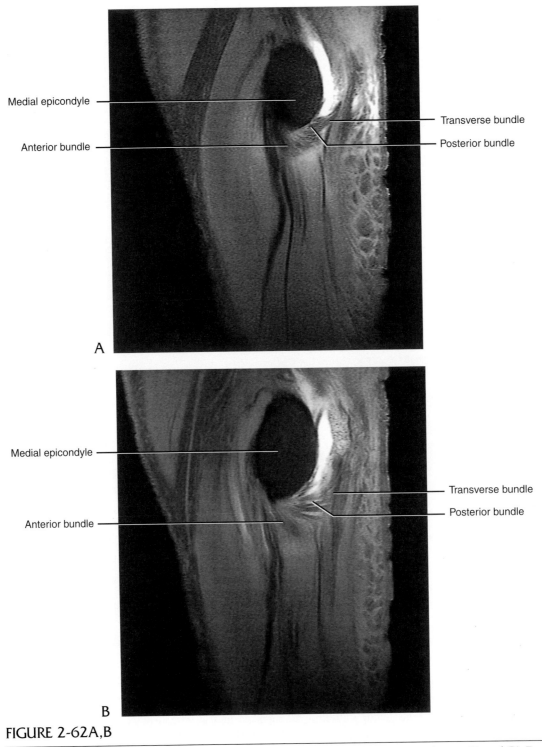

FIGURE 2-62A,B

The anterior, posterior, and transverse bundles of the medial collateral ligament are shown. (**A** and **B**) Fat-suppressed T1-weighted sagittal MR arthrograms (the image in part **A** is more medial than that in part **B**).

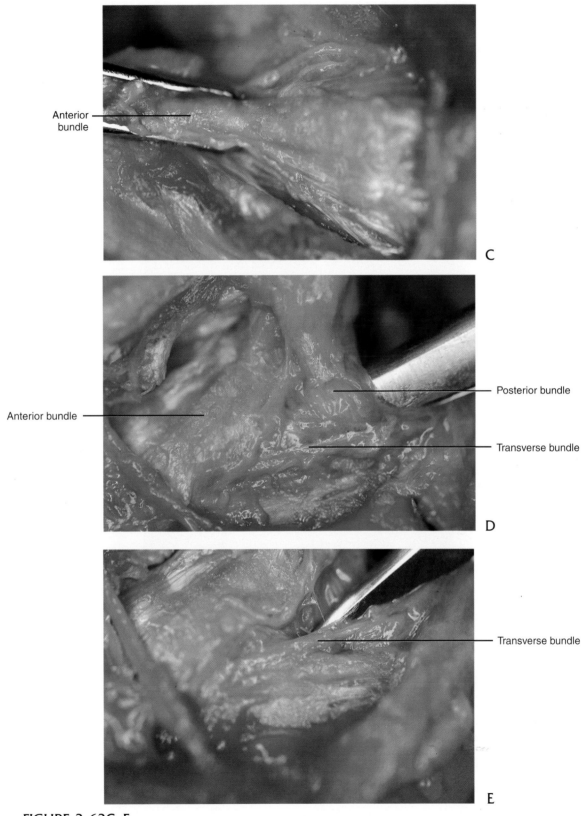

FIGURE 2-62C–E

(**C, D,** and **E**) Corresponding gross dissections showing the anterior bundle (**C**), the posterior bundle (**D**), and the transverse bundle (**E**).

ELBOW: MEDIAL COLLATERAL LIGAMENT

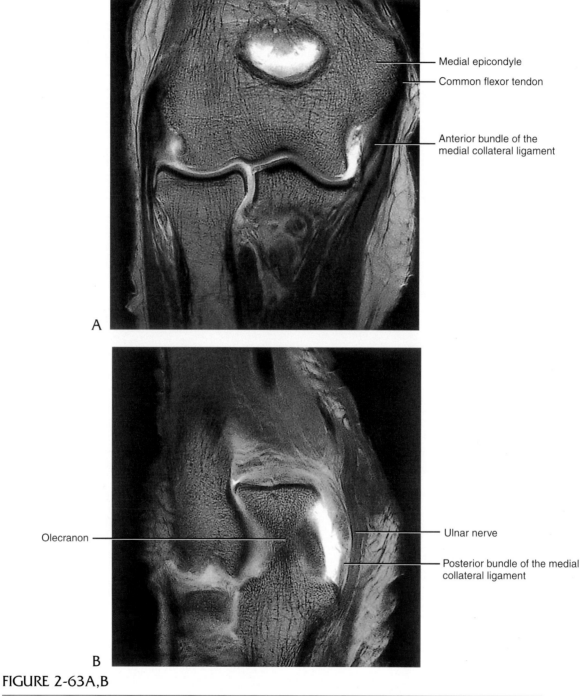

FIGURE 2-63A,B

The anterior **(A)** and posterior **(B)** bundles of the medial collateral ligament complex are shown on T1-weighted coronal MR arthrograms. The corresponding gross dissection identifies the anterior **(C)**, posterior **(D)**, and transverse **(E)** bundles of the medial collateral ligament.

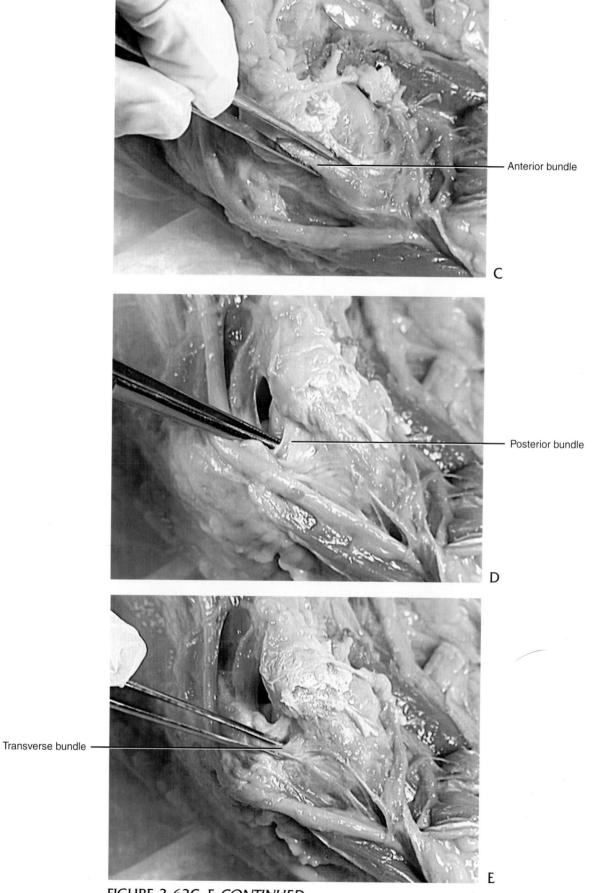

Anterior bundle

C

Posterior bundle

D

Transverse bundle

E

FIGURE 2-63C–E *CONTINUED*

ELBOW: LATERAL COLLATERAL LIGAMENT COMPLEX

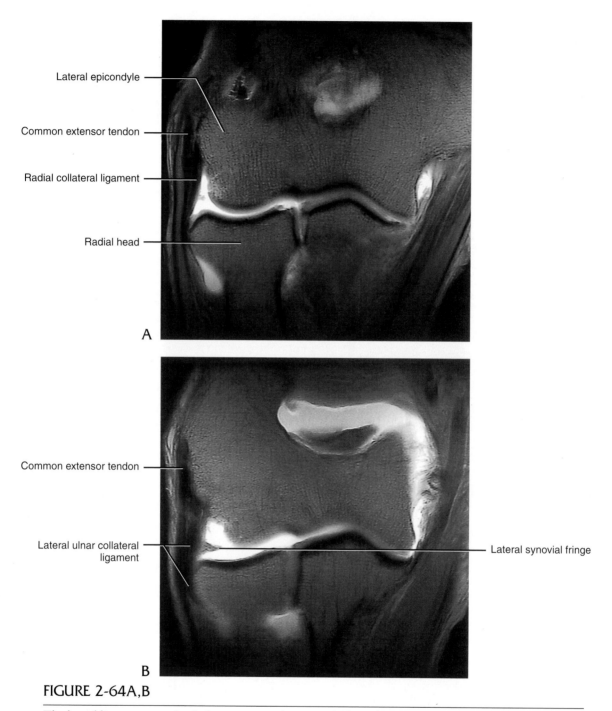

FIGURE 2-64A,B

The lateral ligament complex is shown on anterior coronal **(A)** and posterior coronal **(B)** T1-weighted MR arthrograms. Note the contributions from the radial collateral ligament proper, the lateral ulnar collateral ligament (LUCL), and the annular ligament. **(C, D,** and **E)** Corresponding dissections of the radial collateral ligament proper **(C)**, the LUCL **(D)**, and the annular ligament **(E)**. The normal radial meniscus or synovial fringe is visualized deep to both the radial collateral ligament proper and the LUCL. The LUCL is identified on coronal images posterior to the radial collateral ligament proper.

ELBOW: LATERAL COLLATERAL LIGAMENT COMPLEX

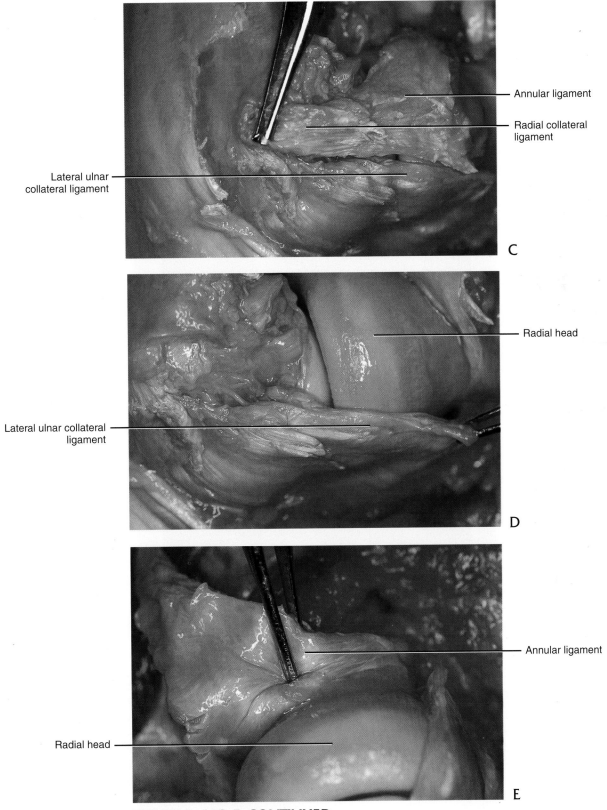

Annular ligament

Radial collateral ligament

Lateral ulnar collateral ligament

C

Radial head

Lateral ulnar collateral ligament

D

Annular ligament

Radial head

E

FIGURE 2-64C–E *CONTINUED*

ELBOW: LATERAL COLLATERAL LIGAMENT COMPLEX

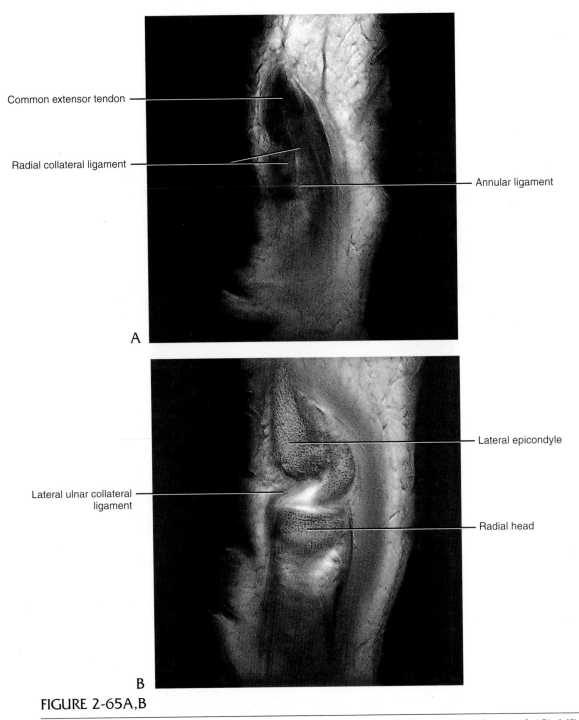

FIGURE 2-65A,B

Visualization of the lateral ligament complex on T1-weighted sagittal (**A** and **B**) and coronal (**C**) MR arthrograms. The lateral ulnar collateral ligament is seen on the posterior coronal image (part **C**) extending from the lateral epicondyle and coursing obliquely and medially about the radial head to attach to the posterolateral aspect of the ulna at the supinator crest. Corresponding gross dissections show the radial collateral ligament proper (**D**) and the distal extent of the lateral ulnar collateral ligament toward the supinator crest (**E**).

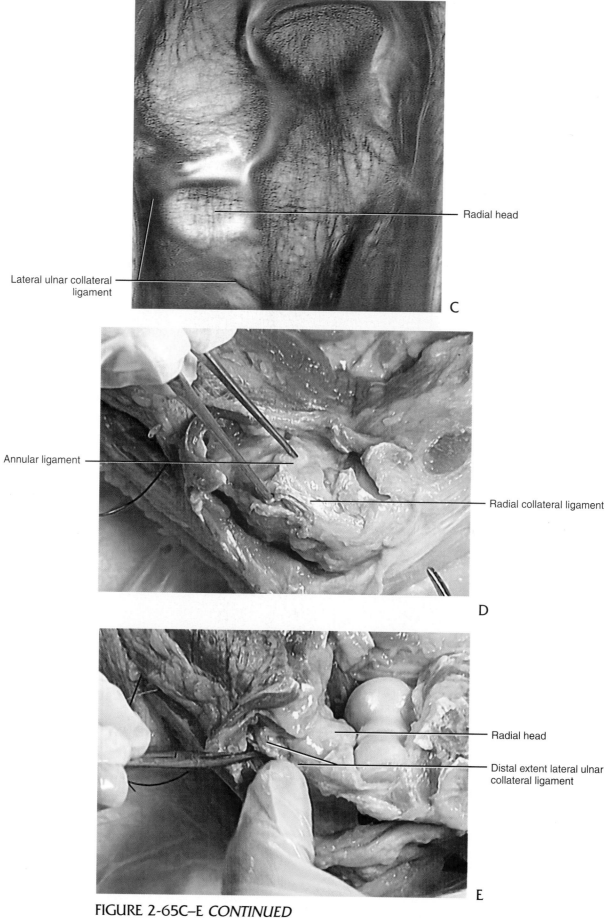

Radial head

Lateral ulnar collateral
ligament

C

Annular ligament

Radial collateral ligament

D

Radial head

Distal extent lateral ulnar
collateral ligament

E

FIGURE 2-65C–E *CONTINUED*

ELBOW: COMMON FLEXOR TENDON

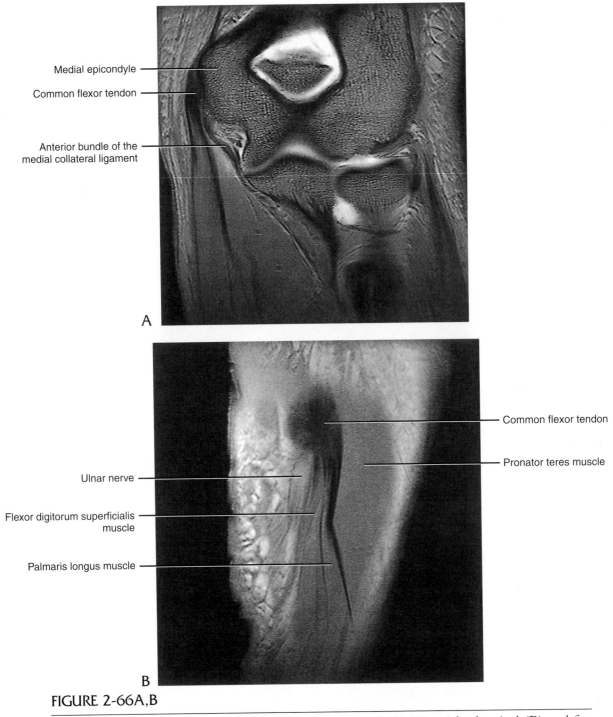

Medial epicondyle

Common flexor tendon

Anterior bundle of the
medial collateral ligament

A

Common flexor tendon

Pronator teres muscle

Ulnar nerve

Flexor digitorum superficialis
muscle

Palmaris longus muscle

B

FIGURE 2-66A,B

The common flexor tendon is shown on T1-weighted coronal **(A)**, T1-weighted sagittal **(B)**, and fat-suppressed T1-weighted axial **(C)** MR arthrograms. **(D)** Corresponding dissections show release of the common flexor tendon from the medial epicondyle. The anterior bundle of the medial collateral ligament is exposed.

ELBOW: COMMON FLEXOR TENDON

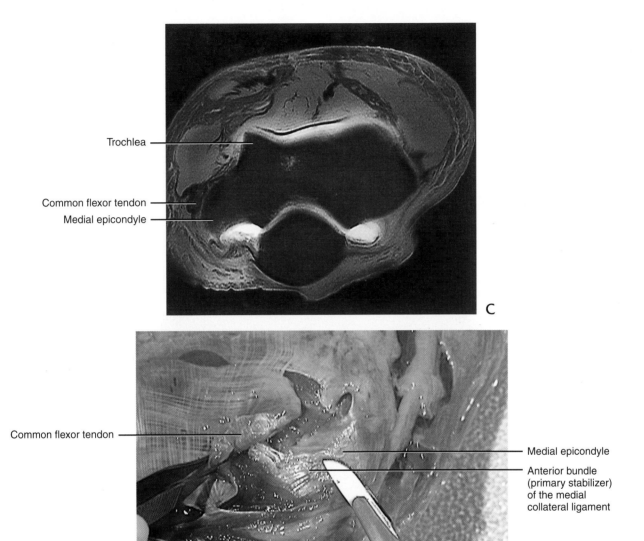

FIGURE 2-66C,D *CONTINUED*

ELBOW: COMMON EXTENSOR TENDON

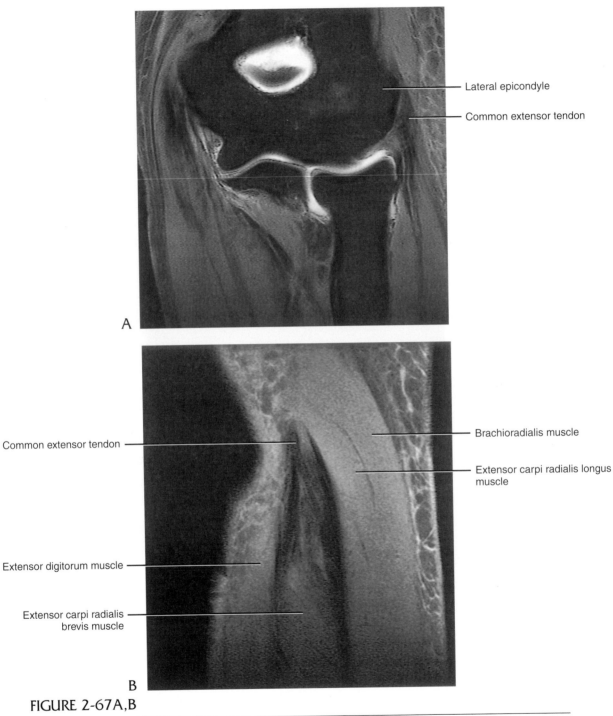

FIGURE 2-67A,B

Fat-suppressed T1-weighted coronal **(A)** and sagittal **(B)** MR arthrograms showing the lateral epicondylar attachment of the common extensor tendon. Corresponding gross dissections demonstrate the superficial landmarks of the lateral aspect of the elbow **(C)** and release of the extensor tendons exposing the underlying lateral ulnar collateral ligament and supinator crest **(D)**.

ELBOW: COMMON EXTENSOR TENDON

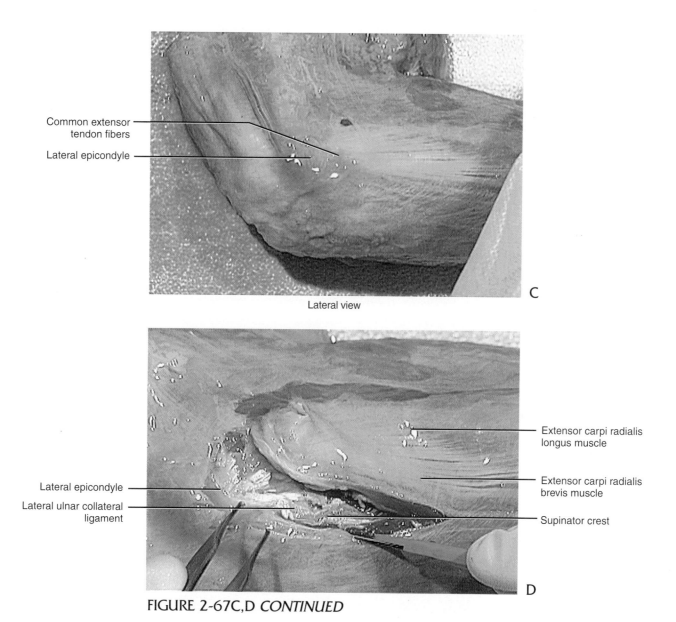

C — Lateral view

Common extensor
tendon fibers

Lateral epicondyle

Extensor carpi radialis
longus muscle

Extensor carpi radialis
brevis muscle

Lateral epicondyle

Lateral ulnar collateral
ligament

Supinator crest

D

FIGURE 2-67C,D *CONTINUED*

ELBOW: PSEUDODEFECT OF THE CAPITELLUM

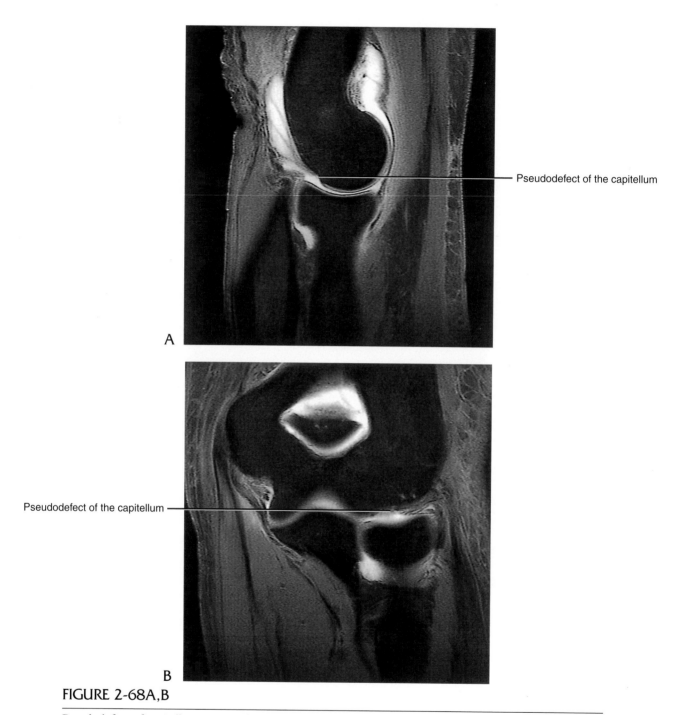

Pseudodefect of the capitellum

Pseudodefect of the capitellum

A

B

FIGURE 2-68A,B

Pseudodefect of capitellum seen on fat-suppressed T1-weighted sagittal **(A)** and posterior coronal **(B)** MR arthrograms. The pseudodefect may be accentuated in extension, during which the lateral aspect of the radial head projects lateral and posterior to the articular surface of the capitellum. The normal groove between the capitellum and the lateral epicondyle produces the pseudodefect on both coronal and sagittal MR images.

ELBOW: PSEUDODEFECT OF THE CAPITELLUM

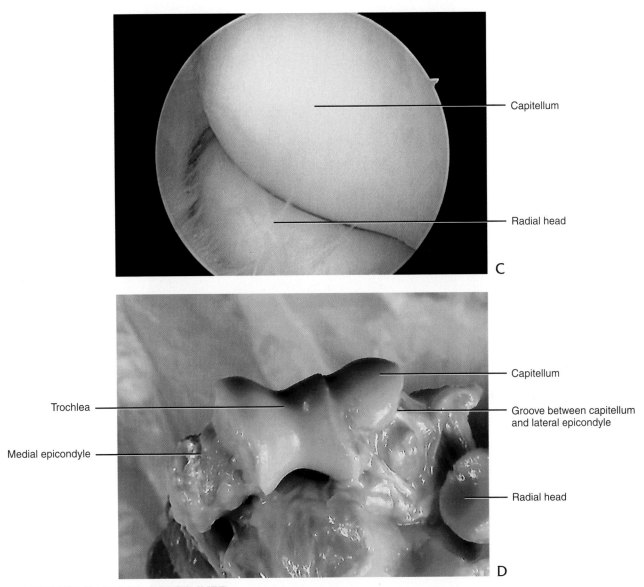

Capitellum

Radial head

C

Trochlea

Medial epicondyle

Capitellum

Groove between capitellum
and lateral epicondyle

Radial head

D

FIGURE 2-68C,D *CONTINUED*

(C) Arthroscopic anterior view of the radiocapitellar joint. **(D)** Anteroinferior view of the dissection showing the rounded eminence of the capitellum and the normal groove, which undercuts the junction between the capitellum and the lateral epicondyle.

ELBOW: ANNULAR LIGAMENT AND PSEUDODEFECT OF THE TROCHLEAR GROOVE

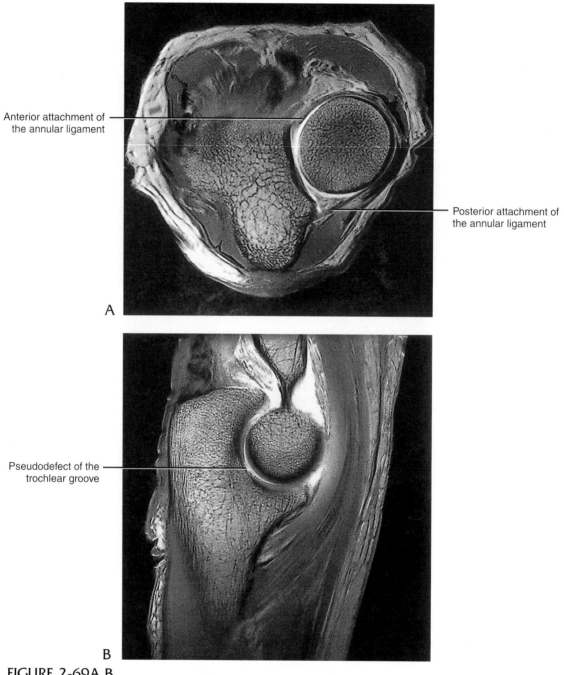

Anterior attachment of
the annular ligament

Posterior attachment of
the annular ligament

Pseudodefect of the
trochlear groove

FIGURE 2-69A,B

(A) T1-weighted axial MR arthrogram showing the anterior and posterior attachments of the annular ligament at the level of the proximal radioulnar joint. **(B)** Pseudodefect of the trochlear groove shown as a focal
defect in the articular surface of the trochlear groove on a T1-weighted sagittal MR arthrogram. The absence of articular cartilage corresponds to normal small cortical notches at the medial and lateral aspects of
the waist of the trochlear groove (on either side of the transverse trochlear ridge). The transverse trochlear
ridge is nonarticular and represents a bare area.

ELBOW: ANNULAR LIGAMENT AND PSEUDODEFECT OF THE TROCHLEAR GROOVE

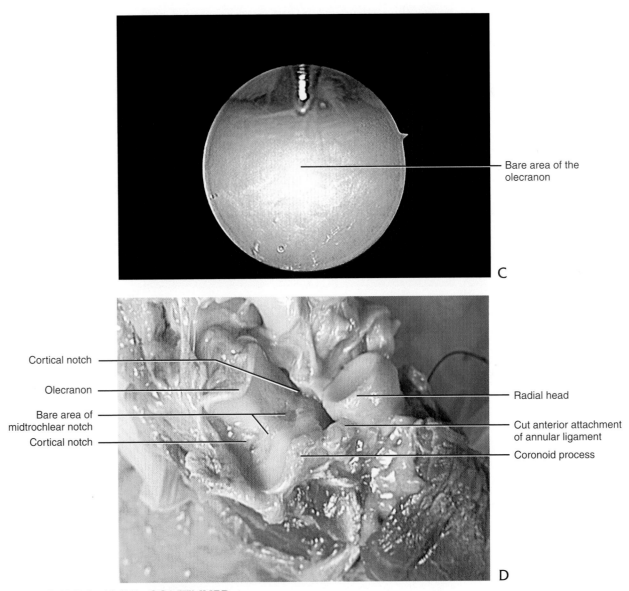

Bare area of the olecranon

C

Cortical notch

Olecranon

Bare area of midtrochlear notch

Cortical notch

Radial head

Cut anterior attachment of annular ligament

Coronoid process

D

FIGURE 2-69C,D *CONTINUED*

(C) Corresponding arthroscopic view of the bare area of the olecranon. **(D)** Gross dissection of the trochlea with the normal bare area devoid of articular cartilage.

ELBOW: HUMEROULNAR JOINT AND TRANSVERSE TROCHLEAR RIDGE

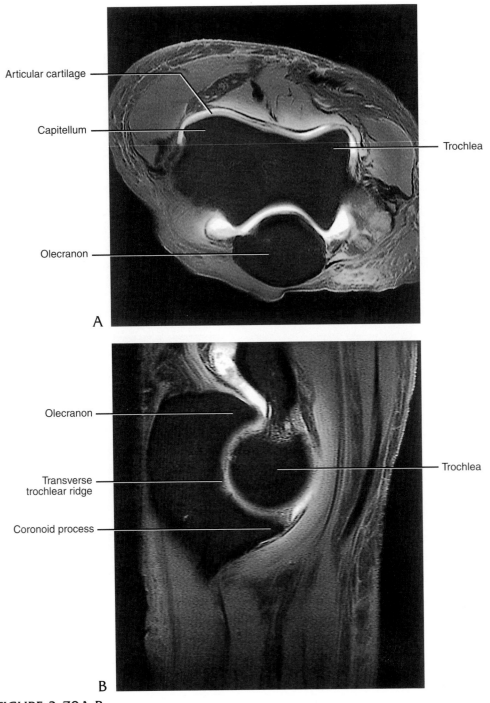

Articular cartilage

Capitellum

Trochlea

Olecranon

A

Olecranon

Transverse trochlear ridge

Trochlea

Coronoid process

B

FIGURE 2-70A,B

Fat-suppressed T1-weighted MR arthrograms of the capitellar and trochlear surfaces in the axial plane **(A)** and the ulnohumeral articulation in the sagittal plane **(B)**. The transverse trochlear ridge may produce a normal prominence in the contour of the trochlear groove on sagittal images. Corresponding arthroscopic view of the coronoid process and trochlea looking medially from the lateral side **(C)** and a gross exposure of the radial head-capitellar articulation and trochlea-coronoid process articulation **(D)**.

ELBOW: HUMEROULNAR JOINT

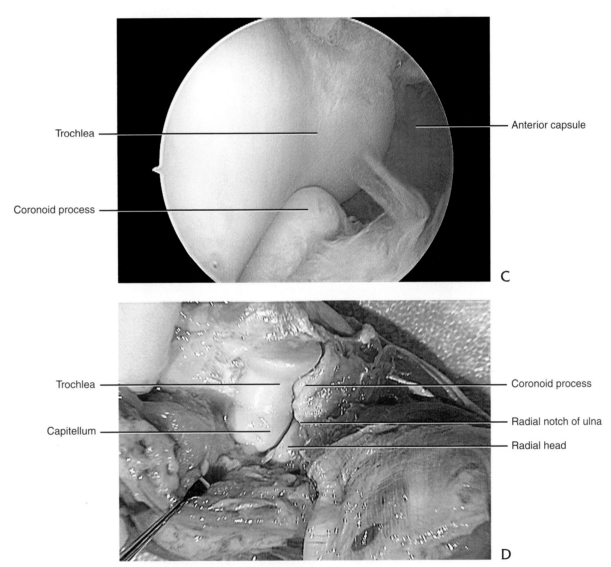

FIGURE 2-70C,D *CONTINUED*

ELBOW: BICEPS AND LACERTUS FIBROSUS

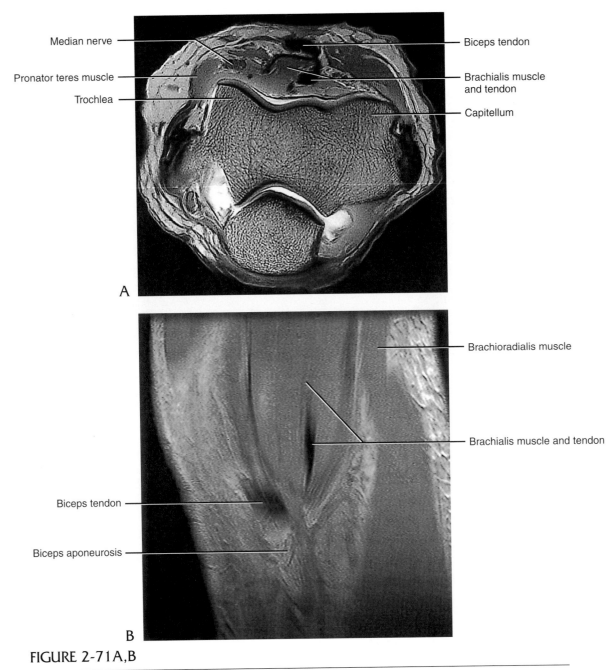

Median nerve

Pronator teres muscle

Trochlea

Biceps tendon

Brachialis muscle
and tendon

Capitellum

A

Brachioradialis muscle

Brachialis muscle and tendon

Biceps tendon

Biceps aponeurosis

B

FIGURE 2-71 A,B

T1–weighted MR arthrograms showing the biceps tendon in the axial **(A)** and coronal **(B** and **C)** planes (the image in part **B** is anterior to the image in part **C**). **(D)** The biceps and lacertus fibrosus are dissected in this corresponding gross specimen. The median nerve may be compressed between the lacertus fibrosus and the origin of the pronator teres. In the pronator syndrome, median nerve entrapment may develop beneath the lacertus fibrosus, the pronator teres, the flexor digitorum superficial arch, or the arcade of vessels. At a more proximal level in the brachium, median nerve entrapment may occur at the level of the supracondylar process and the ligament of Struthers.

ELBOW: BICEPS AND LACERTUS FIBROSUS

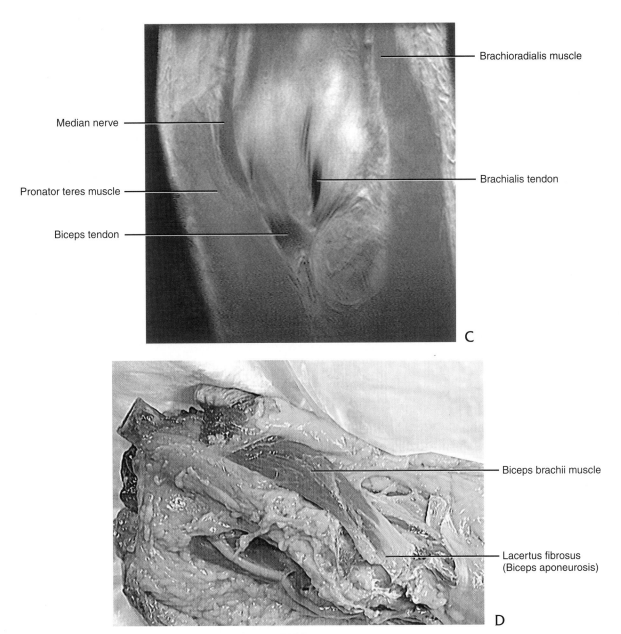

Brachioradialis muscle

Median nerve

Brachialis tendon

Pronator teres muscle

Biceps tendon

C

Biceps brachii muscle

Lacertus fibrosus
(Biceps aponeurosis)

D

FIGURE 2-71C,D *CONTINUED*

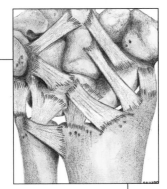

C H A P T E R 3

THE WRIST AND HAND

David W. Stoller
Gordon A. Brody
David M. Lichtman
Salvador Beltran

WRIST ARTHROSCOPY AND DISSECTION
MR NORMAL ANATOMY

COLOR ANATOMIC ILLUSTRATIONS
MR, ARTHROSCOPY, AND SURGICAL CORRELATION

———— WRIST ARTHROSCOPY ————

ARTHROSCOPY OF THE WRIST is facilitated by use of a traction tower with 10 to 12 pounds of distraction. The standard portals include the 3-4 portal (between the extensor pollicis longus of the third extensor compartment and the extensor digitorum communis of the fourth extensor compartment), the 4-5 portal (ulnar to the extensor digitorum communis), and the radial midcarpal portal. Most often, the 3-4 portal is used for arthroscopic visualization and the 4-5 portal is used for instrumentation. The 4-5 portal is used for arthroscopic visualization of the triangular fibrocartilage complex, however, with instrument placement through the 6R (radial) portal. Accessory radiocarpal portals include a 1-2 portal for outflow, the 6R portal for instrumentation, and the 6U (ulnar) portal for outflow. The midcarpal radial portal is used for visualization from the midcarpal joint. The 6R portal is important in the evaluation of the lunotriquetral ligament and the triquetrum.

Proceeding from the radius to the ulna, the arthroscopic structures of the radiocarpal joint include the radial styloid, the radioscaphocapitate ligament, the long radiolunate ligament (also known as the radiolunotriquetral ligament), the proximal pole of the scaphoid, the scaphoid fossa, the scapholunate interosseous ligament, the radioscapholunate ligament (the ligament of Testut), the proximal pole of the lunate, the lunate fossa, the short radiolunate ligament, the triangular fibrocartilage complex, the ulnocarpal ligaments (the ulnolunate and ulnotriquetral ligaments), the lunotriquetral interosseous ligament, and the proximal pole of the triquetrum. A fat pad, more accurately a synovial fold, covers the radioscapholunate ligament. The

221

normal triangular fibrocartilage (TFC) demonstrates the trampoline effect when probed arthroscopically. The prestyloid recess and pisotriquetral space are visualized as two perforations at the ulnar margin of the TFC. The ulnar attachments of the TFC are palpated with a probe. The dorsal attachment of the meniscus homologue may obscure visualization of the peripheral margins of the TFC. Midcarpal arthroscopic portals include the midcarpal radial (the most commonly used), the midcarpal ulnar, and scaphotrapeziotrapezoid. Midcarpal joint arthroscopy is useful in assessing any breaks in the normal carpal arcs, since scapholunate and lunotriquetral alignment is not blocked by torn ligaments. Arthritis of the head of the capitate may be associated with a medial lunate facet and can be visualized through the midcarpal joint. Triscaphe arthritis, which involves the articulation of the scaphoid, trapezium, and the trapezoid, can be evaluated with midcarpal arthroscopy.

SURGICAL DISSECTION OF THE WRIST

Fibrous septa from the deep surface of the extensor retinaculum define the six extensor compartments on the dorsum of the wrist. The first extensor compartment contains the abductor pollicis longus and extensor pollicis brevis. The second compartment contains the extensor carpi radialis brevis and the extensor carpi radialis longus. The third compartment contains the extensor pollicis longus. The extensor pollicis longus courses around the ulnar aspect of Lister's tubercle, on the dorsum of the distal radius. The dorsal surgical approach to the wrist is usually through the floor of the third extensor compartment. The fourth extensor compartment contains the extensor digitorum and extensor indicis (including its separate muscle belly). The fifth extensor compartment contains the extensor digiti minimi. The sixth extensor compartment contains the extensor carpi ulnaris. The carpal bones absorb stress from the palm to the radius and change geometrical shape in response to motion. The proximal carpal row is the intercalary segment. The extrinsic ligaments of the wrist, which connect the radius or ulna to the carpal bones or the metacarpals to the carpal bones, provide gross stability. The extrinsic radiocarpal complex includes the radioscaphocapitate, the long radiolunate, the radioscapholunate, and the short radiolunate ligaments. The intrinsic ligaments include the intercarpal ligaments, which provide intermediate stability, and the interosseous ligaments, which "fine tune" wrist stability. Both the scapholunate and lunotriquetral intrinsic ligaments have dorsal, membranous, and volar components. The dorsal component of the scapholunate ligament is the strongest and thickest portion of the intrinsic scapholunate complex and connects with the dorsal radiocarpal joint capsule. Perforations or tears of the proximal or membranous scapholunate ligament may exist as a normal degenerative finding in older patients. As a result, arthrography of the wrist may not be useful, especially in patients over 35 years of age, because of these communications across the intrinsic interosseous ligaments and the triangular fibrocartilage complex. In normal carpal kinematics, radial deviation of the wrist creates a flexion movement with compression of the scaphotrapeziotrapezoid (STT) joint and proximal row flexion (physiologic volar intercalated segment instability pattern

[VISI]). In ulnar deviation, the extension movement predominates, with interaction at the (triquetrohamate) T-H helicoid slope and proximal row extension (physiologic dorsal intercalated segment instability pattern [DISI]). In the neutral loaded wrist, flexion movements (the radial link) and extension movements (the ulnar link) are balanced. The four stage progression of perilunate injuries includes:

- Stage 1: scapholunate instability
- Stage 2: capitolunate ligament failure
- Stage 3: lunotriquetral instability
- Stage 4: failure of dorsal radiocarpal ligaments associated with volar lunate dislocation or dorsal perilunate dislocation.

Perilunate injuries may involve a disruption of the radial link (e.g., instability, a scaphoid fracture, or a scapholunate tear). In radial link disruptions, the scaphoid flexes and the lunate extends with the triquetrum (i.e., lunate extension in DISI), and the scapholunate angle is increased. In ulnar link disruptions (e.g., a lunotriquetral ligament tear), the triquetrum extends and the scaphoid flexes with the lunate (i.e., lunate flexion in VISI), and the scapholunate angle remains unchanged. Perilunar instabilities may be classified into lesser arc injuries (primarily ligamentous) and greater arc injuries (primarily osseous).

The ulnar head, in the distal radioulnar joint (DRUJ), acts as a guide for rotation of the hand, wrist, and radius. The triangular fibrocartilage complex (TFCC), which attaches at the fovea, is the major stabilizer of the DRUJ. In pronation the distal radius rotates 80° to 90°, shortens, and translates volarly. In supination the distal radius rotates 80° to 90°, lengthens, and translates dorsally. The stabilizers of the DRUJ are the articular disc (the TFC or triangular fibrocartilage represents the articular disc and volar and dorsal radioulnar ligaments), the volar and dorsal radioulnar ligaments, the volar ulnocarpal ligaments, the extensor carpi ulnaris subsheath, the interosseous membrane, the sigmoid notch, and the shape and integrity of the forearm bones. Injuries to the TFCC/DRUJ stabilizers are classified as stable or unstable. Stable injuries include traumatic TFCC tears (central Palmer 1A or radial Palmer 1D), degenerative TFCC tears (central Palmer 2), and ulnocarpal abutment. Partially unstable injuries have incomplete TFCC disruption (peripheral Palmer 1B and distal Palmer 1C). Unstable injuries, with complete TFCC disruption, are associated with a displaced ulnar styloid fracture at the fovea, massive TFCC soft tissue injury, or a displaced distal radius fracture involving the sigmoid notch. Hyperpronation is the mechanism for dorsal dislocation and hypersupination is the mechanism for volar dislocation. Axial compression produces an Essex-Lopresti fracture dislocation.

WRIST: CORONAL

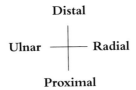

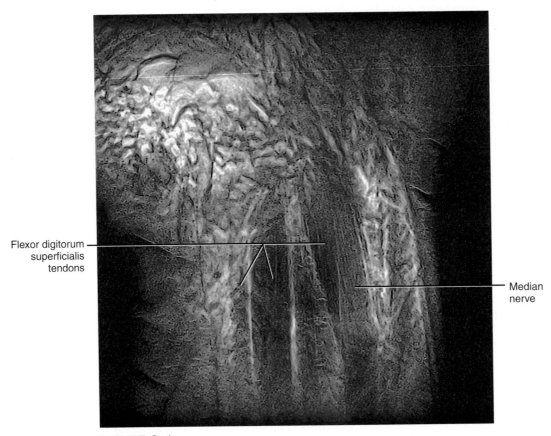

Flexor digitorum
superficialis
tendons

Median
nerve

FIGURE 3-1

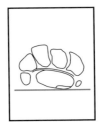

WRIST: CORONAL

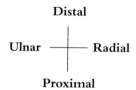

Distal

Ulnar —— Radial

Proximal

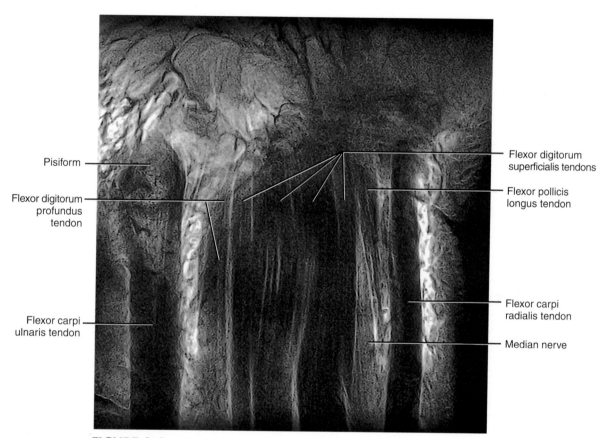

Pisiform

Flexor digitorum
profundus
tendon

Flexor carpi
ulnaris tendon

Flexor digitorum
superficialis tendons

Flexor pollicis
longus tendon

Flexor carpi
radialis tendon

Median nerve

FIGURE 3-2

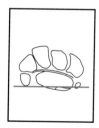

WRIST: CORONAL

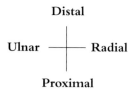

Distal

Ulnar — Radial

Proximal

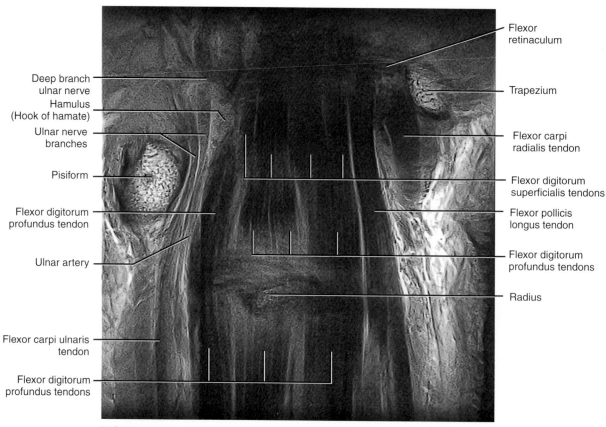

Deep branch ulnar nerve

Hamulus (Hook of hamate)

Ulnar nerve branches

Pisiform

Flexor digitorum profundus tendon

Ulnar artery

Flexor carpi ulnaris tendon

Flexor digitorum profundus tendons

Flexor retinaculum

Trapezium

Flexor carpi radialis tendon

Flexor digitorum superficialis tendons

Flexor pollicis longus tendon

Flexor digitorum profundus tendons

Radius

FIGURE 3-3

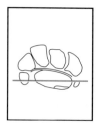

WRIST: CORONAL

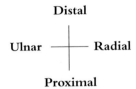

Distal

Ulnar —— Radial

Proximal

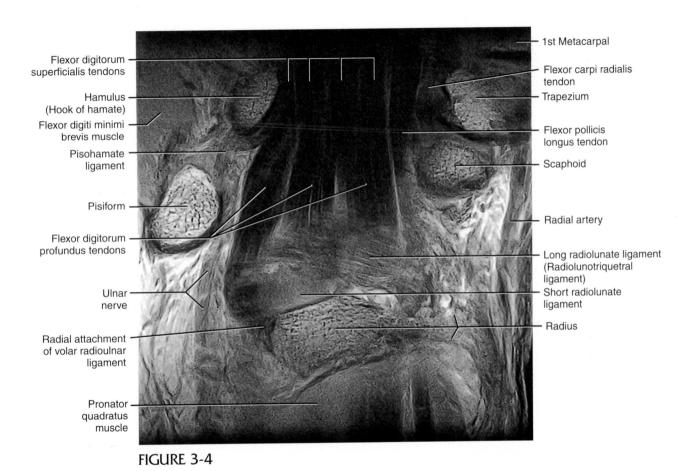

Flexor digitorum
superficialis tendons

Hamulus
(Hook of hamate)

Flexor digiti minimi
brevis muscle

Pisohamate
ligament

Pisiform

Flexor digitorum
profundus tendons

Ulnar
nerve

Radial attachment
of volar radioulnar
ligament

Pronator
quadratus
muscle

1st Metacarpal

Flexor carpi radialis
tendon

Trapezium

Flexor pollicis
longus tendon

Scaphoid

Radial artery

Long radiolunate ligament
(Radiolunotriquetral
ligament)

Short radiolunate
ligament

Radius

FIGURE 3-4

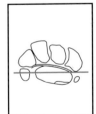

WRIST: CORONAL

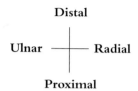

Distal

Ulnar ——|—— Radial

Proximal

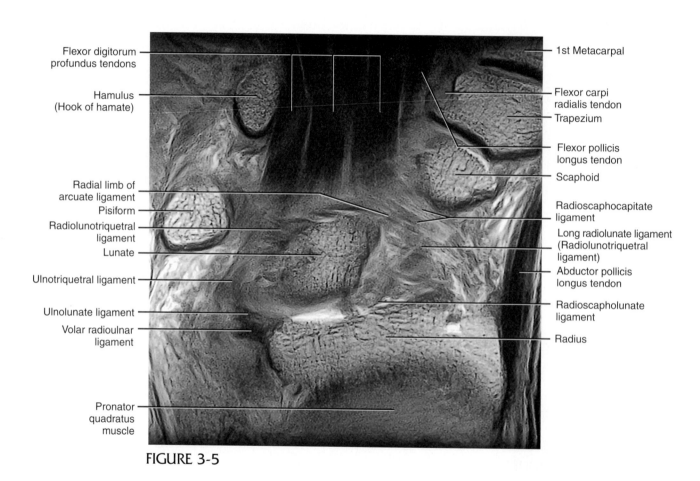

Flexor digitorum profundus tendons

Hamulus (Hook of hamate)

Radial limb of arcuate ligament

Pisiform

Radiolunotriquetral ligament

Lunate

Ulnotriquetral ligament

Ulnolunate ligament

Volar radioulnar ligament

Pronator quadratus muscle

1st Metacarpal

Flexor carpi radialis tendon

Trapezium

Flexor pollicis longus tendon

Scaphoid

Radioscaphocapitate ligament

Long radiolunate ligament (Radiolunotriquetral ligament)

Abductor pollicis longus tendon

Radioscapholunate ligament

Radius

FIGURE 3-5

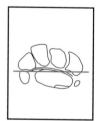

WRIST: CORONAL

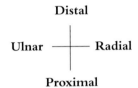

Distal

Ulnar ——┼—— Radial

Proximal

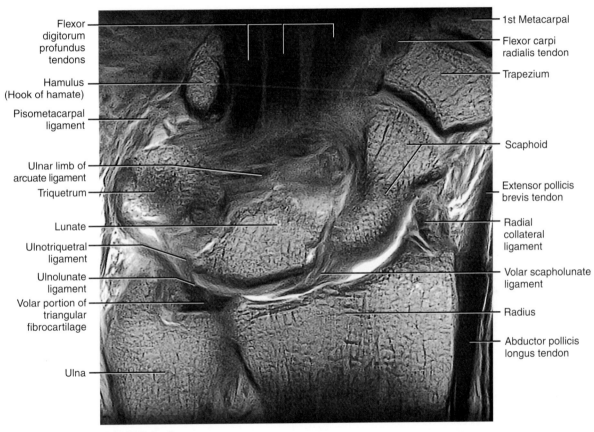

Flexor digitorum profundus tendons

Hamulus (Hook of hamate)

Pisometacarpal ligament

Ulnar limb of arcuate ligament

Triquetrum

Lunate

Ulnotriquetral ligament

Ulnolunate ligament

Volar portion of triangular fibrocartilage

Ulna

1st Metacarpal

Flexor carpi radialis tendon

Trapezium

Scaphoid

Extensor pollicis brevis tendon

Radial collateral ligament

Volar scapholunate ligament

Radius

Abductor pollicis longus tendon

FIGURE 3-6

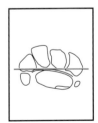

WRIST: CORONAL

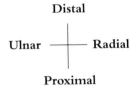

Distal

Ulnar —— Radial

Proximal

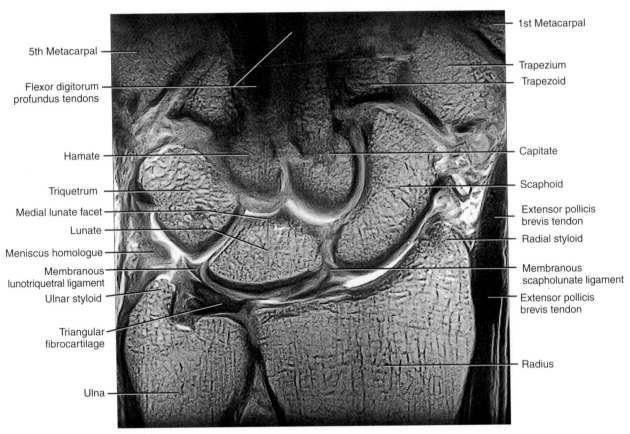

1st Metacarpal

5th Metacarpal

Flexor digitorum
profundus tendons

Trapezium

Trapezoid

Hamate

Capitate

Triquetrum

Scaphoid

Medial lunate facet

Lunate

Extensor pollicis
brevis tendon

Meniscus homologue

Radial styloid

Membranous
lunotriquetral ligament

Ulnar styloid

Membranous
scapholunate ligament

Extensor pollicis
brevis tendon

Triangular
fibrocartilage

Radius

Ulna

FIGURE 3-7

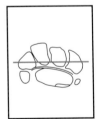

WRIST: CORONAL

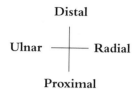

Distal

Ulnar ——|—— Radial

Proximal

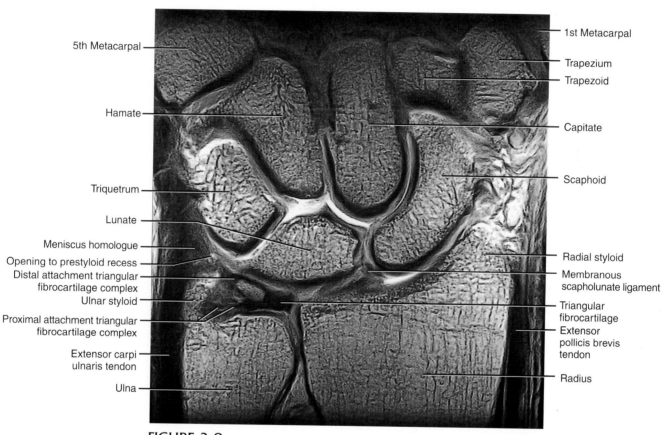

5th Metacarpal

Hamate

Triquetrum

Lunate

Meniscus homologue

Opening to prestyloid recess

Distal attachment triangular fibrocartilage complex

Ulnar styloid

Proximal attachment triangular fibrocartilage complex

Extensor carpi ulnaris tendon

Ulna

1st Metacarpal

Trapezium

Trapezoid

Capitate

Scaphoid

Radial styloid

Membranous scapholunate ligament

Triangular fibrocartilage

Extensor pollicis brevis tendon

Radius

FIGURE 3-8

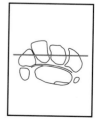

WRIST: CORONAL

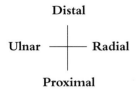

Distal

Ulnar ─┼─ **Radial**

Proximal

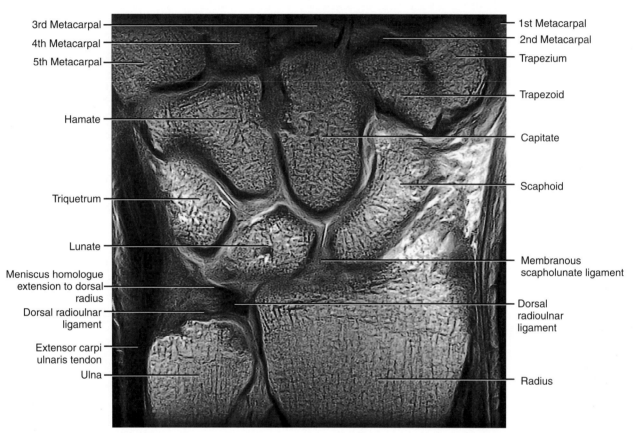

3rd Metacarpal — 1st Metacarpal

4th Metacarpal — 2nd Metacarpal

5th Metacarpal — Trapezium

Hamate — Trapezoid

— Capitate

Triquetrum — Scaphoid

Lunate —

Meniscus homologue extension to dorsal radius — Membranous scapholunate ligament

Dorsal radioulnar ligament — Dorsal radioulnar ligament

Extensor carpi ulnaris tendon —

Ulna — Radius

FIGURE 3-9

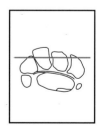

WRIST: CORONAL

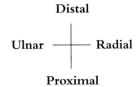

Distal

Ulnar ─┼─ Radial

Proximal

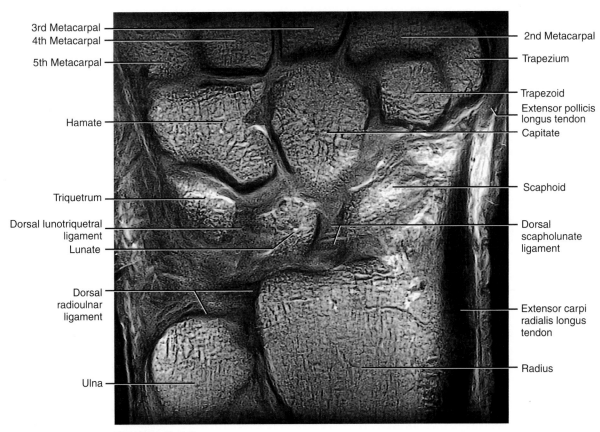

3rd Metacarpal

4th Metacarpal

5th Metacarpal

Hamate

Triquetrum

Dorsal lunotriquetral
ligament

Lunate

Dorsal
radioulnar
ligament

Ulna

2nd Metacarpal

Trapezium

Trapezoid

Extensor pollicis
longus tendon

Capitate

Scaphoid

Dorsal
scapholunate
ligament

Extensor carpi
radialis longus
tendon

Radius

FIGURE 3-10

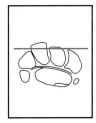

WRIST: CORONAL

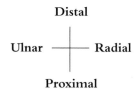

Distal

Ulnar ——|—— Radial

Proximal

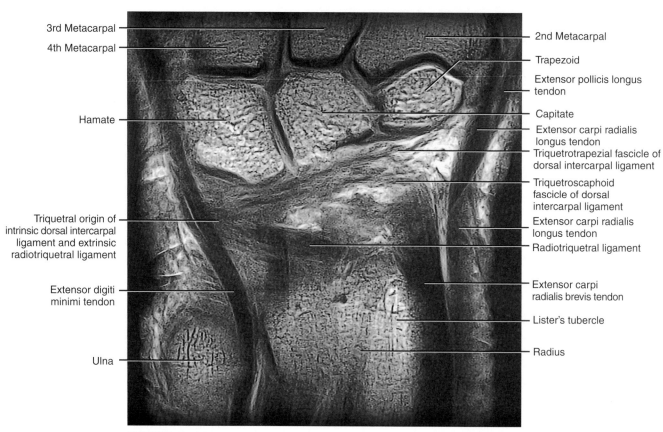

3rd Metacarpal

4th Metacarpal

Hamate

Triquetral origin of
intrinsic dorsal intercarpal
ligament and extrinsic
radiotriquetral ligament

Extensor digiti
minimi tendon

Ulna

2nd Metacarpal

Trapezoid

Extensor pollicis longus
tendon

Capitate

Extensor carpi radialis
longus tendon

Triquetrotrapezial fascicle of
dorsal intercarpal ligament

Triquetroscaphoid
fascicle of dorsal
intercarpal ligament

Extensor carpi radialis
longus tendon

Radiotriquetral ligament

Extensor carpi
radialis brevis tendon

Lister's tubercle

Radius

FIGURE 3-11

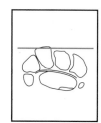

WRIST: CORONAL

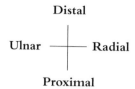

Distal

Ulnar ─┼─ Radial

Proximal

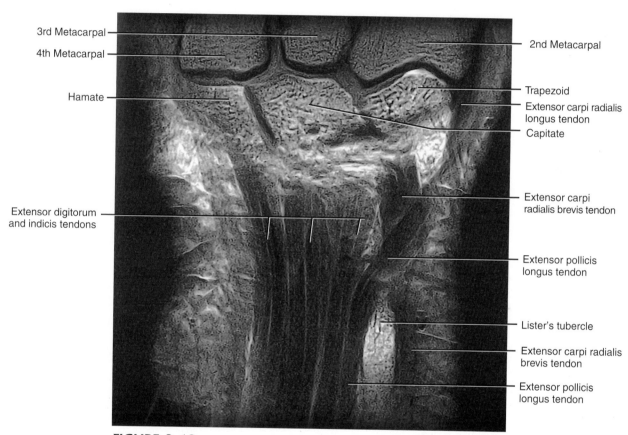

3rd Metacarpal

4th Metacarpal

Hamate

Extensor digitorum
and indicis tendons

2nd Metacarpal

Trapezoid

Extensor carpi radialis
longus tendon

Capitate

Extensor carpi
radialis brevis tendon

Extensor pollicis
longus tendon

Lister's tubercle

Extensor carpi radialis
brevis tendon

Extensor pollicis
longus tendon

FIGURE 3-12

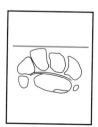

WRIST: AXIAL

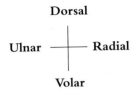

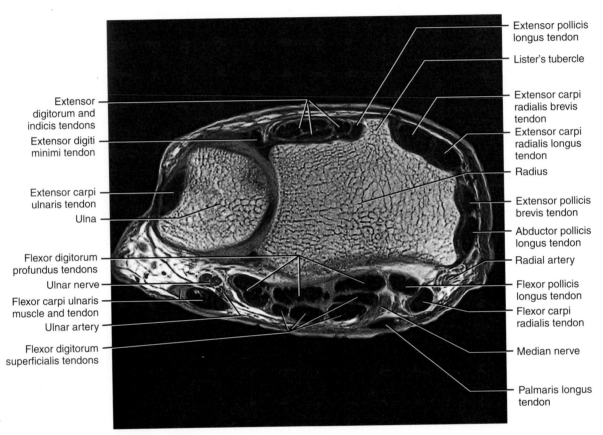

Extensor pollicis
longus tendon

Lister's tubercle

Extensor carpi
radialis brevis
tendon

Extensor carpi
radialis longus
tendon

Radius

Extensor pollicis
brevis tendon

Abductor pollicis
longus tendon

Radial artery

Flexor pollicis
longus tendon

Flexor carpi
radialis tendon

Median nerve

Palmaris longus
tendon

Extensor
digitorum and
indicis tendons

Extensor digiti
minimi tendon

Extensor carpi
ulnaris tendon

Ulna

Flexor digitorum
profundus tendons

Ulnar nerve

Flexor carpi ulnaris
muscle and tendon

Ulnar artery

Flexor digitorum
superficialis tendons

FIGURE 3-13

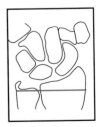

WRIST: AXIAL

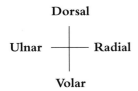

Dorsal

Ulnar —|— Radial

Volar

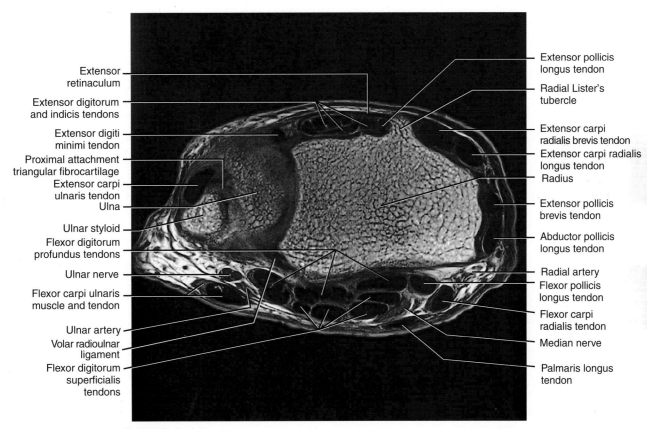

Extensor retinaculum

Extensor digitorum and indicis tendons

Extensor digiti minimi tendon

Proximal attachment triangular fibrocartilage

Extensor carpi ulnaris tendon

Ulna

Ulnar styloid

Flexor digitorum profundus tendons

Ulnar nerve

Flexor carpi ulnaris muscle and tendon

Ulnar artery

Volar radioulnar ligament

Flexor digitorum superficialis tendons

Extensor pollicis longus tendon

Radial Lister's tubercle

Extensor carpi radialis brevis tendon

Extensor carpi radialis longus tendon

Radius

Extensor pollicis brevis tendon

Abductor pollicis longus tendon

Radial artery

Flexor pollicis longus tendon

Flexor carpi radialis tendon

Median nerve

Palmaris longus tendon

FIGURE 3-14

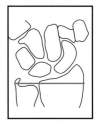

WRIST: AXIAL

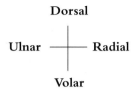

Dorsal

Ulnar ——|—— Radial

Volar

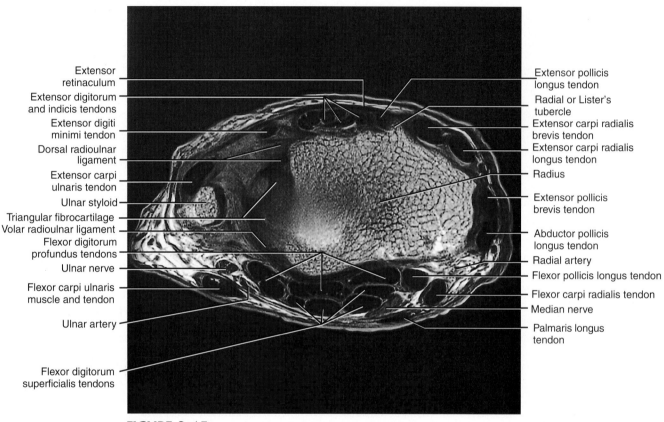

Extensor retinaculum

Extensor digitorum and indicis tendons

Extensor digiti minimi tendon

Dorsal radioulnar ligament

Extensor carpi ulnaris tendon

Ulnar styloid

Triangular fibrocartilage

Volar radioulnar ligament

Flexor digitorum profundus tendons

Ulnar nerve

Flexor carpi ulnaris muscle and tendon

Ulnar artery

Flexor digitorum superficialis tendons

Extensor pollicis longus tendon

Radial or Lister's tubercle

Extensor carpi radialis brevis tendon

Extensor carpi radialis longus tendon

Radius

Extensor pollicis brevis tendon

Abductor pollicis longus tendon

Radial artery

Flexor pollicis longus tendon

Flexor carpi radialis tendon

Median nerve

Palmaris longus tendon

FIGURE 3-15

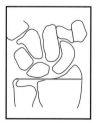

WRIST: AXIAL

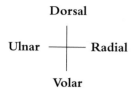

Dorsal

Ulnar —— Radial

Volar

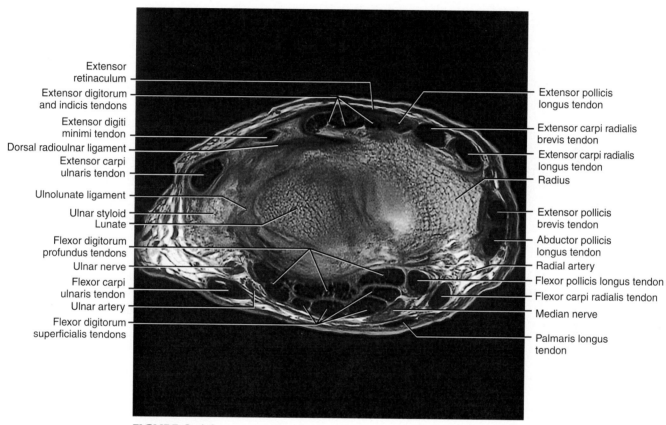

Extensor
retinaculum

Extensor digitorum
and indicis tendons

Extensor digiti
minimi tendon

Dorsal radioulnar ligament

Extensor carpi
ulnaris tendon

Ulnolunate ligament

Ulnar styloid
Lunate

Flexor digitorum
profundus tendons

Ulnar nerve

Flexor carpi
ulnaris tendon

Ulnar artery

Flexor digitorum
superficialis tendons

Extensor pollicis
longus tendon

Extensor carpi radialis
brevis tendon

Extensor carpi radialis
longus tendon

Radius

Extensor pollicis
brevis tendon

Abductor pollicis
longus tendon

Radial artery

Flexor pollicis longus tendon

Flexor carpi radialis tendon

Median nerve

Palmaris longus
tendon

FIGURE 3-16

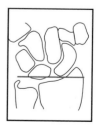

WRIST: AXIAL

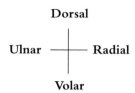

Dorsal

Ulnar ——|—— Radial

Volar

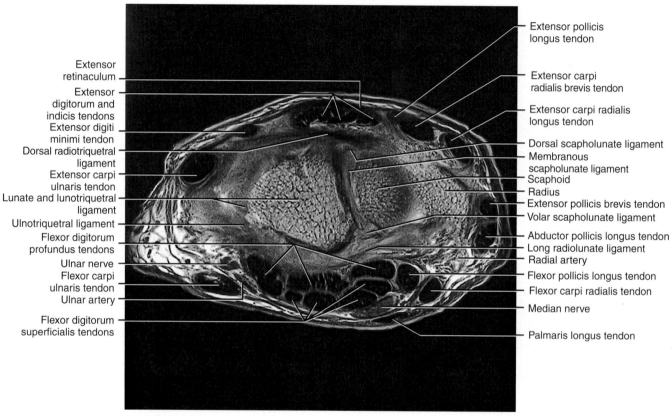

Extensor retinaculum
Extensor digitorum and indicis tendons
Extensor digiti minimi tendon
Dorsal radiotriquetral ligament
Extensor carpi ulnaris tendon
Lunate and lunotriquetral ligament
Ulnotriquetral ligament
Flexor digitorum profundus tendons
Ulnar nerve
Flexor carpi ulnaris tendon
Ulnar artery
Flexor digitorum superficialis tendons

Extensor pollicis longus tendon
Extensor carpi radialis brevis tendon
Extensor carpi radialis longus tendon
Dorsal scapholunate ligament
Membranous scapholunate ligament
Scaphoid
Radius
Extensor pollicis brevis tendon
Volar scapholunate ligament
Abductor pollicis longus tendon
Long radiolunate ligament
Radial artery
Flexor pollicis longus tendon
Flexor carpi radialis tendon
Median nerve
Palmaris longus tendon

FIGURE 3-17

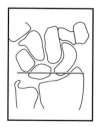

WRIST: AXIAL

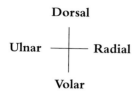

Dorsal

Ulnar ——┼—— Radial

Volar

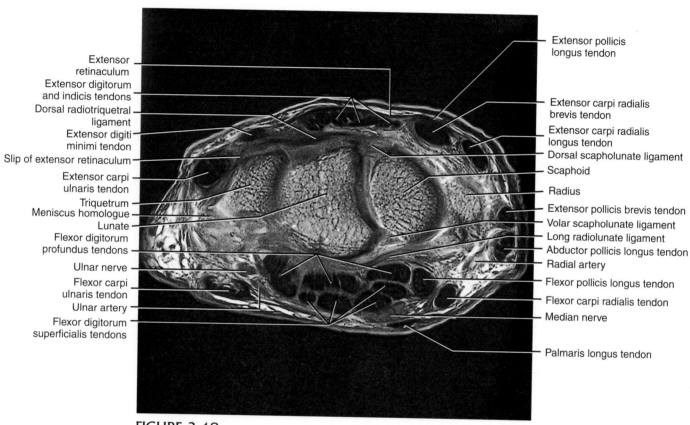

Extensor retinaculum

Extensor digitorum and indicis tendons

Dorsal radiotriquetral ligament

Extensor digiti minimi tendon

Slip of extensor retinaculum

Extensor carpi ulnaris tendon

Triquetrum

Meniscus homologue

Lunate

Flexor digitorum profundus tendons

Ulnar nerve

Flexor carpi ulnaris tendon

Ulnar artery

Flexor digitorum superficialis tendons

Extensor pollicis longus tendon

Extensor carpi radialis brevis tendon

Extensor carpi radialis longus tendon

Dorsal scapholunate ligament

Scaphoid

Radius

Extensor pollicis brevis tendon

Volar scapholunate ligament

Long radiolunate ligament

Abductor pollicis longus tendon

Radial artery

Flexor pollicis longus tendon

Flexor carpi radialis tendon

Median nerve

Palmaris longus tendon

FIGURE 3-18

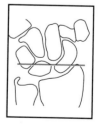

WRIST: AXIAL

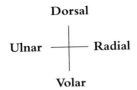

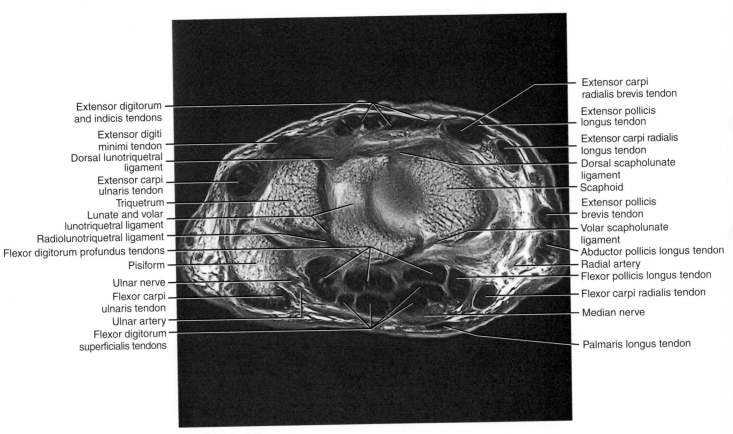

Extensor digitorum
and indicis tendons

Extensor digiti
minimi tendon

Dorsal lunotriquetral
ligament

Extensor carpi
ulnaris tendon

Triquetrum

Lunate and volar
lunotriquetral ligament

Radiolunotriquetral ligament

Flexor digitorum profundus tendons

Pisiform

Ulnar nerve

Flexor carpi
ulnaris tendon

Ulnar artery

Flexor digitorum
superficialis tendons

Extensor carpi
radialis brevis tendon

Extensor pollicis
longus tendon

Extensor carpi radialis
longus tendon

Dorsal scapholunate
ligament

Scaphoid

Extensor pollicis
brevis tendon

Volar scapholunate
ligament

Abductor pollicis longus tendon

Radial artery

Flexor pollicis longus tendon

Flexor carpi radialis tendon

Median nerve

Palmaris longus tendon

FIGURE 3-19

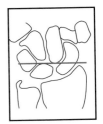

WRIST: AXIAL

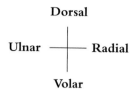

Dorsal

Ulnar —— Radial

Volar

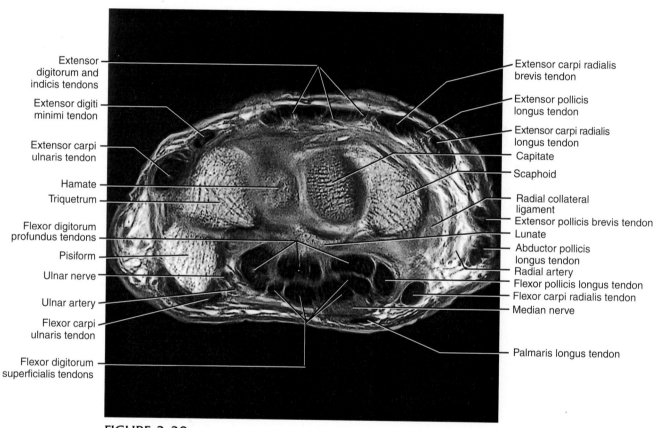

Extensor digitorum and indicis tendons

Extensor digiti minimi tendon

Extensor carpi ulnaris tendon

Hamate

Triquetrum

Flexor digitorum profundus tendons

Pisiform

Ulnar nerve

Ulnar artery

Flexor carpi ulnaris tendon

Flexor digitorum superficialis tendons

Extensor carpi radialis brevis tendon

Extensor pollicis longus tendon

Extensor carpi radialis longus tendon

Capitate

Scaphoid

Radial collateral ligament

Extensor pollicis brevis tendon

Lunate

Abductor pollicis longus tendon

Radial artery

Flexor pollicis longus tendon

Flexor carpi radialis tendon

Median nerve

Palmaris longus tendon

FIGURE 3-20

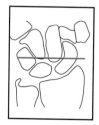

WRIST: AXIAL

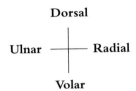

Dorsal

Ulnar —|— Radial

Volar

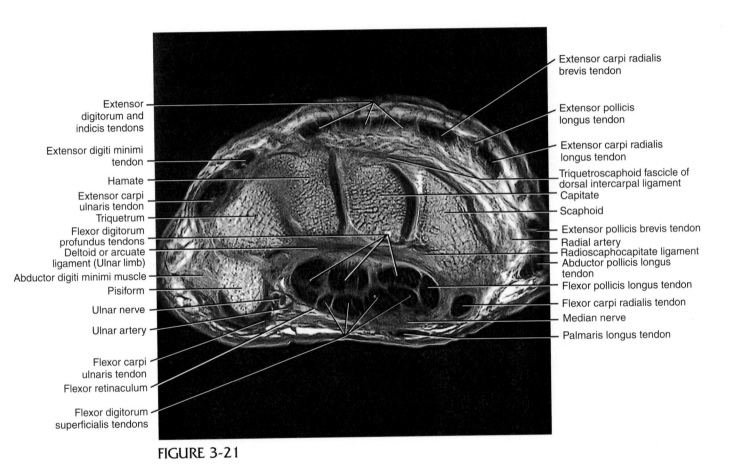

Extensor
digitorum and
indicis tendons

Extensor digiti minimi
tendon

Hamate

Extensor carpi
ulnaris tendon

Triquetrum

Flexor digitorum
profundus tendons

Deltoid or arcuate
ligament (Ulnar limb)

Abductor digiti minimi muscle

Pisiform

Ulnar nerve

Ulnar artery

Flexor carpi
ulnaris tendon

Flexor retinaculum

Flexor digitorum
superficialis tendons

Extensor carpi radialis
brevis tendon

Extensor pollicis
longus tendon

Extensor carpi radialis
longus tendon

Triquetroscaphoid fascicle of
dorsal intercarpal ligament

Capitate

Scaphoid

Extensor pollicis brevis tendon

Radial artery

Radioscaphocapitate ligament

Abductor pollicis longus
tendon

Flexor pollicis longus tendon

Flexor carpi radialis tendon

Median nerve

Palmaris longus tendon

FIGURE 3-21

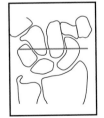

WRIST: AXIAL

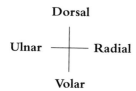

Dorsal

Ulnar ——┼—— Radial

Volar

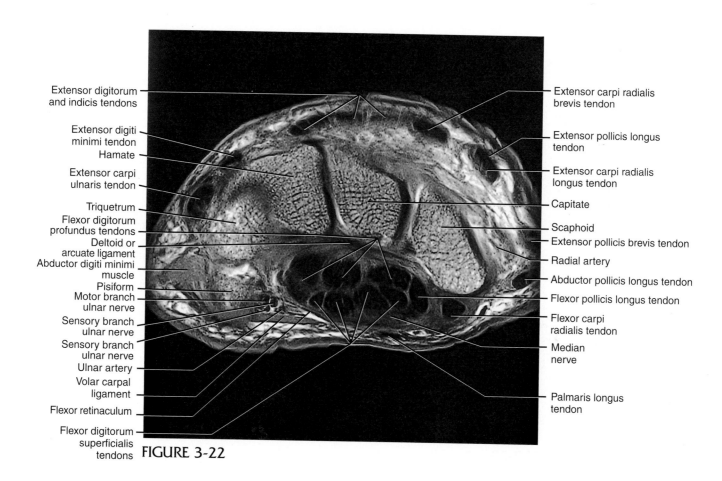

Extensor digitorum
and indicis tendons

Extensor digiti
minimi tendon

Hamate

Extensor carpi
ulnaris tendon

Triquetrum

Flexor digitorum
profundus tendons

Deltoid or
arcuate ligament

Abductor digiti minimi
muscle

Pisiform

Motor branch
ulnar nerve

Sensory branch
ulnar nerve

Sensory branch
ulnar nerve

Ulnar artery

Volar carpal
ligament

Flexor retinaculum

Flexor digitorum
superficialis
tendons

Extensor carpi radialis
brevis tendon

Extensor pollicis longus
tendon

Extensor carpi radialis
longus tendon

Capitate

Scaphoid

Extensor pollicis brevis tendon

Radial artery

Abductor pollicis longus tendon

Flexor pollicis longus tendon

Flexor carpi
radialis tendon

Median
nerve

Palmaris longus
tendon

FIGURE 3-22

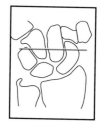

WRIST: AXIAL

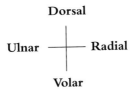

Dorsal

Ulnar —|— Radial

Volar

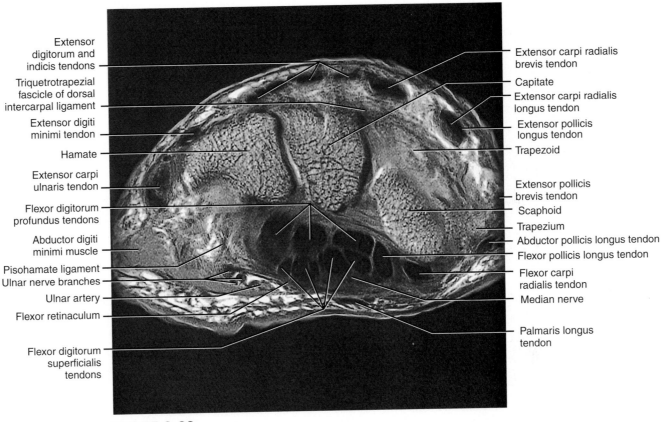

Extensor
digitorum and
indicis tendons

Triquetrotrapezial
fascicle of dorsal
intercarpal ligament

Extensor digiti
minimi tendon

Hamate

Extensor carpi
ulnaris tendon

Flexor digitorum
profundus tendons

Abductor digiti
minimi muscle

Pisohamate ligament
Ulnar nerve branches

Ulnar artery

Flexor retinaculum

Flexor digitorum
superficialis
tendons

Extensor carpi radialis
brevis tendon

Capitate

Extensor carpi radialis
longus tendon

Extensor pollicis
longus tendon

Trapezoid

Extensor pollicis
brevis tendon

Scaphoid

Trapezium

Abductor pollicis longus tendon

Flexor pollicis longus tendon

Flexor carpi
radialis tendon

Median nerve

Palmaris longus
tendon

FIGURE 3-23

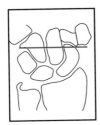

WRIST: AXIAL

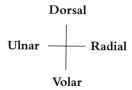

Dorsal

Ulnar —— Radial

Volar

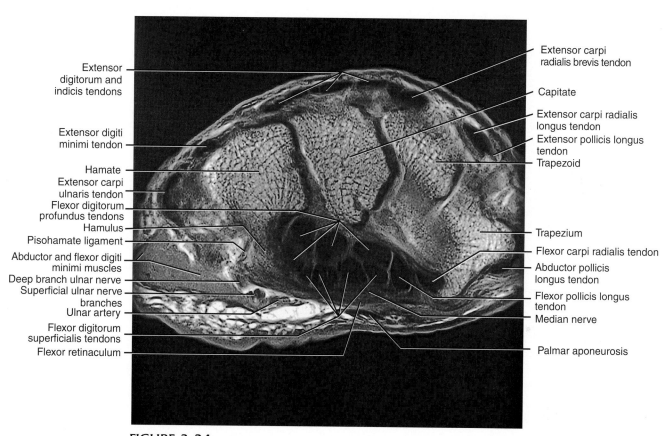

Extensor
digitorum and
indicis tendons

Extensor digiti
minimi tendon

Hamate

Extensor carpi
ulnaris tendon

Flexor digitorum
profundus tendons

Hamulus

Pisohamate ligament

Abductor and flexor digiti
minimi muscles

Deep branch ulnar nerve

Superficial ulnar nerve
branches

Ulnar artery

Flexor digitorum
superficialis tendons

Flexor retinaculum

Extensor carpi
radialis brevis tendon

Capitate

Extensor carpi radialis
longus tendon

Extensor pollicis longus
tendon

Trapezoid

Trapezium

Flexor carpi radialis tendon

Abductor pollicis
longus tendon

Flexor pollicis longus
tendon

Median nerve

Palmar aponeurosis

FIGURE 3-24

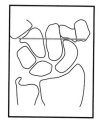

WRIST: AXIAL

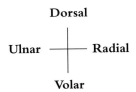

Dorsal

Ulnar —┼— Radial

Volar

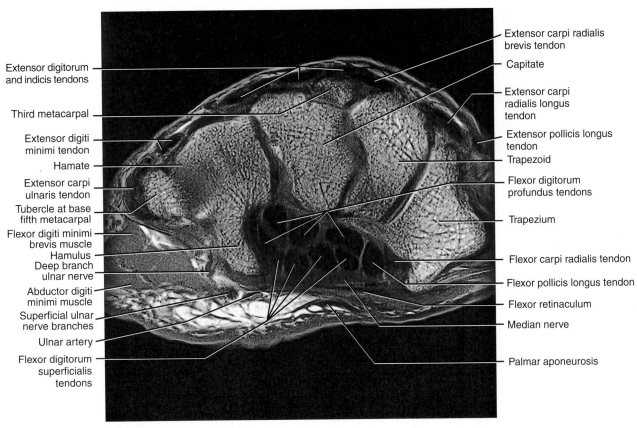

Extensor carpi radialis brevis tendon

Capitate

Extensor carpi radialis longus tendon

Extensor pollicis longus tendon

Trapezoid

Flexor digitorum profundus tendons

Trapezium

Flexor carpi radialis tendon

Flexor pollicis longus tendon

Flexor retinaculum

Median nerve

Palmar aponeurosis

Extensor digitorum and indicis tendons

Third metacarpal

Extensor digiti minimi tendon

Hamate

Extensor carpi ulnaris tendon

Tubercle at base fifth metacarpal

Flexor digiti minimi brevis muscle

Hamulus

Deep branch ulnar nerve

Abductor digiti minimi muscle

Superficial ulnar nerve branches

Ulnar artery

Flexor digitorum superficialis tendons

FIGURE 3-25

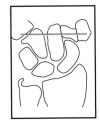

WRIST: AXIAL

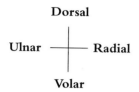

Dorsal

Ulnar ─┼─ Radial

Volar

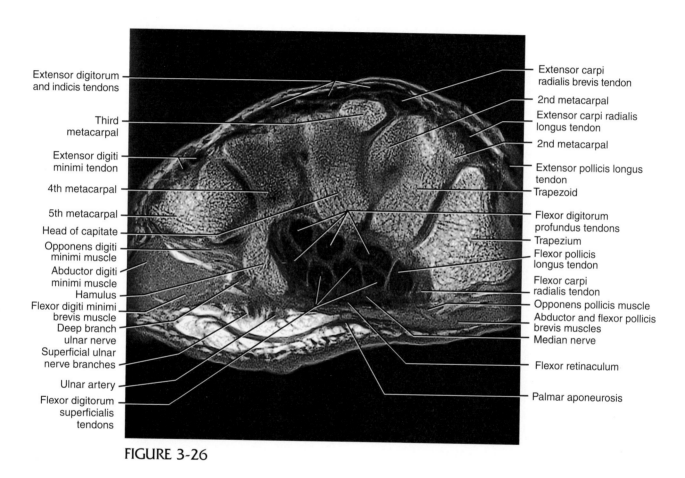

Extensor digitorum and indicis tendons

Third metacarpal

Extensor digiti minimi tendon

4th metacarpal

5th metacarpal

Head of capitate

Opponens digiti minimi muscle

Abductor digiti minimi muscle

Hamulus

Flexor digiti minimi brevis muscle

Deep branch ulnar nerve

Superficial ulnar nerve branches

Ulnar artery

Flexor digitorum superficialis tendons

Extensor carpi radialis brevis tendon

2nd metacarpal

Extensor carpi radialis longus tendon

2nd metacarpal

Extensor pollicis longus tendon

Trapezoid

Flexor digitorum profundus tendons

Trapezium

Flexor pollicis longus tendon

Flexor carpi radialis tendon

Opponens pollicis muscle

Abductor and flexor pollicis brevis muscles

Median nerve

Flexor retinaculum

Palmar aponeurosis

FIGURE 3-26

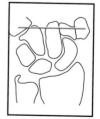

WRIST: SAGITTAL

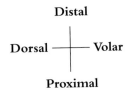

Distal

Dorsal ——|—— Volar

Proximal

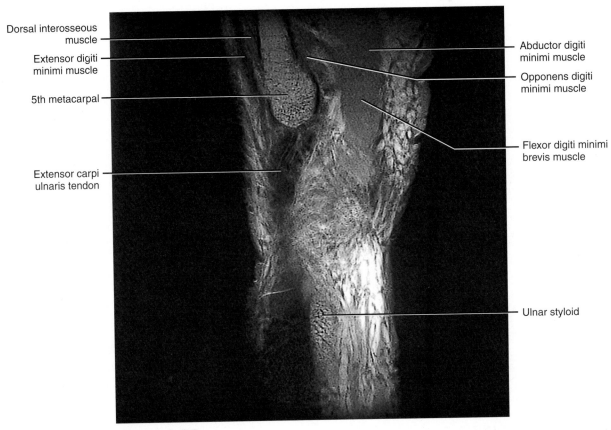

Dorsal interosseous
muscle

Extensor digiti
minimi muscle

5th metacarpal

Extensor carpi
ulnaris tendon

Abductor digiti
minimi muscle

Opponens digiti
minimi muscle

Flexor digiti minimi
brevis muscle

Ulnar styloid

FIGURE 3-27

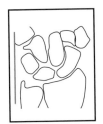

WRIST: SAGITTAL

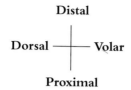

Distal

Dorsal ——|—— Volar

Proximal

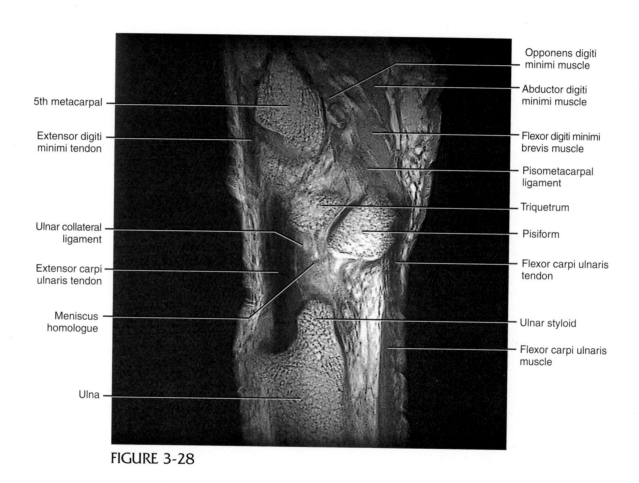

5th metacarpal

Extensor digiti
minimi tendon

Ulnar collateral
ligament

Extensor carpi
ulnaris tendon

Meniscus
homologue

Ulna

Opponens digiti
minimi muscle

Abductor digiti
minimi muscle

Flexor digiti minimi
brevis muscle

Pisometacarpal
ligament

Triquetrum

Pisiform

Flexor carpi ulnaris
tendon

Ulnar styloid

Flexor carpi ulnaris
muscle

FIGURE 3-28

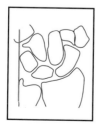

WRIST: SAGITTAL

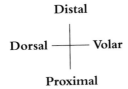

Distal

Dorsal ── ──Volar

Proximal

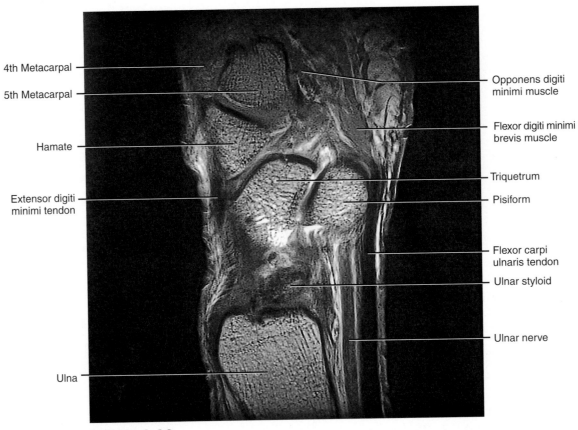

4th Metacarpal

5th Metacarpal

Hamate

Extensor digiti
minimi tendon

Ulna

Opponens digiti
minimi muscle

Flexor digiti minimi
brevis muscle

Triquetrum

Pisiform

Flexor carpi
ulnaris tendon

Ulnar styloid

Ulnar nerve

FIGURE 3-29

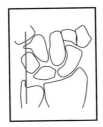

WRIST: SAGITTAL

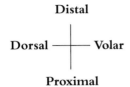

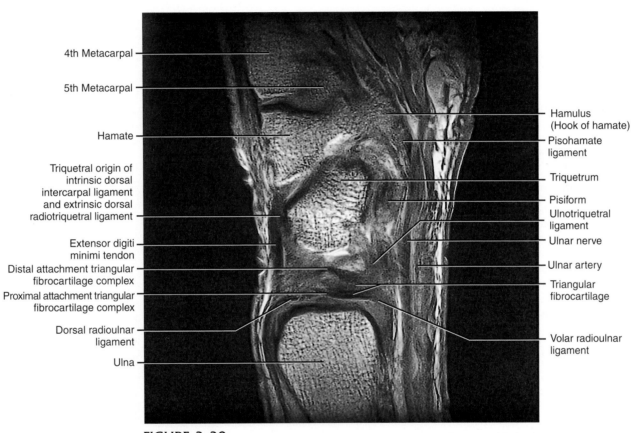

4th Metacarpal

5th Metacarpal

Hamate

Triquetral origin of
intrinsic dorsal
intercarpal ligament
and extrinsic dorsal
radiotriquetral ligament

Extensor digiti
minimi tendon

Distal attachment triangular
fibrocartilage complex

Proximal attachment triangular
fibrocartilage complex

Dorsal radioulnar
ligament

Ulna

Hamulus
(Hook of hamate)

Pisohamate
ligament

Triquetrum

Pisiform

Ulnotriquetral
ligament

Ulnar nerve

Ulnar artery

Triangular
fibrocartilage

Volar radioulnar
ligament

FIGURE 3-30

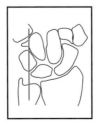

WRIST: SAGITTAL

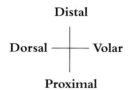

Distal

Dorsal ——— Volar

Proximal

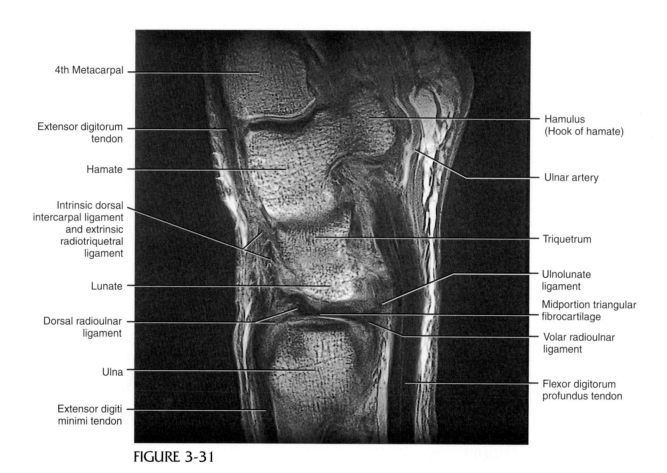

4th Metacarpal

Extensor digitorum tendon

Hamate

Intrinsic dorsal intercarpal ligament and extrinsic radiotriquetral ligament

Lunate

Dorsal radioulnar ligament

Ulna

Extensor digiti minimi tendon

Hamulus (Hook of hamate)

Ulnar artery

Triquetrum

Ulnolunate ligament

Midportion triangular fibrocartilage

Volar radioulnar ligament

Flexor digitorum profundus tendon

FIGURE 3-31

WRIST: SAGITTAL

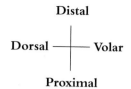

Distal

Dorsal —— Volar

Proximal

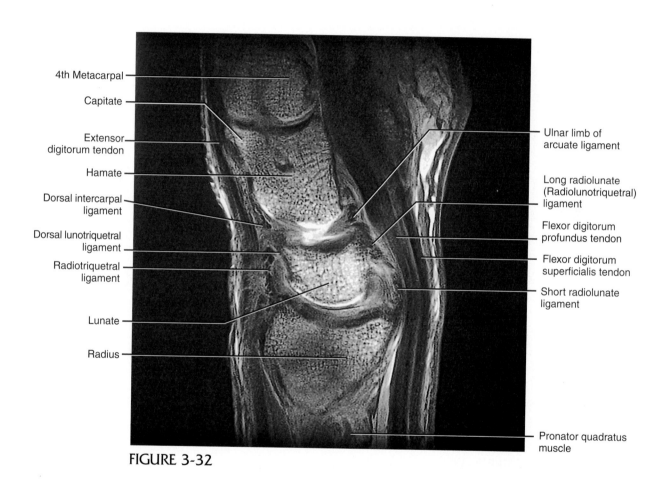

4th Metacarpal

Capitate

Extensor digitorum tendon

Hamate

Dorsal intercarpal ligament

Dorsal lunotriquetral ligament

Radiotriquetral ligament

Lunate

Radius

Ulnar limb of arcuate ligament

Long radiolunate (Radiolunotriquetral) ligament

Flexor digitorum profundus tendon

Flexor digitorum superficialis tendon

Short radiolunate ligament

Pronator quadratus muscle

FIGURE 3-32

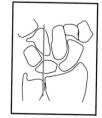

WRIST: SAGITTAL

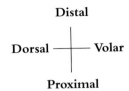

Distal

Dorsal —|— Volar

Proximal

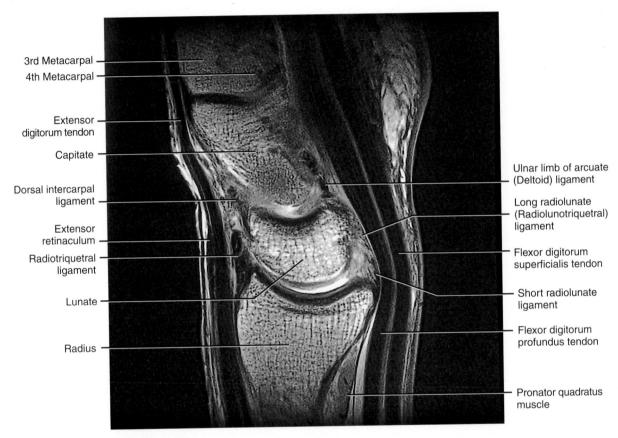

3rd Metacarpal

4th Metacarpal

Extensor digitorum tendon

Capitate

Dorsal intercarpal ligament

Extensor retinaculum

Radiotriquetral ligament

Lunate

Radius

Ulnar limb of arcuate (Deltoid) ligament

Long radiolunate (Radiolunotriquetral) ligament

Flexor digitorum superficialis tendon

Short radiolunate ligament

Flexor digitorum profundus tendon

Pronator quadratus muscle

FIGURE 3-33

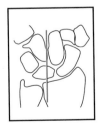

WRIST: SAGITTAL

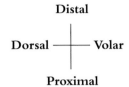

Distal

Dorsal —— Volar

Proximal

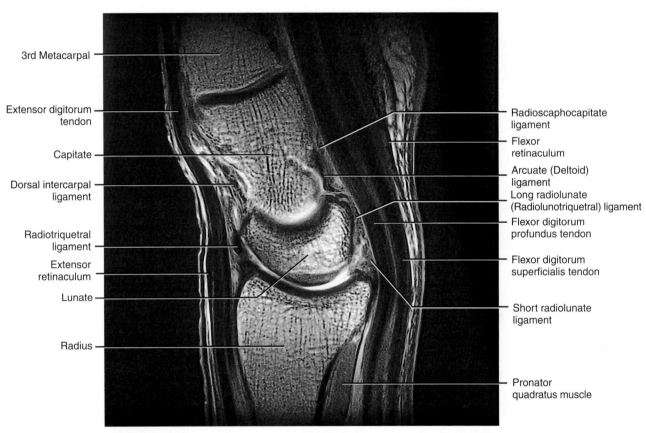

3rd Metacarpal

Extensor digitorum
tendon

Capitate

Dorsal intercarpal
ligament

Radiotriquetral
ligament

Extensor
retinaculum

Lunate

Radius

Radioscaphocapitate
ligament

Flexor
retinaculum

Arcuate (Deltoid)
ligament

Long radiolunate
(Radiolunotriquetral) ligament

Flexor digitorum
profundus tendon

Flexor digitorum
superficialis tendon

Short radiolunate
ligament

Pronator
quadratus muscle

FIGURE 3-34

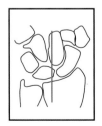

WRIST: SAGITTAL

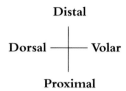

Distal

Dorsal ——|—— Volar

Proximal

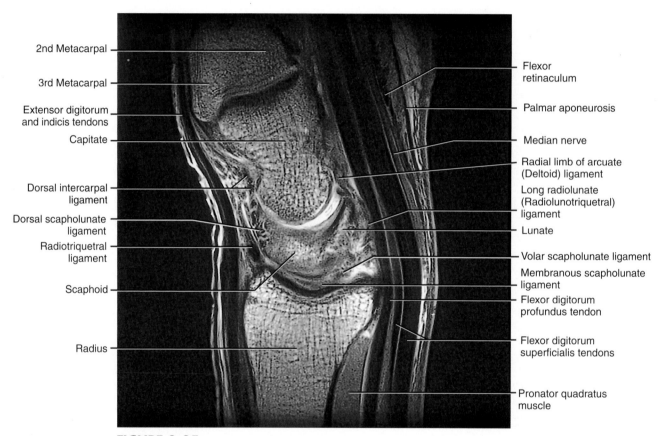

2nd Metacarpal

3rd Metacarpal

Extensor digitorum
and indicis tendons

Capitate

Dorsal intercarpal
ligament

Dorsal scapholunate
ligament

Radiotriquetral
ligament

Scaphoid

Radius

Flexor
retinaculum

Palmar aponeurosis

Median nerve

Radial limb of arcuate
(Deltoid) ligament

Long radiolunate
(Radiolunotriquetral)
ligament

Lunate

Volar scapholunate ligament

Membranous scapholunate
ligament

Flexor digitorum
profundus tendon

Flexor digitorum
superficialis tendons

Pronator quadratus
muscle

FIGURE 3-35

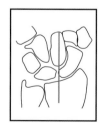

WRIST: SAGITTAL

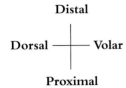

Distal

Dorsal ──┼── Volar

Proximal

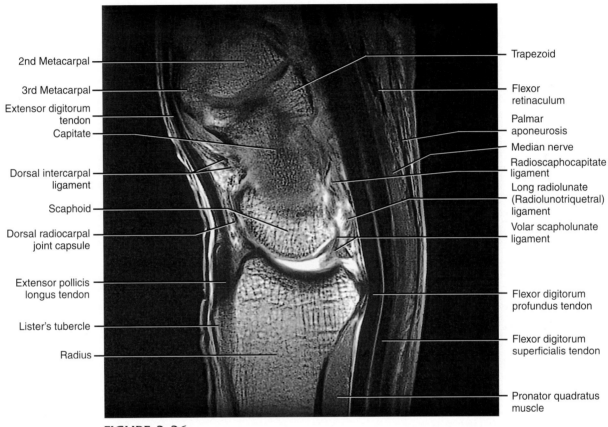

2nd Metacarpal

3rd Metacarpal

Extensor digitorum tendon

Capitate

Dorsal intercarpal ligament

Scaphoid

Dorsal radiocarpal joint capsule

Extensor pollicis longus tendon

Lister's tubercle

Radius

Trapezoid

Flexor retinaculum

Palmar aponeurosis

Median nerve

Radioscaphocapitate ligament

Long radiolunate (Radiolunotriquetral) ligament

Volar scapholunate ligament

Flexor digitorum profundus tendon

Flexor digitorum superficialis tendon

Pronator quadratus muscle

FIGURE 3-36

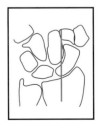

WRIST: SAGITTAL

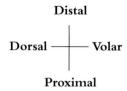

Distal

Dorsal — Volar

Proximal

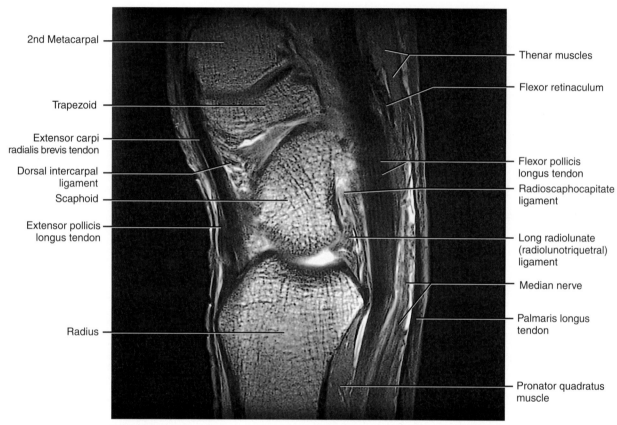

2nd Metacarpal

Trapezoid

Extensor carpi
radialis brevis tendon

Dorsal intercarpal
ligament

Scaphoid

Extensor pollicis
longus tendon

Radius

Thenar muscles

Flexor retinaculum

Flexor pollicis
longus tendon

Radioscaphocapitate
ligament

Long radiolunate
(radiolunotriquetral)
ligament

Median nerve

Palmaris longus
tendon

Pronator quadratus
muscle

FIGURE 3-37

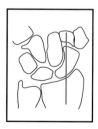

WRIST: SAGITTAL

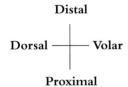

Distal

Dorsal —|— Volar

Proximal

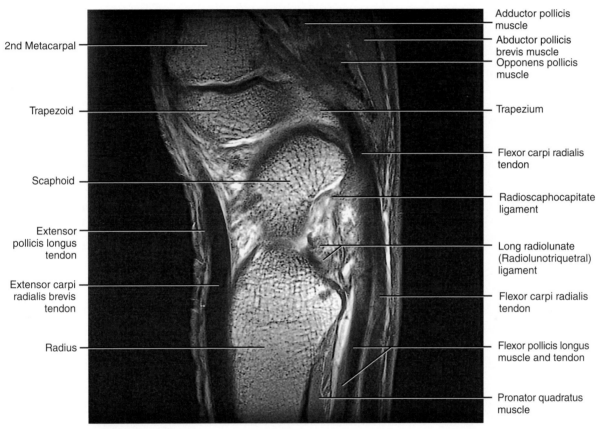

2nd Metacarpal

Trapezoid

Scaphoid

Extensor pollicis longus tendon

Extensor carpi radialis brevis tendon

Radius

Adductor pollicis muscle

Abductor pollicis brevis muscle

Opponens pollicis muscle

Trapezium

Flexor carpi radialis tendon

Radioscaphocapitate ligament

Long radiolunate (Radiolunotriquetral) ligament

Flexor carpi radialis tendon

Flexor pollicis longus muscle and tendon

Pronator quadratus muscle

FIGURE 3-38

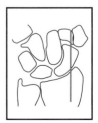

WRIST: SAGITTAL

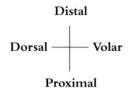

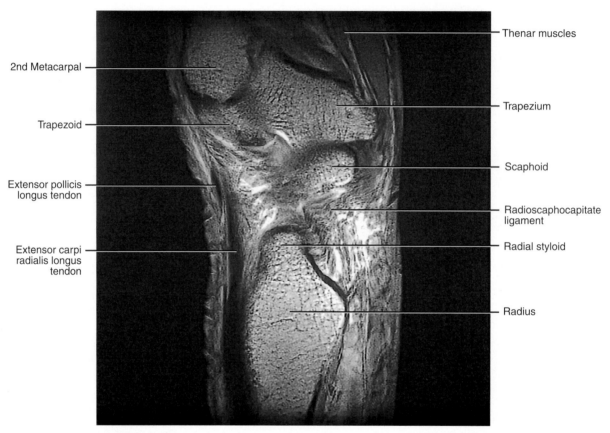

2nd Metacarpal

Trapezoid

Extensor pollicis
longus tendon

Extensor carpi
radialis longus
tendon

Thenar muscles

Trapezium

Scaphoid

Radioscaphocapitate
ligament

Radial styloid

Radius

FIGURE 3-39

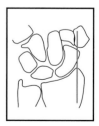

WRIST: SAGITTAL

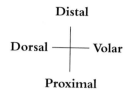

Distal

Dorsal ——— Volar

Proximal

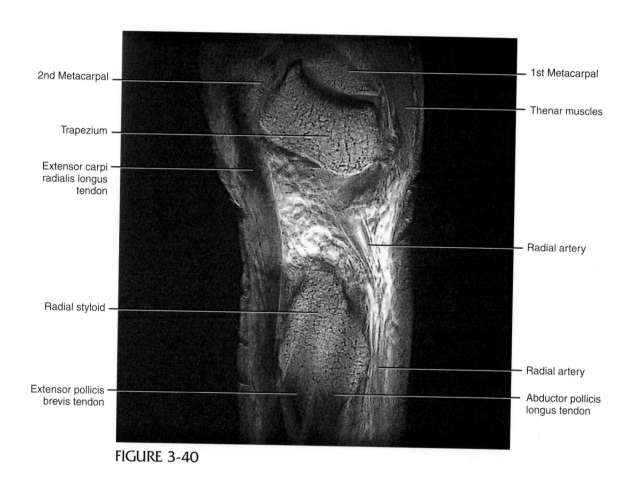

2nd Metacarpal

Trapezium

Extensor carpi
radialis longus
tendon

Radial styloid

Extensor pollicis
brevis tendon

1st Metacarpal

Thenar muscles

Radial artery

Radial artery

Abductor pollicis
longus tendon

FIGURE 3-40

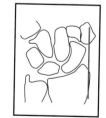

WRIST: SAGITTAL

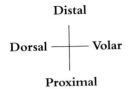

Distal

Dorsal —┼— Volar

Proximal

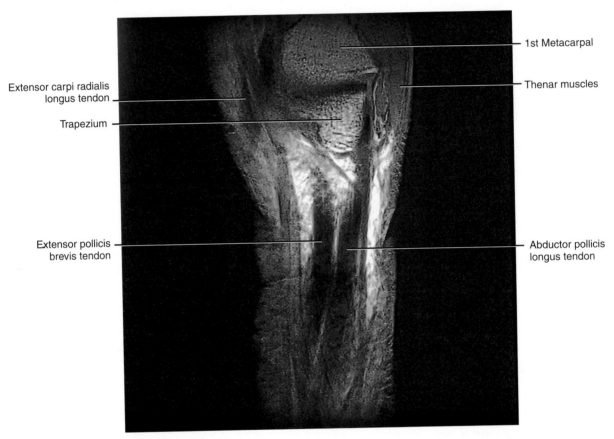

Extensor carpi radialis
longus tendon

Trapezium

Extensor pollicis
brevis tendon

1st Metacarpal

Thenar muscles

Abductor pollicis
longus tendon

FIGURE 3-41

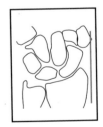

WRIST: LIGAMENTS OF THE WRIST, VOLAR VIEW

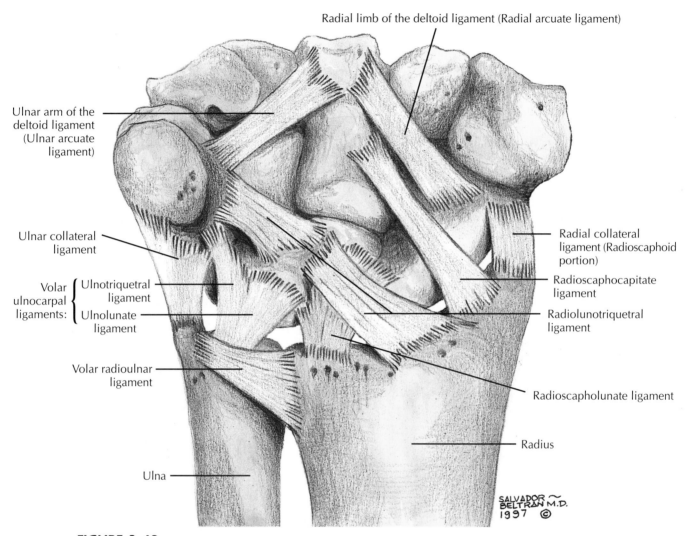

Radial limb of the deltoid ligament (Radial arcuate ligament)

Ulnar arm of the deltoid ligament (Ulnar arcuate ligament)

Ulnar collateral ligament

Volar ulnocarpal ligaments: { Ulnotriquetral ligament / Ulnolunate ligament }

Volar radioulnar ligament

Ulna

Radial collateral ligament (Radioscaphoid portion)

Radioscaphocapitate ligament

Radiolunotriquetral ligament

Radioscapholunate ligament

Radius

SALVADOR BELTRAN M.D. 1997 ©

FIGURE 3-42

The volar intrinsic and extrinsic carpal ligaments. The extrinsic ligaments include the following: (1) Radiocarpal ligaments: the radioscaphocapitate ligament, the radiolunotriquetral (the long radiolunate) ligament, the radioscapholunate ligament (ligament of Testut and Kuenz), and the radial collateral ligament; and (2) Ulnocarpal ligaments: the medial collateral (ulnar collateral) ligament, the ulnotriquetral and ulnolunate volar ulnocarpal ligaments, and the volar radioulnar ligament. The intrinsic ligaments include: Arcuate (deltoid) ligaments: the radial arcuate ligament and the ulnar arcuate ligament. The scapholunate and lunotriquetral intrinsic ligaments are not shown. The space of Poirier is over the volar aspect of the capitolunate joint. For related MR, arthroscopy, and surgical anatomy images see Figures 3-55 through 3-64.

WRIST: LIGAMENTS OF THE WRIST, DORSAL VIEW

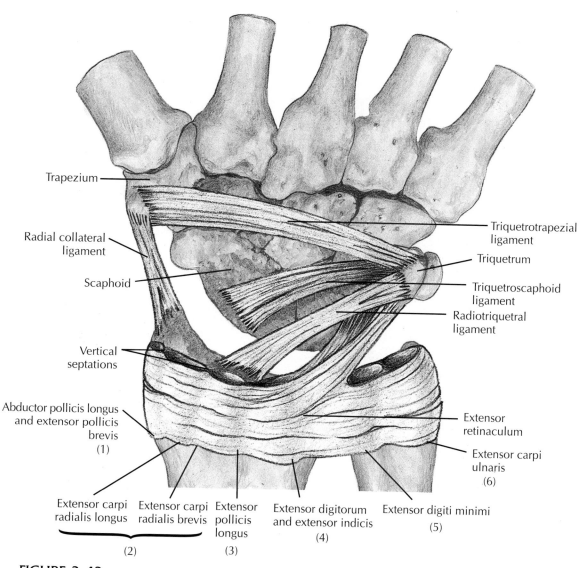

Trapezium

Radial collateral ligament

Scaphoid

Vertical septations

Abductor pollicis longus and extensor pollicis brevis (1)

Extensor carpi radialis longus

Extensor carpi radialis brevis

Extensor pollicis longus

Extensor digitorum and extensor indicis (4)

Extensor digiti minimi (5)

(2)

(3)

Triquetrotrapezial ligament

Triquetrum

Triquetroscaphoid ligament

Radiotriquetral ligament

Extensor retinaculum

Extensor carpi ulnaris (6)

FIGURE 3-43

The extensor retinaculum and dorsal carpal ligaments. The radiotriquetral ligament (an extrinsic dorsal capsular ligament) and the dorsal intercarpal ligament (an intrinsic dorsal capsular ligament) are illustrated. The dorsal intercarpal ligament is composed of separate triquetroscaphoid and triquetrotrapezial fasicles. The radial collateral ligament and the bilaminar extensor retinaculum are also shown. The vertical septations of the extensor retinaculum define the six extensor compartments (1–6). A slip of the extensor retinaculum attaches to the dorsal triquetrum. For related MR, arthroscopy, and surgical anatomy images see Figure 3-53.

WRIST: TRIANGULAR FIBROCARTILAGE COMPLEX

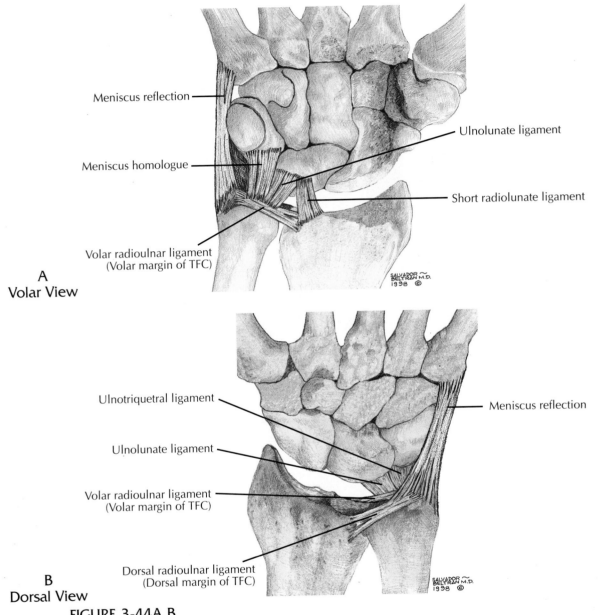

Meniscus reflection

Meniscus homologue

Volar radioulnar ligament
(Volar margin of TFC)

Ulnolunate ligament

Short radiolunate ligament

A
Volar View

Ulnotriquetral ligament

Ulnolunate ligament

Volar radioulnar ligament
(Volar margin of TFC)

Dorsal radioulnar ligament
(Dorsal margin of TFC)

Meniscus reflection

B
Dorsal View

FIGURE 3-44A,B

Triangular fibrocartilage complex. **(A)** Volar view of the ligaments of the ulnar side of the carpus. The meniscus homologue and meniscus reflection are shown. The meniscus homologue inserts into the volar surface of the triquetrum. The meniscus homologue shares a common origin from the dorsal ulnar corner of the radius with the triangular fibrocartilage. The triangular fibrocartilage extends in a volar direction from the meniscus homologue to the base of the ulnar styloid. The ulnolunate component of the ulnocarpal ligament is considered to be part of or a continuation of the short radiolunate ligament. **(B)** In this dorsal view, the ulnar and dorsal aspect of the triangular fibrocartilage complex (TFCC) is invested by a thin ligamentous layer (the meniscus reflection) with proximal attachment to the TFCC and ulna and distal attachment to the base of the fifth metacarpal. For related MR, arthroscopy, and surgical anatomy images see Figures 3-65 through 3-68.

WRIST: TRIANGULAR FIBROCARTILAGE COMPLEX

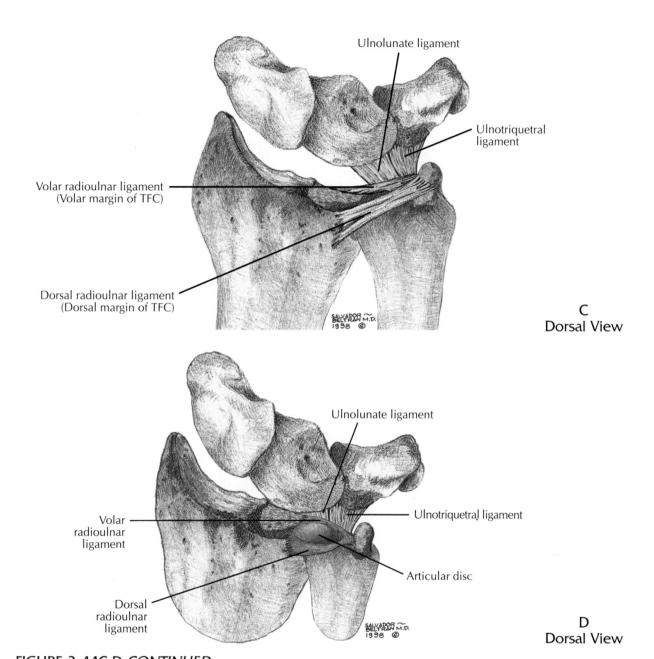

Ulnolunate ligament

Ulnotriquetral ligament

Volar radioulnar ligament
(Volar margin of TFC)

Dorsal radioulnar ligament
(Dorsal margin of TFC)

C
Dorsal View

Ulnolunate ligament

Ulnotriquetral ligament

Volar radioulnar ligament

Articular disc

Dorsal radioulnar ligament

D
Dorsal View

FIGURE 3-44C,D *CONTINUED*

The dorsal views of the triangular fibrocartilage complex (TFCC) show the dorsal and volar radioulnar ligaments as separate from the articular disc of the triangular fibrocartilage. The term TFC or triangular fibrocartilage refers to the central horizontal articular disc and adjoining volar and dorsal radioulnar ligaments. The triangular fibrocartilage complex refers to the triangular fibrocartilage and any additional ulnar ligamentous structures, such as the meniscus homologue, ulnar collateral ligaments, subsheath of the extensor carpi ulnaris tendon, and the ulnolunate and ulnotriquetral ligaments. For related MR, arthroscopy, and surgical anatomy images see Figures 3-65 through 3-68.

WRIST: FLEXOR RETINACULUM, VOLAR VIEW

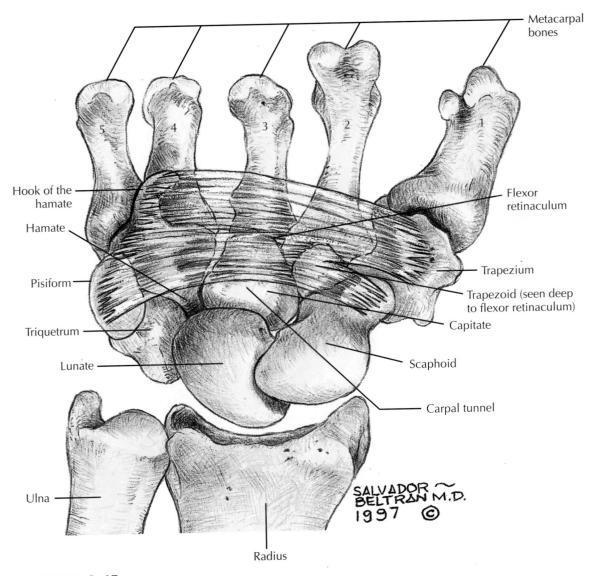

FIGURE 3-45

Flexor retinaculum. The concave volar surface of the carpus and the flexor retinaculum form the anatomic boundaries of the carpal tunnel (for passage of the long flexor tendons of the fingers and thumb). Medially, the flexor retinaculum is attached to the pisiform and hook of the hamate and laterally, to the tuberosities of the scaphoid and trapezium.

WRIST: SUPERFICIAL PALMAR ARTERIAL ARCH, VOLAR VIEW

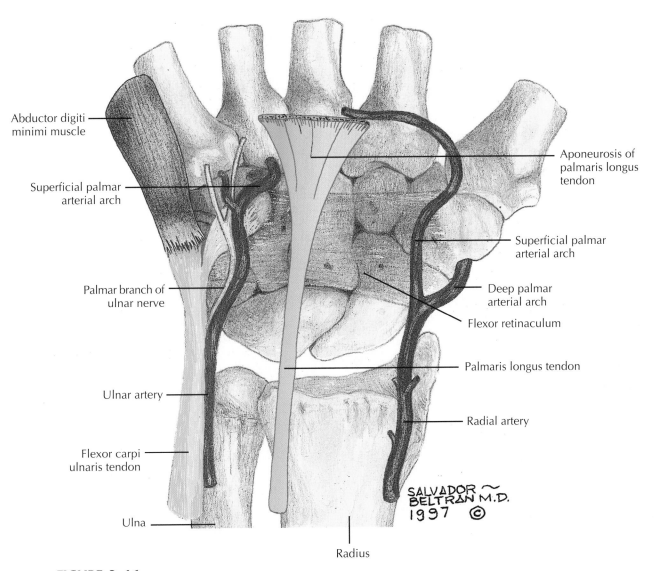

Abductor digiti
minimi muscle

Superficial palmar
arterial arch

Palmar branch of
ulnar nerve

Ulnar artery

Flexor carpi
ulnaris tendon

Ulna

Aponeurosis of
palmaris longus
tendon

Superficial palmar
arterial arch

Deep palmar
arterial arch

Flexor retinaculum

Palmaris longus tendon

Radial artery

Radius

SALVADOR ~
BELTRAN M.D.
1997 ©

FIGURE 3-46

The flexor retinaculum and palmar aponeurosis represent thickened deep fascia of the wrist. The radial and more principal ulnar arterial contributions to the superficial palmar arterial arch are shown. The palmar branch of the ulnar nerve is superficial to the flexor retinaculum. For related MR, arthroscopy, and surgical anatomy image see Figure 3-54.

WRIST: HYPOTHENAR MUSCLES, VOLAR VIEW

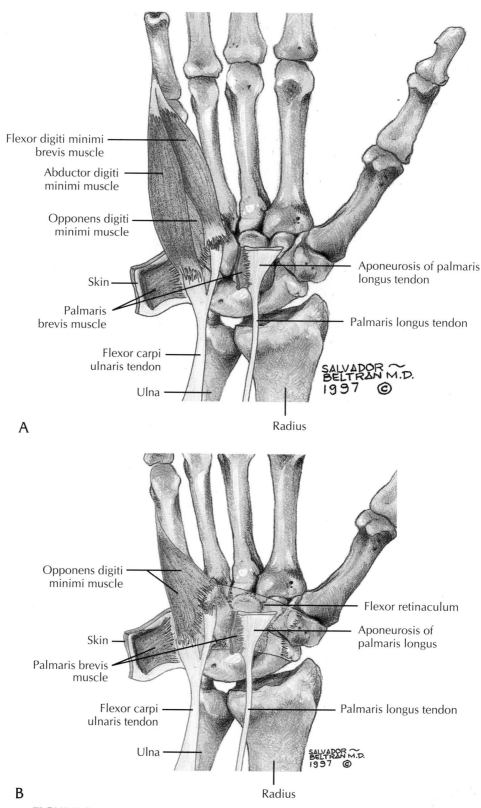

Flexor digiti minimi brevis muscle

Abductor digiti minimi muscle

Opponens digiti minimi muscle

Skin

Palmaris brevis muscle

Flexor carpi ulnaris tendon

Ulna

Aponeurosis of palmaris longus tendon

Palmaris longus tendon

Radius

A

Opponens digiti minimi muscle

Skin

Palmaris brevis muscle

Flexor carpi ulnaris tendon

Ulna

Flexor retinaculum

Aponeurosis of palmaris longus

Palmaris longus tendon

Radius

B

FIGURE 3-47A,B

Hypothenar muscles of the hand. Superficial dissection (**A**) and deep dissection (**B**).

WRIST: THENAR MUSCLES, VOLAR VIEW

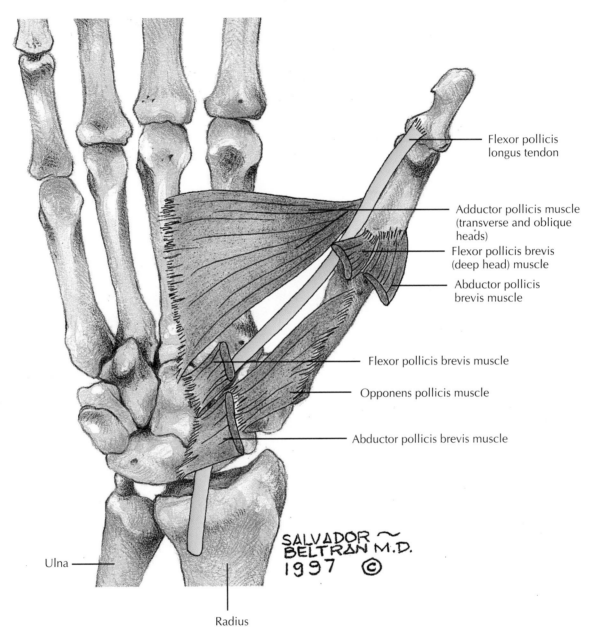

Flexor pollicis
longus tendon

Adductor pollicis muscle
(transverse and oblique
heads)

Flexor pollicis brevis
(deep head) muscle

Abductor pollicis
brevis muscle

Flexor pollicis brevis muscle

Opponens pollicis muscle

Abductor pollicis brevis muscle

Ulna

Radius

SALVADOR ~
BELTRAN M.D.
1997 ©

FIGURE 3-48

Thenar muscles of the hand include the abductor pollicis brevis, the opponens pollicis, the flexor pollicis brevis, and the adductor pollicis. The flexor pollicis brevis has a superficial and a deep head origin. The adductor pollicis has an oblique and a transverse head origin.

WRIST: FLEXOR POLLICIS LONGUS TENDON, VOLAR VIEW

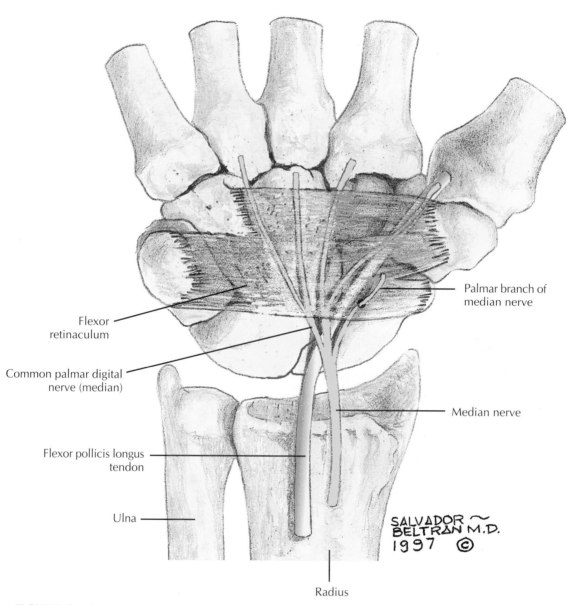

Palmar branch of
median nerve

Flexor
retinaculum

Common palmar digital
nerve (median)

Median nerve

Flexor pollicis longus
tendon

Ulna

Radius

SALVADOR
BELTRAN M.D.
1997 ©

FIGURE 3-49

The insertion of the flexor pollicis longus attaches to the base of the distal phalanx of the thumb. The palmar branch of the median nerve to the lateral palm and common digitals are also illustrated. For related MR, arthroscopy, and surgical anatomy image see Figure 3-54.

WRIST: FLEXOR CARPI RADIALIS TENDON, VOLAR VIEW

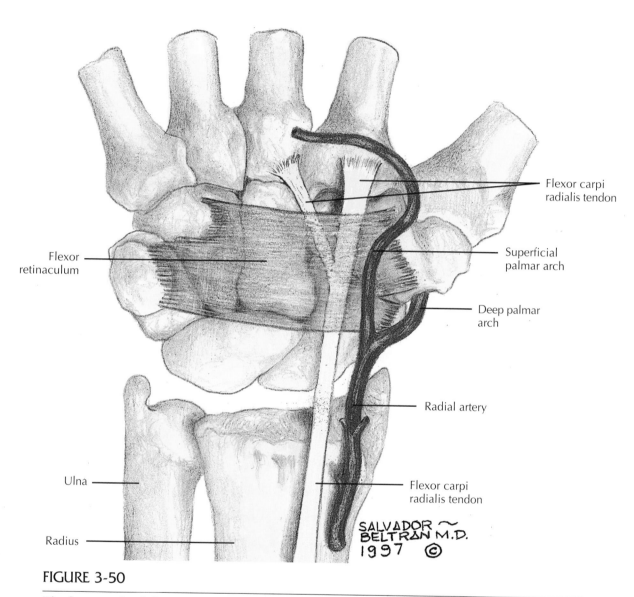

Flexor carpi
radialis tendon

Superficial
palmar arch

Deep palmar
arch

Radial artery

Flexor carpi
radialis tendon

Flexor
retinaculum

Ulna

Radius

FIGURE 3-50

The flexor carpi radialis inserts on the base of the second and third metacarpal bones.

WRIST: FLEXOR DIGITORUM SUPERFICIALIS AND PROFUNDUS TENDONS, VOLAR VIEW

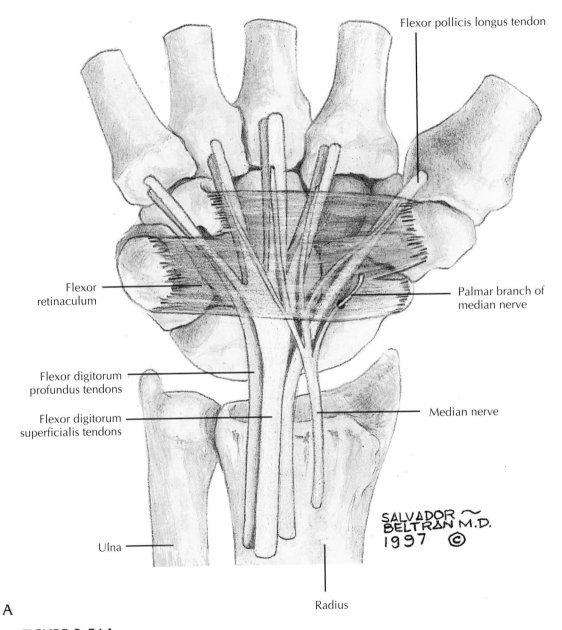

Flexor pollicis longus tendon

Flexor retinaculum

Palmar branch of median nerve

Flexor digitorum profundus tendons

Flexor digitorum superficialis tendons

Median nerve

Ulna

Radius

SALVADOR
BELTRAN M.D.
1997 ©

A

FIGURE 3-51A

(A) The tendons of the flexor digitorum superficialis are arranged with the middle and ring fingers superficial to the index and little fingers at the level of the wrist. The tendons of the flexor digitorum profundus are arranged in a single plane in order from side to side, deep to the flexor digitorum superficialis.

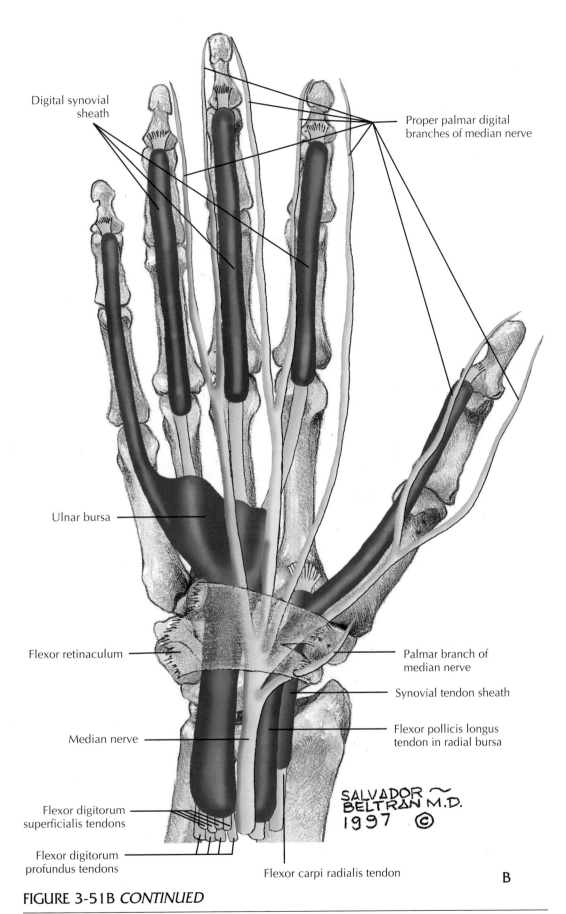

Digital synovial sheath

Proper palmar digital branches of median nerve

Ulnar bursa

Flexor retinaculum

Palmar branch of median nerve

Synovial tendon sheath

Median nerve

Flexor pollicis longus tendon in radial bursa

Flexor digitorum superficialis tendons

Flexor digitorum profundus tendons

Flexor carpi radialis tendon

SALVADOR ~
BELTRAN M.D.
1997 ©

B

FIGURE 3-51B *CONTINUED*

(B) The common synovial sheath (ulnar bursa), which contains the flexor tendons, and the radial bursa, which contains the flexor pollicis longus tendon, are illustrated. The palmar digital branches (off the common digital branches of the median nerve) extend to the first, second, third, and radial side of the fourth (ring) digit. For related MR, arthroscopy, and surgical anatomy image see Figure 3-54.

WRIST: EXTENSOR TENDONS, DORSAL VIEW

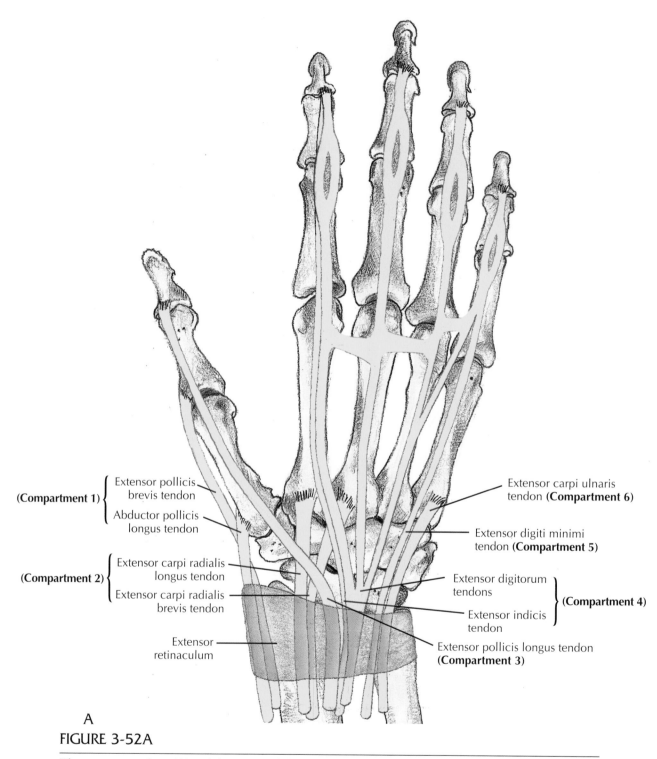

(Compartment 1) { Extensor pollicis brevis tendon

Abductor pollicis longus tendon

(Compartment 2) { Extensor carpi radialis longus tendon

Extensor carpi radialis brevis tendon

Extensor retinaculum

Extensor carpi ulnaris tendon **(Compartment 6)**

Extensor digiti minimi tendon **(Compartment 5)**

Extensor digitorum tendons

Extensor indicis tendon } **(Compartment 4)**

Extensor pollicis longus tendon **(Compartment 3)**

A

FIGURE 3-52A

The extensor tendons **(A)** and their synovial sheaths **(B)** are arranged into six compartments on the dorsum of the wrist. For related MR, arthroscopy, and surgical anatomy image see Figure 3-53.

WRIST: EXTENSOR TENDONS, DORSAL VIEW

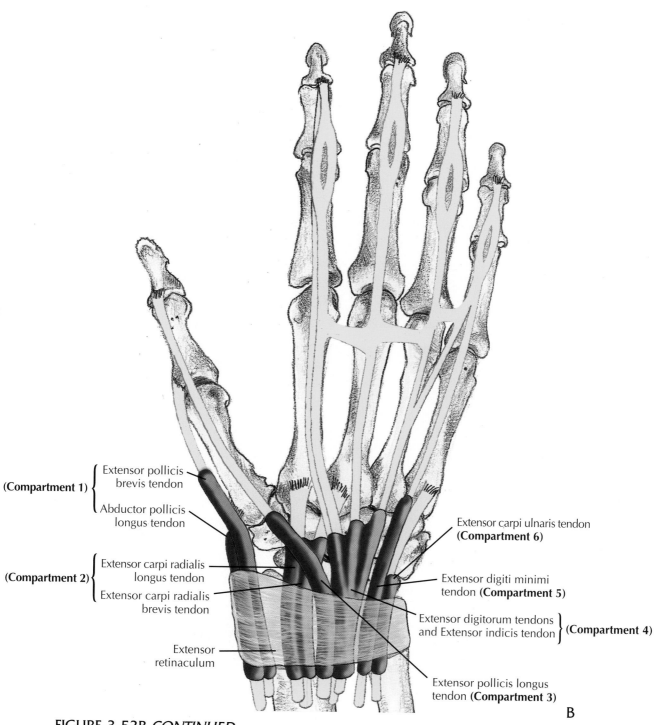

(Compartment 1) { Extensor pollicis brevis tendon

Abductor pollicis longus tendon

(Compartment 2) { Extensor carpi radialis longus tendon

Extensor carpi radialis brevis tendon

Extensor retinaculum

Extensor carpi ulnaris tendon (Compartment 6)

Extensor digiti minimi tendon (Compartment 5)

Extensor digitorum tendons and Extensor indicis tendon } (Compartment 4)

Extensor pollicis longus tendon (Compartment 3)

B

FIGURE 3-52B *CONTINUED*

WRIST: EXTENSOR TENDONS

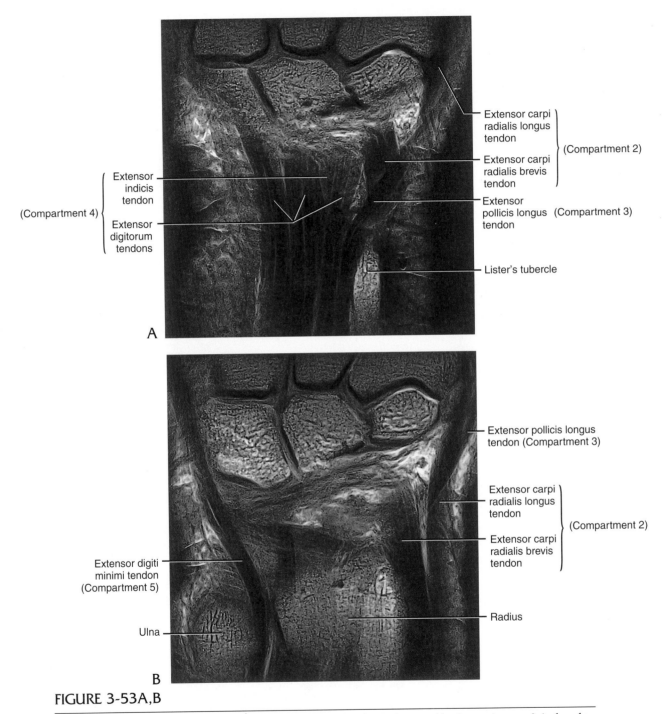

FIGURE 3-53A,B

(**A** and **B**) Extensor tendon anatomy on T1-weighted coronal MR images (the image in part **A** is dorsal to the image in part **B**). (**C, D,** and **E**) Corresponding dissections of the six extensor compartments. Radio-carpal joint arthroscopy is initiated with the arthroscope in the 3-4 portal (located between the extensor pollicis longus [the third compartment] and the extensor digitorum communis [the fourth compartment]). The 4-5 portal, ulnar to the extensor digitorum communis, is used to evaluate the triangular fibrocartilage.

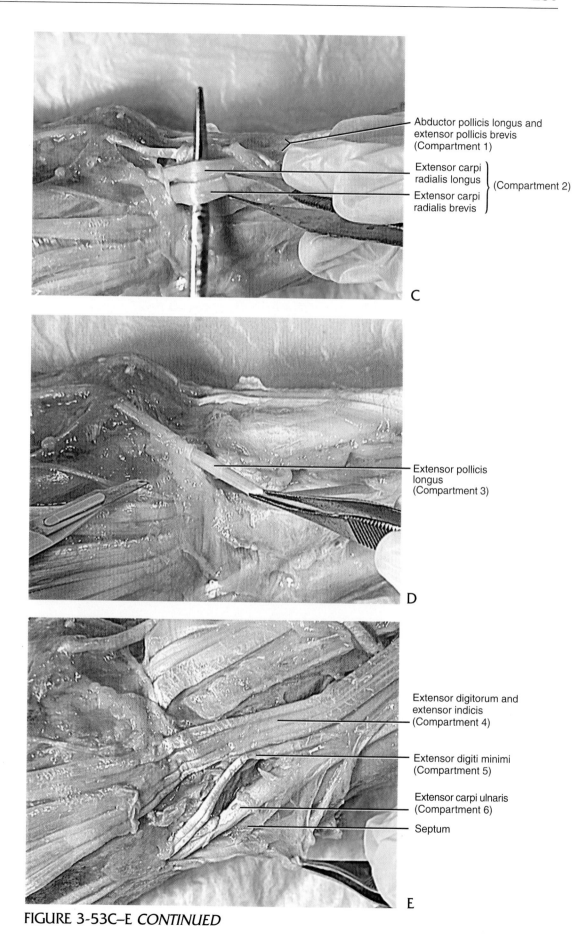

Abductor pollicis longus and
extensor pollicis brevis
(Compartment 1)

Extensor carpi
radialis longus

Extensor carpi
radialis brevis } (Compartment 2)

C

Extensor pollicis
longus
(Compartment 3)

D

Extensor digitorum and
extensor indicis
(Compartment 4)

Extensor digiti minimi
(Compartment 5)

Extensor carpi ulnaris
(Compartment 6)

Septum

E

FIGURE 3-53C–E CONTINUED

WRIST: MEDIAN AND ULNAR NERVES

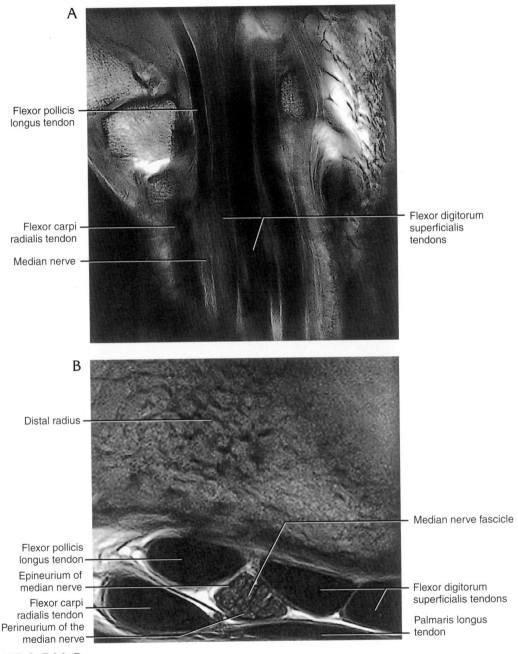

Flexor pollicis
longus tendon

Flexor digitorum
superficialis
tendons

Flexor carpi
radialis tendon

Median nerve

Distal radius

Median nerve fascicle

Flexor pollicis
longus tendon

Epineurium of
median nerve

Flexor digitorum
superficialis tendons

Flexor carpi
radialis tendon
Perineurium of the
median nerve

Palmaris longus
tendon

FIGURE 3-54A,B

Median nerve anatomy. (**A, B,** and **C**) T1-weighted coronal (**A**) and axial images at the level of the distal radius (**B**) and proximal carpal row (**C**). MR distinguishes multiple fascicles bounded by the nerve sheath. (**D**) Guyon's canal containing the ulnar nerve and artery at the level of the distal carpal row (T1-weighted axial image). Guyon's canal is formed by the pisiform bone, the flexor retinaculum, and a volar carpal ligament. The separate motor and sensory branches of the ulnar nerve are seen in zone I, deep to the volar carpal ligament. Division into the deep motor branch constitutes zone II, and the superficial sensory branch constitutes zone III. Compression of the ulnar nerve in zones I and III produces sensory findings, whereas compression in zones I and II produces motor findings.

WRIST: MEDIAN AND ULNAR NERVES

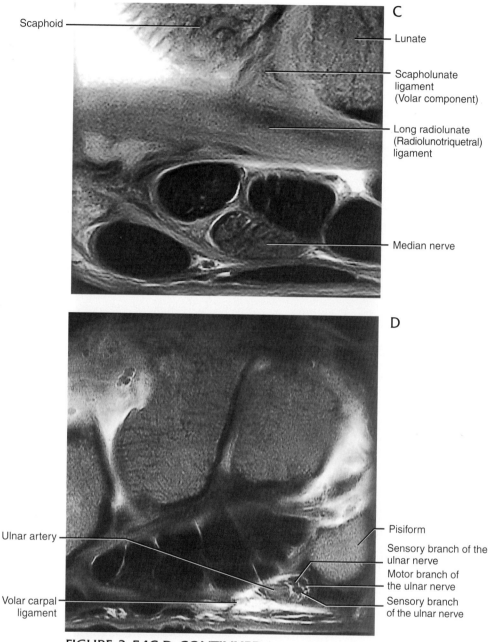

Scaphoid

Lunate

Scapholunate ligament (Volar component)

Long radiolunate (Radiolunotriquetral) ligament

Median nerve

C

D

Ulnar artery

Volar carpal ligament

Pisiform

Sensory branch of the ulnar nerve

Motor branch of the ulnar nerve

Sensory branch of the ulnar nerve

FIGURE 3-54C,D *CONTINUED*

WRIST: VOLAR RADIOCARPAL LIGAMENTS

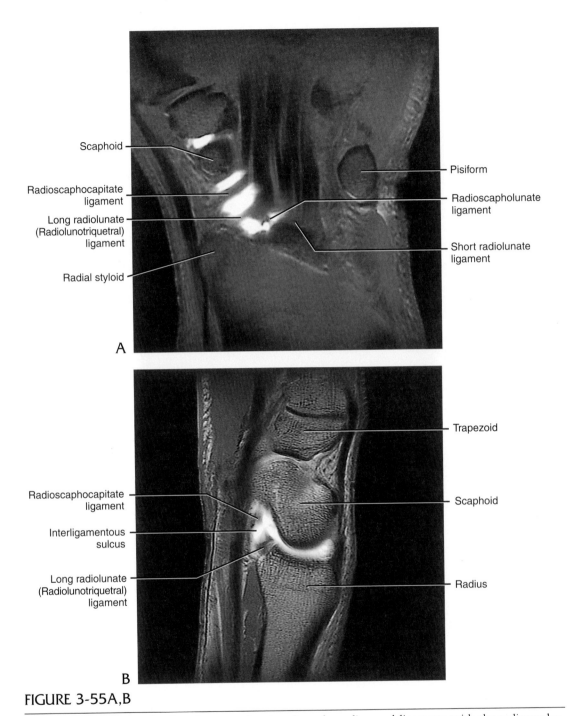

FIGURE 3-55A,B

(A) T1-weighted coronal MR arthrogram showing the volar radiocarpal ligaments with the radioscapho-capitate, radiolunotriquetral (long radiolunate), and radioscapholunate ligaments. There is partial visualiza-tion of the short radiolunate ligament, which is separate from the radiolunotriquetral ligament. The radiol-unotriquetral ligament can be seen extending from the volar lip of the distal radius to insert on the volar pole of the lunate. **(B)** T1-weighted sagittal MR arthrogram showing the radioscaphocapitate and radiol-unotriquetral ligaments.

WRIST: VOLAR RADIOCARPAL LIGAMENTS

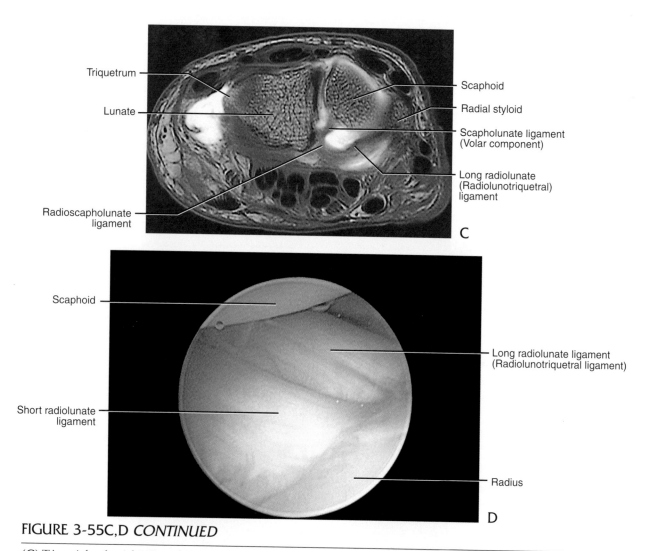

Triquetrum

Lunate

Radioscapholunate ligament

Scaphoid

Radial styloid

Scapholunate ligament (Volar component)

Long radiolunate (Radiolunotriquetral) ligament

C

Scaphoid

Short radiolunate ligament

Long radiolunate ligament (Radiolunotriquetral ligament)

Radius

D

FIGURE 3-55C,D *CONTINUED*

(C) T1-weighted axial MR arthrogram demonstrating the radiolunotriquetral ligament extending from the radial styloid to the lunate and blending with the volar portion of the interosseous lunotriquetral ligament. **(D)** Arthroscopic view of the radiolunotriquetral and short radiolunate ligaments.

WRIST: VOLAR RADIOCARPAL LIGAMENTS

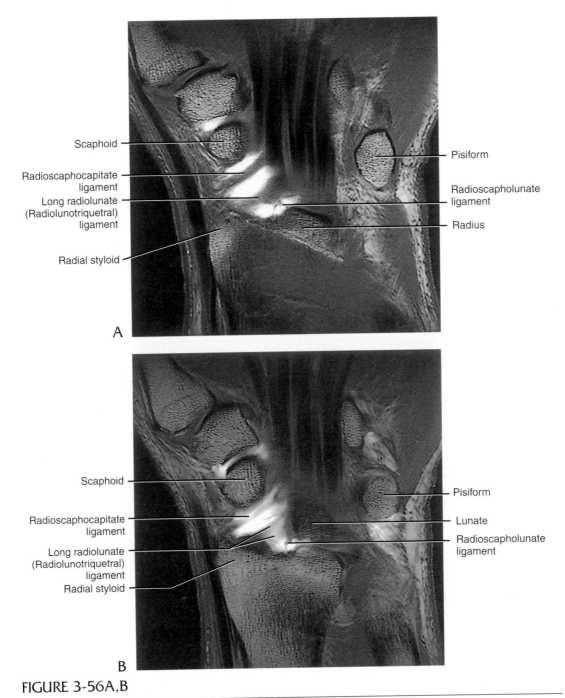

FIGURE 3-56A,B

(**A** and **B**) The radioscaphocapitate, radiolunotriquetral (long radiolunate), and radioscapholunate ligaments on T1-weighted coronal MR arthrograms (the image in part **A** is volar to the image in part **B**). (**C** and **D**) Corresponding arthroscopic views show the radioscaphocapitate (**C**) and radioscapholunate (**D**) ligaments. The radioscapholunate ligament (also referred to as the ligament of Testut) provides a vascular supply to the scapholunate interosseous ligament and is not biomechanically important. A fat pad covers the radioscapholunate ligament at the base of the scapholunate ligament. (**E**) Dissection showing (from a dorsal to volar perspective) the intraarticular anatomy of the radioscaphocapitate, radioscapholunate, and interosseous scapholunate ligaments.

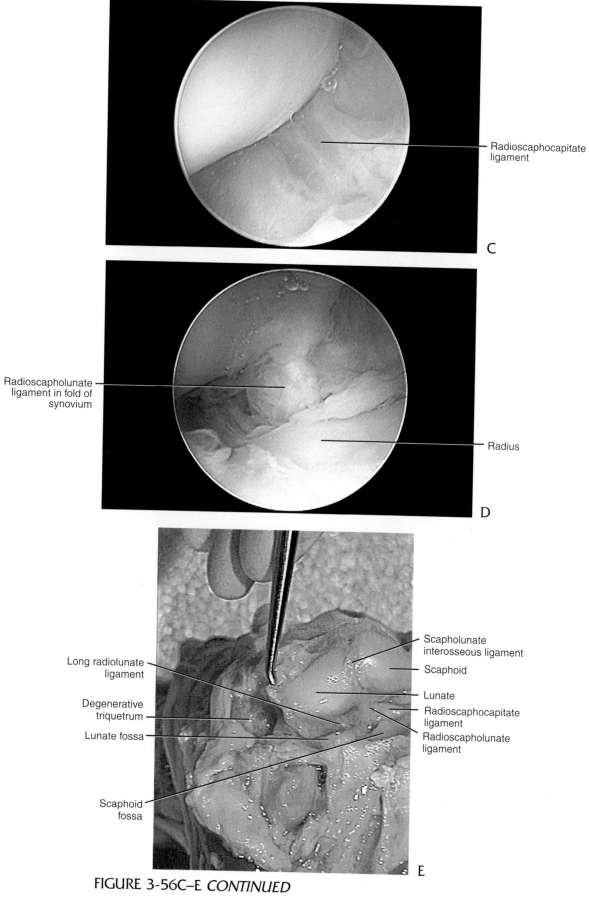

C

Radioscaphocapitate
ligament

D

Radioscapholunate
ligament in fold of
synovium

Radius

Long radiolunate
ligament

Degenerative
triquetrum

Lunate fossa

Scaphoid
fossa

Scapholunate
interosseous ligament

Scaphoid

Lunate

Radioscaphocapitate
ligament

Radioscapholunate
ligament

E

FIGURE 3-56C–E *CONTINUED*

WRIST: SCAPHOLUNATE LIGAMENT

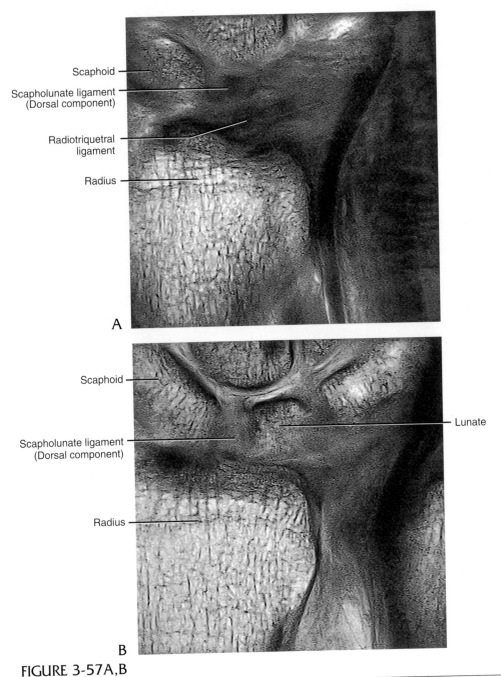

FIGURE 3-57A,B

(**A** and **B**) T1–weighted coronal images showing the band-like fibers of the thick dorsal portion of the scapholunate ligament (the image in part **A** is dorsal to the image in part **B**).

WRIST: SCAPHOLUNATE LIGAMENT

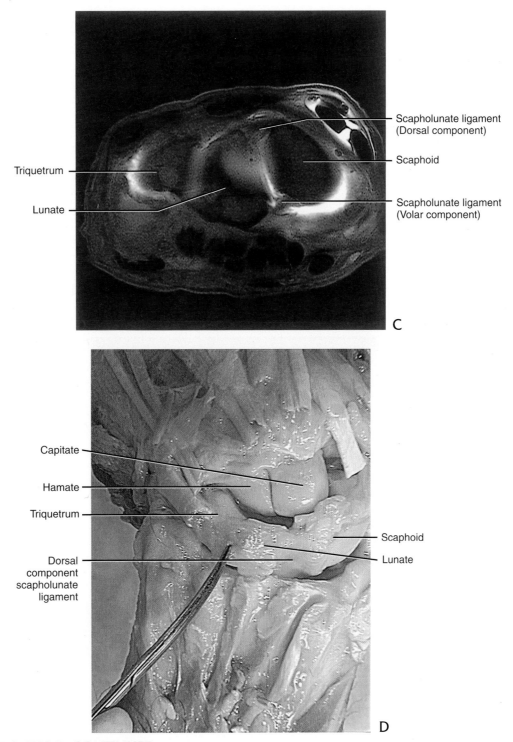

FIGURE 3-57C,D *CONTINUED*

(C) The scapholunate ligament on a fat-suppressed T1-weighted axial MR arthrogram. **(D)** Corresponding gross dissection showing the intact dorsal fibers of the scapholunate ligament. The probe is directed at the lunotriquetral ligament.

WRIST: SCAPHOLUNATE LIGAMENT

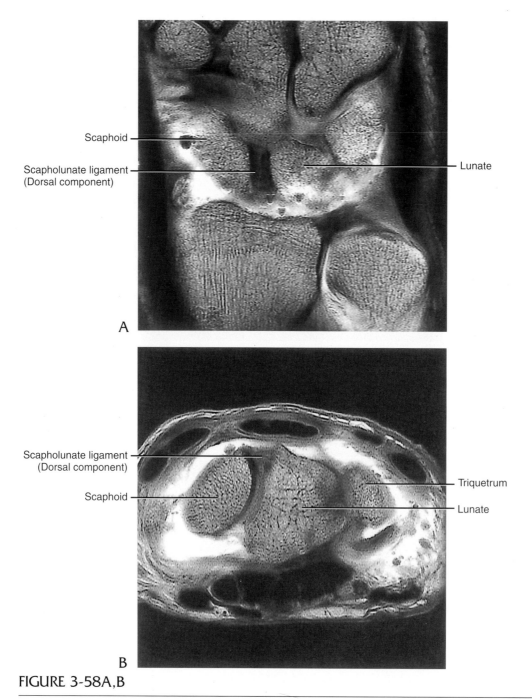

FIGURE 3-58A,B

(**A** and **B**) T1-weighted coronal (**A**) and axial (**B**) MR arthrograms showing that the dorsal fibers of the scapholunate ligament have a transverse orientation and form a thick bundle perpendicular to the scapholunate joint.

WRIST: SCAPHOLUNATE LIGAMENT

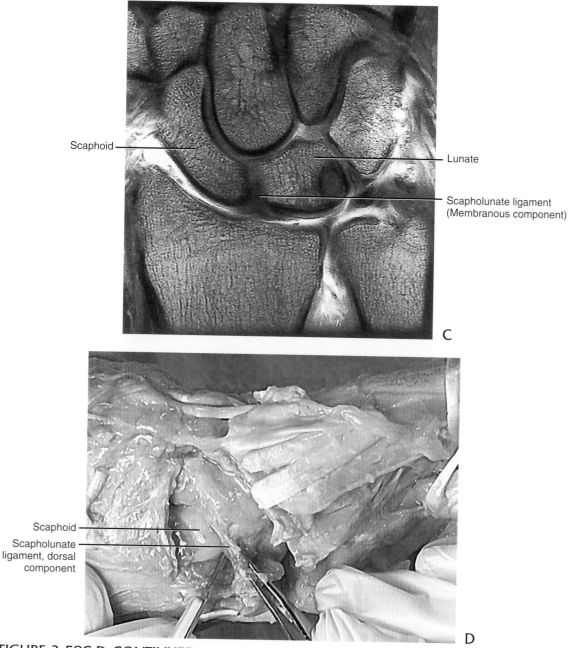

Scaphoid

Lunate

Scapholunate ligament
(Membranous component)

C

Scaphoid
Scapholunate
ligament, dorsal
component

D

FIGURE 3-58C,D *CONTINUED*

(C) T1-weighted coronal MR arthrogram showing that the membranous portion of the scapholunate ligament has a triangular shape and peripheral attachment. **(D)** The normal dorsal thickening of the scapholunate ligament is shown on gross dissection. The biomechanically stronger dorsal fibers of the scapholunate
ligament hinge the dorsum of the scapholunate interval, which allows mobility or opening of the volar aspect of the joint.

WRIST: SCAPHOLUNATE LIGAMENT

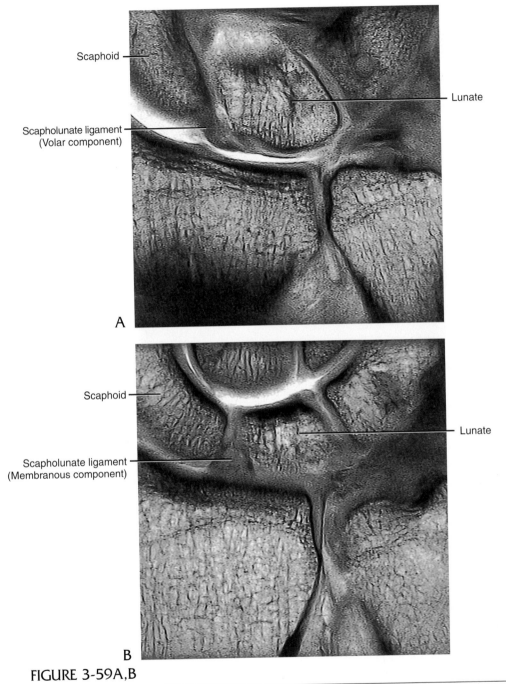

Scaphoid

Lunate

Scapholunate ligament
(Volar component)

A

Scaphoid

Lunate

Scapholunate ligament
(Membranous component)

B

FIGURE 3-59A,B

(**A** and **B**) T1-weighted coronal MR arthrograms showing volar (**A**) and membranous (**B**) portions of the scapholunate ligament (the image in part **A** is volar to the image in part **B**). There is a small linear collection of contrast material, superficial to the lunate articular cartilage which extends to the volar scapholunate ligament at the site of a previous tear. The normal membranous attachments of the scapholunate ligament are to the articular cartilage surfaces of the scaphoid and lunate. The membranous component of the scapholunate ligament does not directly attach to the distal radius, although volarly it merges with the extrinsic radioscapholunate ligament.

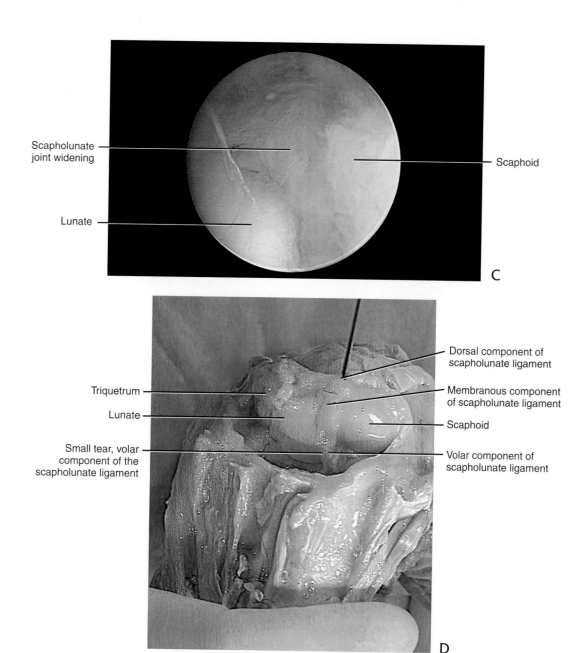

Scapholunate joint widening

Scaphoid

Lunate

C

Dorsal component of scapholunate ligament

Membranous component of scapholunate ligament

Scaphoid

Volar component of scapholunate ligament

Triquetrum

Lunate

Small tear, volar component of the scapholunate ligament

D

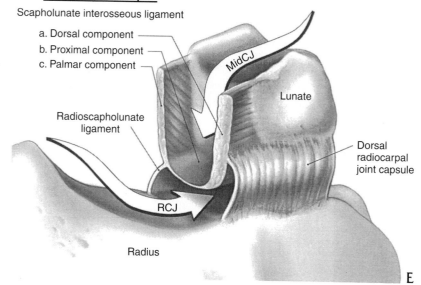

**Intrinsic
Scapholunate Complex**

Scapholunate interosseous ligament

  a. Dorsal component

  b. Proximal component

  c. Palmar component

Radioscapholunate ligament

MidCJ

Lunate

Dorsal radiocarpal joint capsule

RCJ

Radius

E

FIGURE 3-59C–E *CONTINUED*

(C) Corresponding arthroscopic view shows mild widening of the scapholunate interval. **(D)** A shotgun dorsal view demonstrates intact dorsal and membranous portions of the scapholunate ligament. A small volar tear was confirmed. **(E)** The scapholunate ligament forms a C-shaped complex, which is open distally at the level of the midcarpal joint. The membranous or proximal component forms the base of this C-shaped complex. The dorsal radiocarpal joint capsule inserts proximally into the dorsal component. The proximal aspect of the dorsal and volar components merge with the membranous component. Volarly, the radioscapholunate ligament inserts at the junction of the volar and membranous components of the scapholunate ligament.

WRIST: SCAPHOLUNATE LIGAMENT

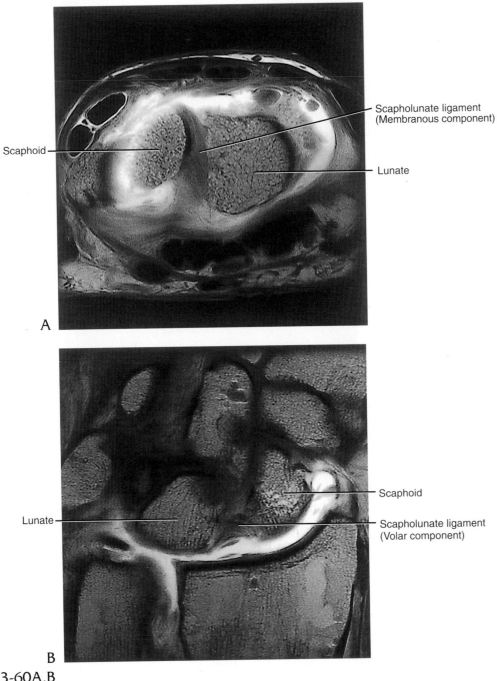

FIGURE 3-60A,B

(A and B) T1-weighted axial (A) and coronal (B) MR arthrograms showing the scapholunate ligament with intact membranous portion on part A and intact volar portion on part B.

WRIST: SCAPHOLUNATE LIGAMENT

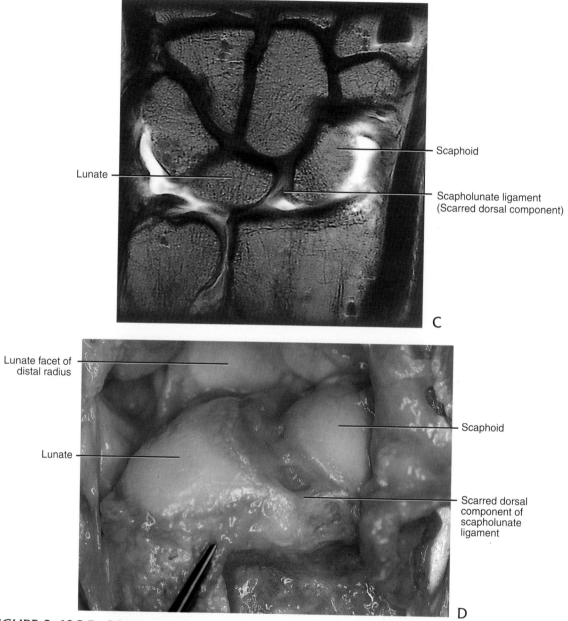

Lunate

Scaphoid

Scapholunate ligament
(Scarred dorsal component)

C

Lunate facet of
distal radius

Scaphoid

Lunate

Scarred dorsal
component of
scapholunate
ligament

D

FIGURE 3-60C,D *CONTINUED*

(C) An abnormally attenuated dorsal portion of the scapholunate ligament is shown on a T1–weighted coronal MR arthrogram. **(D)** Corresponding dorsal view of the opened radiocarpal joint demonstrates the scarred dorsal component of the scapholunate ligament and interval widening. Note the normal oblique direction of fibers from the membranous component extending downward from the scaphoid to the lunate in part **A**.

WRIST: SCAPHOLUNATE LIGAMENT

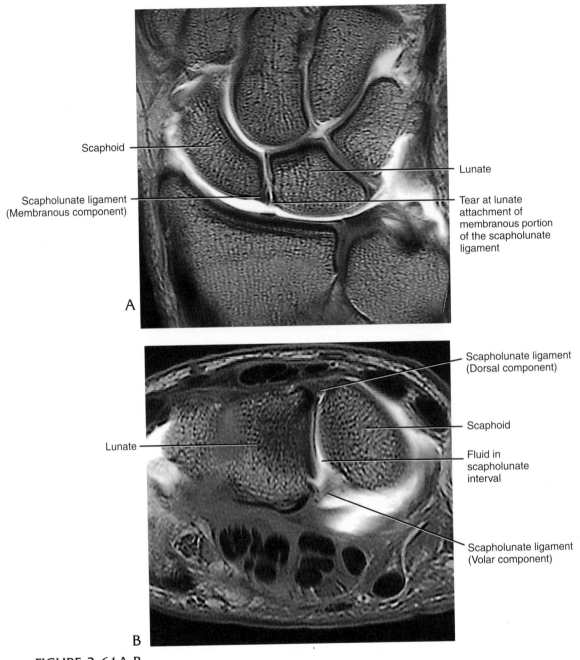

Scaphoid

Scapholunate ligament
(Membranous component)

Lunate

Tear at lunate
attachment of
membranous portion
of the scapholunate
ligament

A

Scapholunate ligament
(Dorsal component)

Scaphoid

Lunate

Fluid in
scapholunate
interval

Scapholunate ligament
(Volar component)

B

FIGURE 3-61A,B

(A) T1-weighted coronal MR arthrogram demonstrating a membranous tear of the scapholunate ligament at its lunate attachment. **(B)** T1-weighted axial MR arthrogram illustrating the fluid communicating across the torn membranous portion of the scapholunate ligament. These fibers would normally course peripherally and obliquely across the scapholunate interval. Note the intact dorsal and volar portions of the scapholunate ligament.

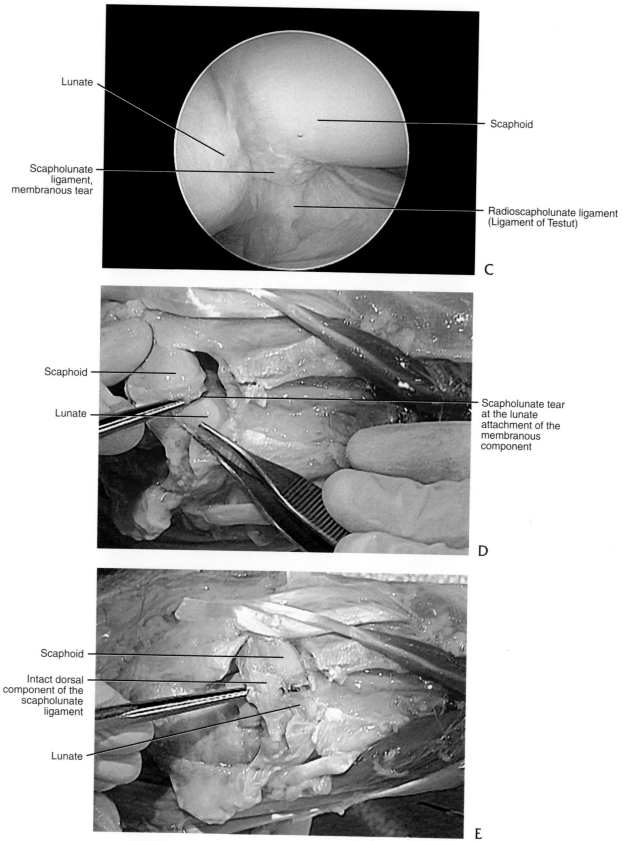

Lunate

Scaphoid

Scapholunate
ligament,
membranous tear

Radioscapholunate ligament
(Ligament of Testut)

C

Scaphoid

Lunate

Scapholunate tear
at the lunate
attachment of the
membranous
component

D

Scaphoid

Intact dorsal
component of the
scapholunate
ligament

Lunate

E

FIGURE 3-61C–E *CONTINUED*

(C and **D)** Corresponding arthroscopic view **(C)** and dissection **(D)** demonstrating the torn membranous scapholunate ligament. The continuity between the radioscapholunate ligament with the membranous component of the scapholunate ligament can also be appreciated on the arthroscopic view (part **C**). **(E)** The stronger dorsal portion of the scapholunate ligament is intact on corresponding arthrotomy of the dorsum of the wrist.

WRIST: LUNOTRIQUETRAL LIGAMENT

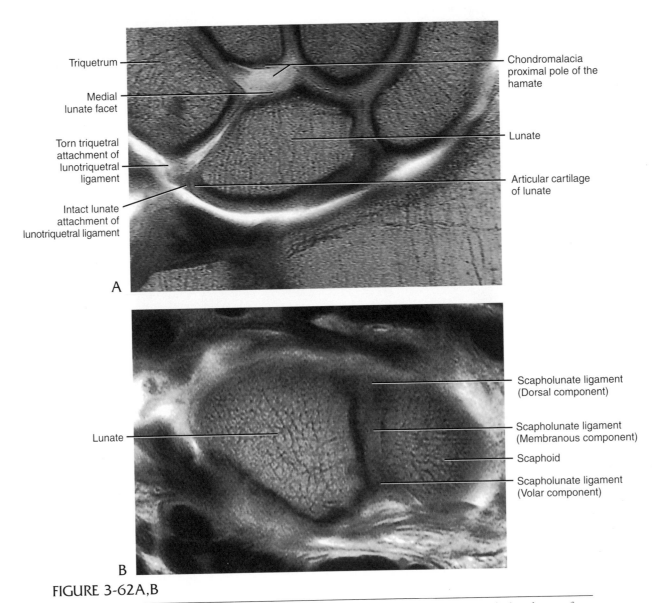

Triquetrum

Chondromalacia proximal pole of the hamate

Medial lunate facet

Torn triquetral attachment of lunotriquetral ligament

Lunate

Intact lunate attachment of lunotriquetral ligament

Articular cartilage of lunate

A

Lunate

Scapholunate ligament (Dorsal component)

Scapholunate ligament (Membranous component)

Scaphoid

Scapholunate ligament (Volar component)

B

FIGURE 3-62A,B

(A) T1-weighted coronal MR arthrogram illustrating a lunotriquetral ligament tear with detachment from the proximal surface of the triquetrum. There is loss of continuity of the normal proximal carpal row arc at the level of the lunotriquetral interval. In addition, this specimen has a medial lunate facet and proximal hamate chondral erosion. **(B)** T1-weighted axial MR arthrogram displaying the scapholunate ligament, intact in its volar, membranous, and dorsal fibers. The torn triquetral attachment of the lunotriquetral ligament is surrounded by fluid.

WRIST: LUNOTRIQUETRAL LIGAMENT

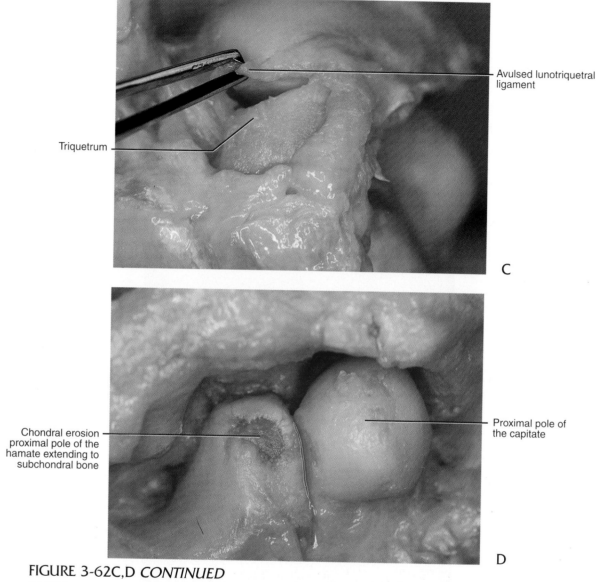

FIGURE 3-62C,D *CONTINUED*

(**C** and **D**) Corresponding gross dissections (dorsal view) of the avulsed lunotriquetral ligament in part **C** and of the hamate erosion as shown in the dorsal view of the opened midcarpal joint in part **D**.

WRIST: LUNOTRIQUETRAL LIGAMENT

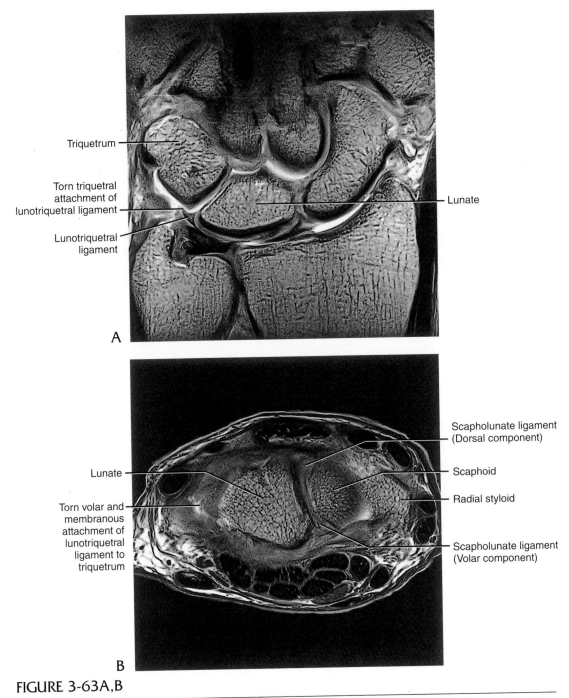

FIGURE 3-63A,B

(A and **B)** Flap tear of the lunotriquetral ligament on T1–weighted coronal **(A)** and axial **(B)** MR arthrograms.

WRIST: LUNOTRIQUETRAL LIGAMENT

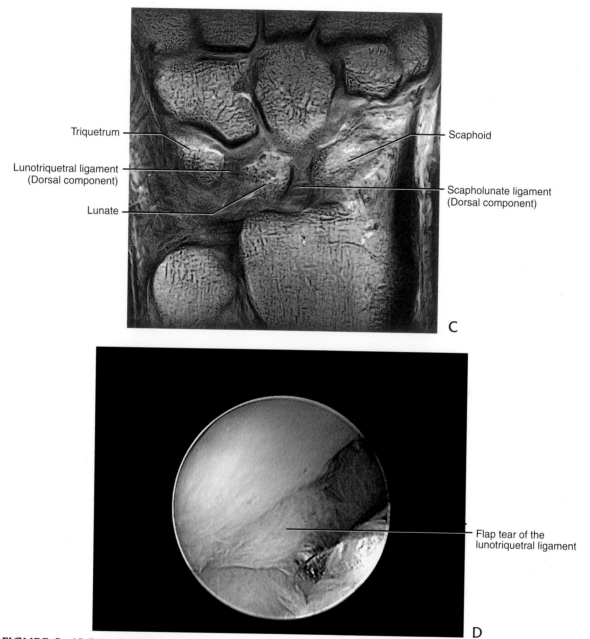

Triquetrum

Lunotriquetral ligament
(Dorsal component)

Lunate

Scaphoid

Scapholunate ligament
(Dorsal component)

C

Flap tear of the
lunotriquetral ligament

D

FIGURE 3-63C,D *CONTINUED*

(C) A T1-weighted dorsal coronal MR image shows the intact dorsal component of the lunotriquetral and scapholunate ligaments. Unlike the dorsal component of the scapholunate ligament, it is the volar portion of the lunotriquetral ligament that has the highest tensile strength. **(D)** Corresponding arthroscopic view of the lunotriquetral flap tear. Lunotriquetral dissociations may present with either normal carpal bone alignment, a dynamic volar intercalated segment instability (VISI) pattern, or a static VISI pattern. A static VISI pattern requires involvement of the membranous and volar lunotriquetral ligament and dorsal radiocarpal ligaments.

WRIST: LUNOTRIQUETRAL LIGAMENT

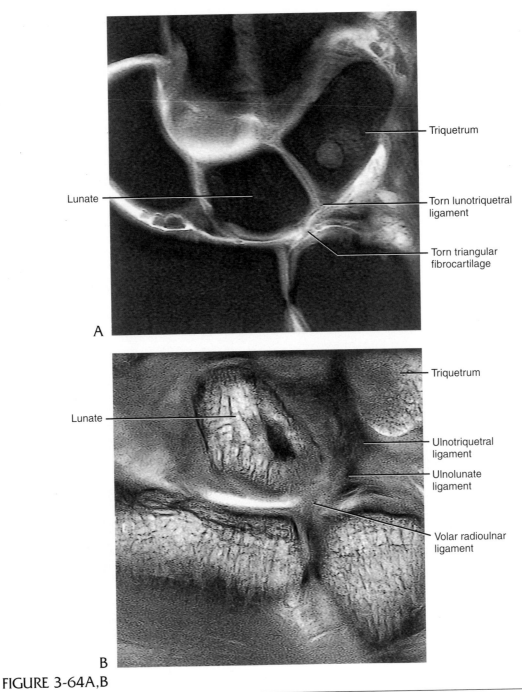

FIGURE 3-64A,B

(A) Lunotriquetral ligament tear without visualized fibers on a fat–suppressed T1-weighted coronal MR arthrogram. (B) A more volar T1-weighted coronal MR arthrogram shows the ulnocarpal ligament layer volar to the lunotriquetral interval.

WRIST: LUNOTRIQUETRAL LIGAMENT

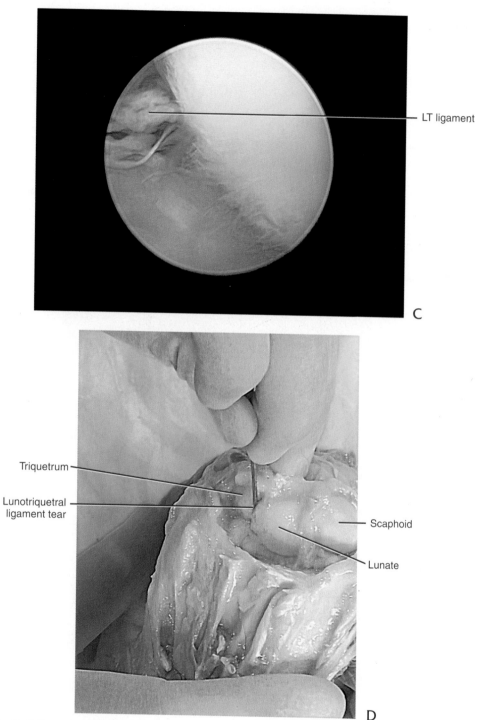

FIGURE 3-64C,D *CONTINUED*

(**C** and **D**) An incompetent lunotriquetral ligament is shown on corresponding arthroscopic view (**C**) and open dissection (**D**).

WRIST: TRIANGULAR FIBROCARTILAGE

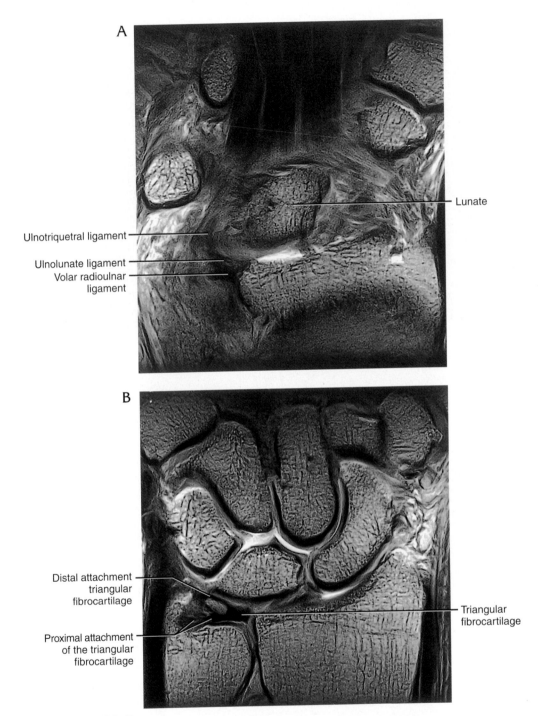

FIGURE 3-65A,B

(A and **B)** T1-weighted coronal MR arthrograms displaying normal volar ulnocarpal ligaments (ulnolunate and ulnotriquetral) **(A)** and intact triangular fibrocartilage disc **(B)**. The ulnar insertion of the triangular fibrocartilage complex is shown as a proximal and distal band of tissue.

WRIST: TRIANGULAR FIBROCARTILAGE

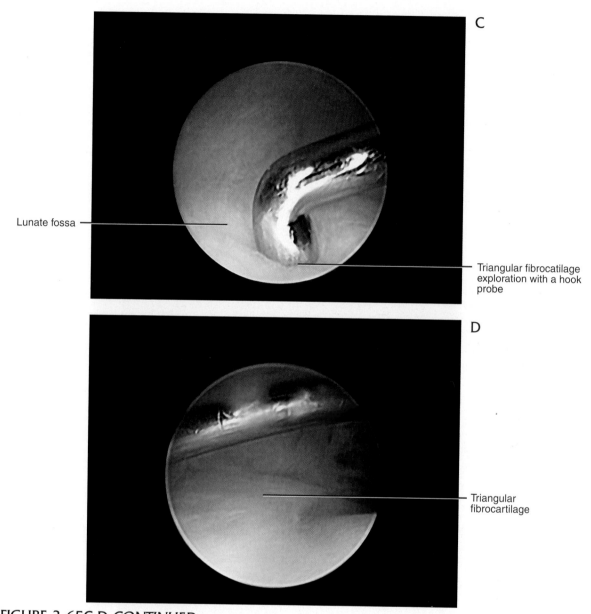

C

Lunate fossa

Triangular fibrocatilage
exploration with a hook
probe

D

Triangular
fibrocartilage

FIGURE 3-65C,D *CONTINUED*

(**C** and **D**) Triangular fibrocartilage shown as palpated with a probe. The normal triangular fibrocartilage should demonstrate a "trampoline" effect—or resilience—in the absence of a tear. The prestyloid recess (lateral) and pisotriquetral space (volar) are normal perforations that exist in the ulnar margins of the triangular fibrocartilage. Arthroscopic confirmation of intact ulnolunate and ulnotriquetral ligaments can be performed at their origin at the base of the ulnar styloid.

WRIST: TRIANGULAR FIBROCARTILAGE

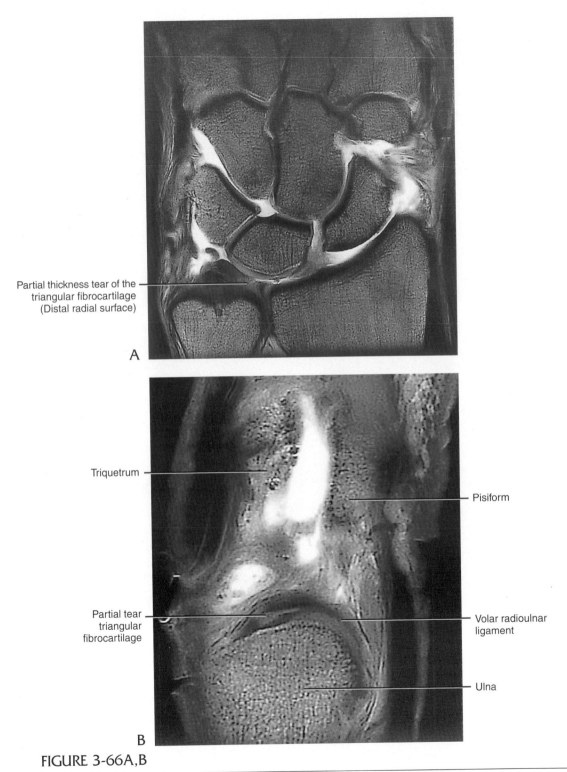

Partial thickness tear of the triangular fibrocartilage (Distal radial surface)

A

Triquetrum

Pisiform

Partial tear triangular fibrocartilage

Volar radioulnar ligament

Ulna

B

FIGURE 3-66A,B

(**A** and **B**) Partial thickness distal triangular fibrocartilage tear on T1-weighted coronal (**A**) and sagittal (**B**) MR arthrograms.

WRIST: TRIANGULAR FIBROCARTILAGE

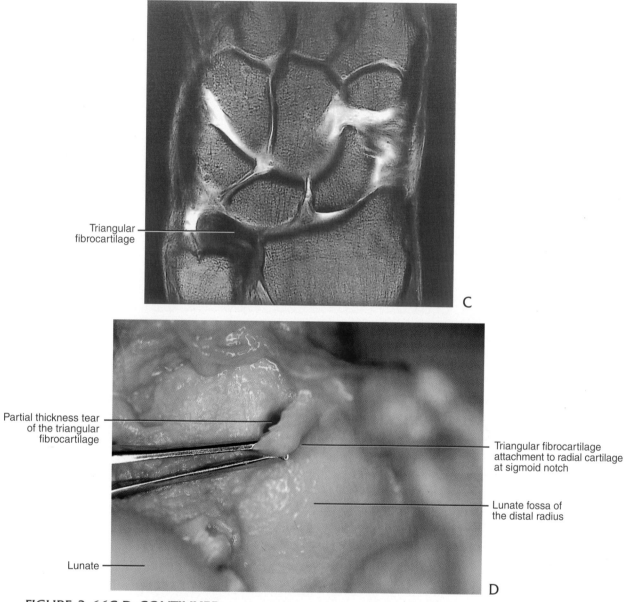

Triangular fibrocartilage

C

Partial thickness tear of the triangular fibrocartilage

Triangular fibrocartilage attachment to radial cartilage at sigmoid notch

Lunate fossa of the distal radius

Lunate

D

FIGURE 3-66C,D *CONTINUED*

(C) A more dorsal T1–weighted coronal MR image shows a normal distal triangular fibrocartilage surface. **(D)** Corresponding dissection shows the partial triangular fibrocartilage tear in a dorsal view of the opened radiocarpal joint.

WRIST: TRIANGULAR FIBROCARTILAGE

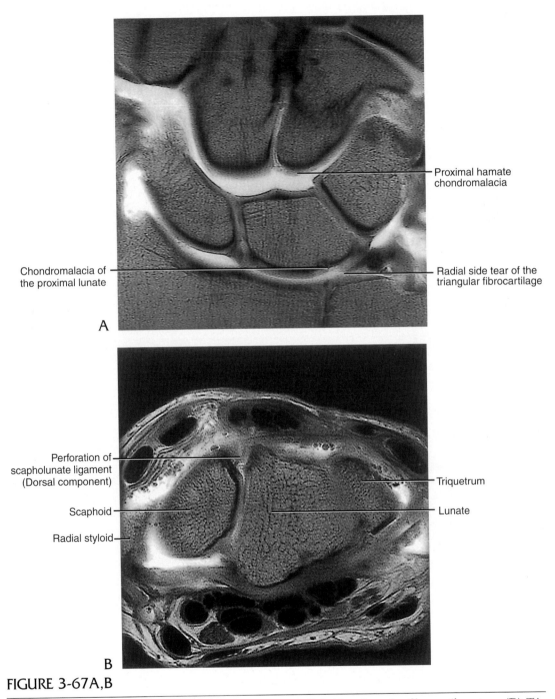

Proximal hamate chondromalacia

Chondromalacia of the proximal lunate

Radial side tear of the triangular fibrocartilage

A

Perforation of scapholunate ligament (Dorsal component)

Scaphoid

Radial styloid

Triquetrum

Lunate

B

FIGURE 3-67A,B

(A) T1-weighted coronal MR arthrogram illustrating a radial side triangular fibrocartilage tear. **(B)** T1-weighted axial MR arthrogram showing dorsal perforation of the scapholunate ligament.

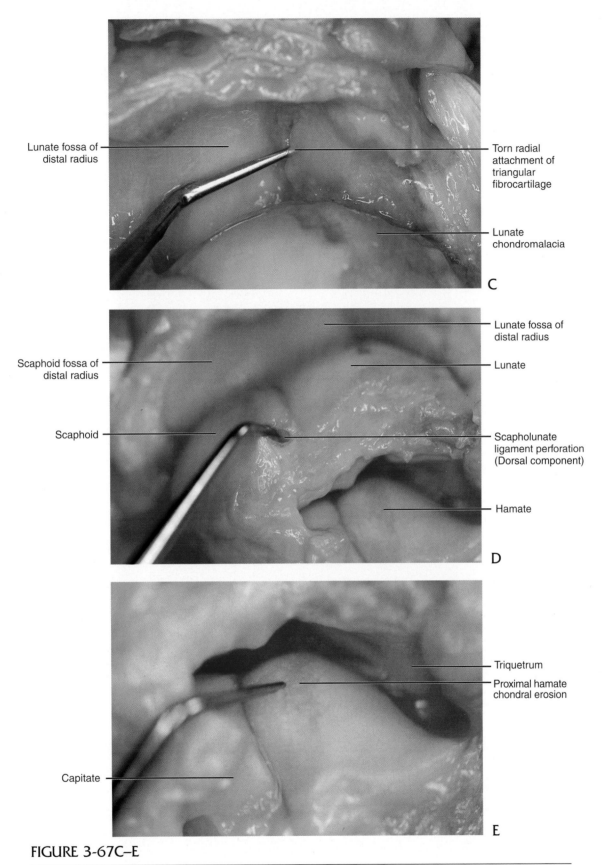

Lunate fossa of distal radius

Torn radial attachment of triangular fibrocartilage

Lunate chondromalacia

C

Scaphoid fossa of distal radius

Lunate fossa of distal radius

Lunate

Scaphoid

Scapholunate ligament perforation (Dorsal component)

Hamate

D

Triquetrum

Proximal hamate chondral erosion

Capitate

E

FIGURE 3-67C–E

(C, D, and **E)** Corresponding dissections (dorsal view) with triangular fibrocartilage detachment and associated lunate chondromalacia **(C)**, scapholunate perforation **(D)**, and proximal hamate chondromalacia **(E)**.

WRIST: TRIANGULAR FIBROCARTILAGE

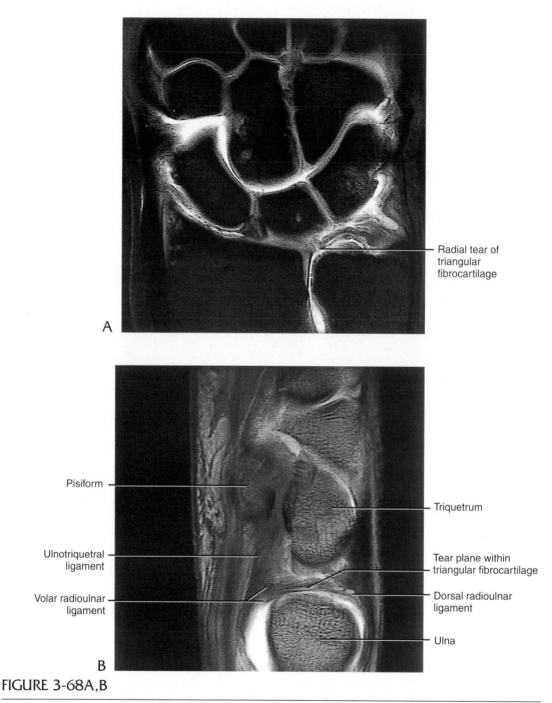

FIGURE 3-68A,B

(A) Fat-suppressed T1-weighted coronal MR arthrogram demonstrating a triangular fibrocartilage tear with communication of contrast material across the radial aspect of the articular disc. **(B)** T1-weighted sagittal MR arthrogram demonstrating abnormal morphology of the triangular fibrocartilage disc, although the volar and dorsal radioulnar ligaments are intact. Contrast material can be seen within the substance of the triangular fibrocartilage. **(C and D)** Arthroscopic views showing probing of the triangular fibrocartilage tear **(C)** and the exposed surface of the ulna **(D)**. **(E)** Open exposure of the wrist confirms a radial-sided tear of the triangular fibrocartilage.

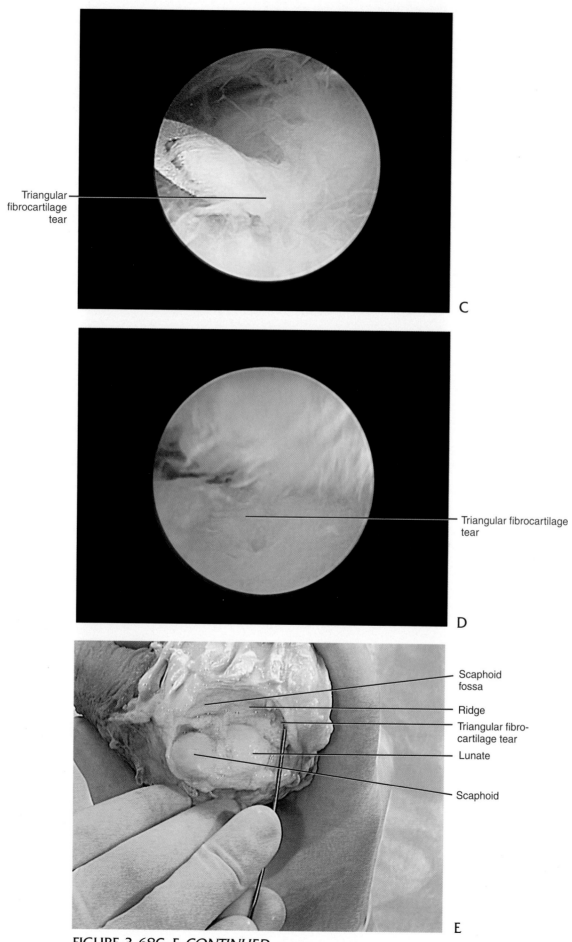

Triangular fibrocartilage tear

C

Triangular fibrocartilage tear

D

Scaphoid fossa

Ridge

Triangular fibro-cartilage tear

Lunate

Scaphoid

E

FIGURE 3-68C–E *CONTINUED*

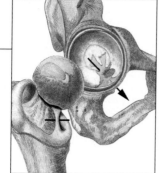

C H A P T E R 4

THE HIP

David W. Stoller
Robert J. Gilbert
James M. Glick
Salvador Beltran

| HIP ARTHROSCOPY AND DISSECTION | COLOR ANATOMIC ILLUSTRATIONS |
| MR NORMAL ANATOMY | MR, ARTHROSCOPY, AND SURGICAL CORRELATION |

HIP ARTHROSCOPY

THERE ARE A NUMBER OF INDICATIONS FOR HIP ARTHROSCOPY, including:

- Evaluation and treatment of arthritis in a young individual, including the planning of more definitive treatment such as an osteotomy or a joint replacement
- Removal of loose bodies, including synovial chondromatosis, and following a hip dislocation
- Removal of foreign bodies, such as bullets or cement from a hip replacement
- Removal of a torn acetabular labrum
- Synovectomy in rheumatoid arthritis or pigmented villonodular synovitis
- Incision and drainage in infections
- Biopsy
- Evaluation of pediatric conditions such as Legg-Calvé-Perthes disease
- Evaluation of undiagnosed hip pain
- Release of the iliopsoas tendon for a snapping hip
- Buroscopy and bursectomy for trochanteric bursitis

Arthroscopy of the hip is performed with the patient in the lateral decubitus position, with the involved hip upward. Traction with 25 to 50 pounds is performed to achieve up to 1 cm of distraction. The leg is abducted (at 45°) and flexed forward (at 10°). Three portals are established, including anterior and posterior peri-trochanteric portals. The arthroscope is initially placed in the anterior peri-trochanteric portal and the shaver is placed in the posterior peri-trochanteric portal. A 15 gauge spinal needle is placed within the hip joint from an anterior portal off the edge of the anterior superior iliac spine (ASIS), using both the ASIS and greater trochanter as landmarks. An image intensifier is used to confirm the initial entry into the hip joint. With the arthroscope the lunate surface of the acetabulum, the acetabular fossa, the ligamentum teres, and the acetabular labrum in its anterior, posterior, and lateral portions can be visualized. Except for the femoral head below the ligamentum teres, the majority of the weight bearing chondral surface of the femoral head can be viewed. With the anterior peritrochanteric (anterolateral portal) approach, the anterior labrum and anterior acetabulum wall are visualized. Both the anterior and posterior labrum and posterior acetabular wall are best seen through the posterior peritrochanteric (posterolateral portal) approach. The lateral femoral cutaneous nerve is closest to the anterior portal and the sciatic nerve is closest to the posterior peri-trochanteric portal.

A stellate crease, or bare area, exists above the anterosuperior margin of the acetabular fossa within the articular area of the acetabulum. Arthroscopically, three distinct gutters can be identified peripheral to the labrum. These include a perilabral sulcus and the anterior and posterior synovial gutters, which are the margins of the hip joint. The insertion of the ligamentum teres onto the fovea represents a bare area, devoid of articular cartilage. Arthroscopically, the zona orbicularis (formed by deep circular fibers from the ischiofemoral ligament) may be mistaken for the acetabular labrum.

SURGICAL DISSECTION OF THE HIP

Surgical landmarks include the anterior superior iliac spine, the iliac crest, the inguinal ligament, and the greater trochanter. In an adult, a posterior surgical approach is used. In a child, the approach is anterior because the blood supply is posterosuperior. The trochanteric anastomosis provides the main blood supply for the femoral head. The descending branch of the superior gluteal artery and the ascending branches of the lateral and medial circumflex femoral arteries form the anastomosis near the trochanteric fossa. To use the internervous plane, the interval between the sartorius and tensor fascia femoris must be identified. The superior gluteal nerve supplies the gluteus medius, gluteus minimus, and tensor fasciae latae muscles. The muscular branch of the femoral nerve supplies the pectineus, sartorius, and quadriceps muscles. The rectus femoris muscle has its origin from the anterior inferior iliac spine (straight head) and the acetabular rim (reflected head). A shiny or glistening aponeurosis can be seen superiorly, on the surface of the rectus femoris. The sartorius has its origin from the anterior superior iliac spine. The origin of the tensor fasciae latae is from the anterior iliac crest and anterior superior and anterior inferior iliac spines.

The piriformis muscle is an important landmark for understanding the posterior gluteal region. The origin of the piriformis is from the anterior sacrum and greater sciatic notch. The piriformis inserts onto the upper border of the greater trochanter. The superior gluteal nerve and vessels emerge superior to the upper border of the piriformis. The inferior gluteal nerve and vessels, the pudendal nerve and vessels, the nerve to the obturator internus, and the large sciatic nerve are identified inferior to the lower border of the piriformis. The posterior femoral cutaneous nerve and the nerve to the quadratus femoris are superior and deep, respectively, in relationship to the sciatic nerve. In 85% of cases, the sciatic nerve originates from under the piriformis muscle. The piriformis, the obturator internus, the gemelli, the obturator externus, and the quadratus femoris, as well as the gluteus maximus and adductors, contribute to lateral rotation.

The femoral head is a multiaxial, synovial, ball-and-socket joint. The acetabulum, which provides bony coverage of 40% of the femoral head, has a horseshoe-shaped lunate articular surface. The acetabular fossa lies in the inferomedial portion of the acetabulum. This region is occupied by the pulvinar (fat pad) and round ligament (ligamentum teres). The dense fibrocartilaginous labrum of the acetabulum increases the depth of the acetabular notch. The fovea capitus, a small depression on the medial femoral head, is the site of attachment of the ligamentum teres, which originates in the acetabular fossa. There is no articular cartilage over the fovea capitus. The transverse acetabular ligament bridges the notch at the inferolateral acetabulum. The inelastic fibrous capsule of the hip is reinforced by the iliofemoral, pubofemoral, and ischiofemoral ligaments (thickenings of the hip capsule). Twisting and shortening of the capsule limit full hip extension. The main hip abductors, the gluteus minimus and gluteus medius, insert on the greater trochanter. The iliopsoas tendon, a major hip flexor, passes anterior to the hip joint and attaches to the lesser trochanter.

HIP: CORONAL

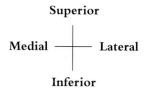

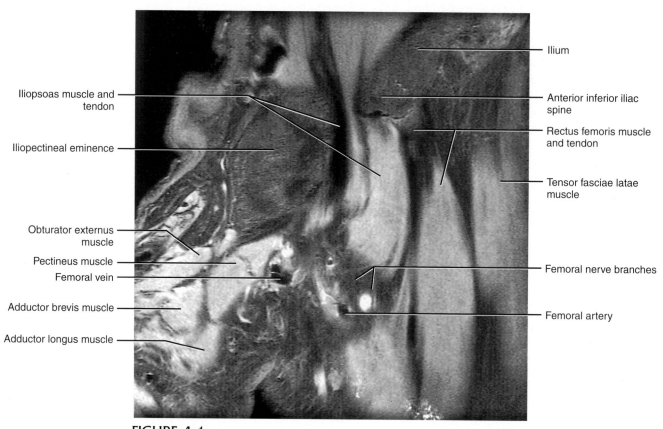

Ilium

Anterior inferior iliac spine

Rectus femoris muscle and tendon

Tensor fasciae latae muscle

Femoral nerve branches

Femoral artery

Iliopsoas muscle and tendon

Iliopectineal eminence

Obturator externus muscle

Pectineus muscle

Femoral vein

Adductor brevis muscle

Adductor longus muscle

FIGURE 4-1

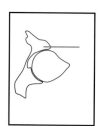

HIP: CORONAL

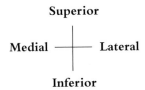

Superior

Medial ——+—— Lateral

Inferior

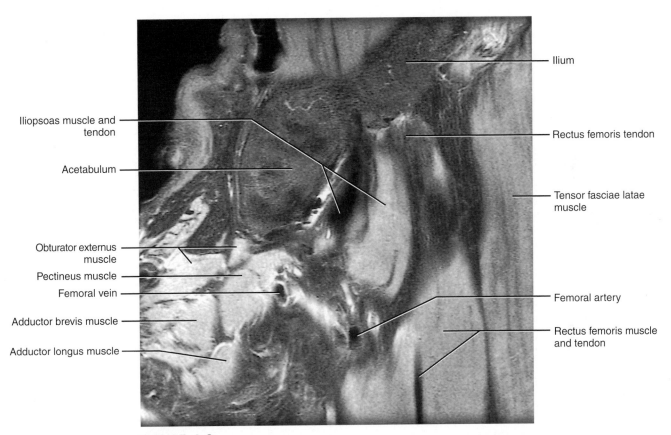

Iliopsoas muscle and tendon

Acetabulum

Obturator externus muscle

Pectineus muscle

Femoral vein

Adductor brevis muscle

Adductor longus muscle

Ilium

Rectus femoris tendon

Tensor fasciae latae muscle

Femoral artery

Rectus femoris muscle and tendon

FIGURE 4-2

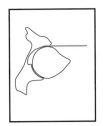

HIP: CORONAL

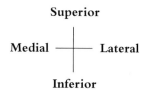

Superior

Medial —┼— Lateral

Inferior

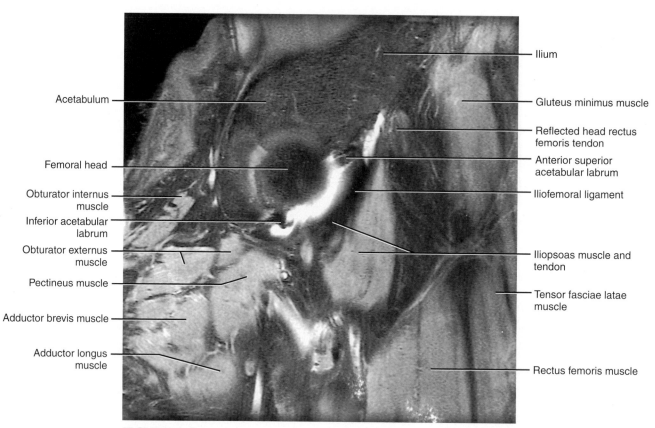

Acetabulum

Femoral head

Obturator internus
muscle

Inferior acetabular
labrum

Obturator externus
muscle

Pectineus muscle

Adductor brevis muscle

Adductor longus
muscle

Ilium

Gluteus minimus muscle

Reflected head rectus
femoris tendon

Anterior superior
acetabular labrum

Iliofemoral ligament

Iliopsoas muscle and
tendon

Tensor fasciae latae
muscle

Rectus femoris muscle

FIGURE 4-3

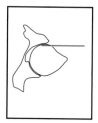

HIP: CORONAL

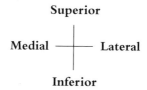

Superior

Medial — Lateral

Inferior

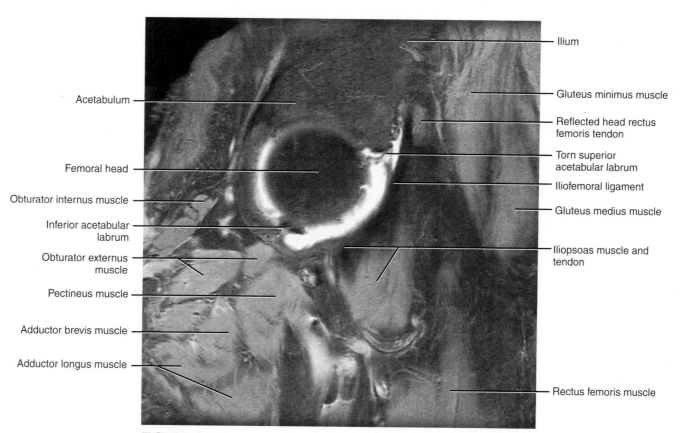

Acetabulum

Femoral head

Obturator internus muscle

Inferior acetabular labrum

Obturator externus muscle

Pectineus muscle

Adductor brevis muscle

Adductor longus muscle

Ilium

Gluteus minimus muscle

Reflected head rectus femoris tendon

Torn superior acetabular labrum

Iliofemoral ligament

Gluteus medius muscle

Iliopsoas muscle and tendon

Rectus femoris muscle

FIGURE 4-4

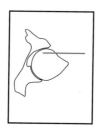

HIP: CORONAL

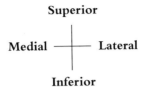

Superior

Medial ——|—— Lateral

Inferior

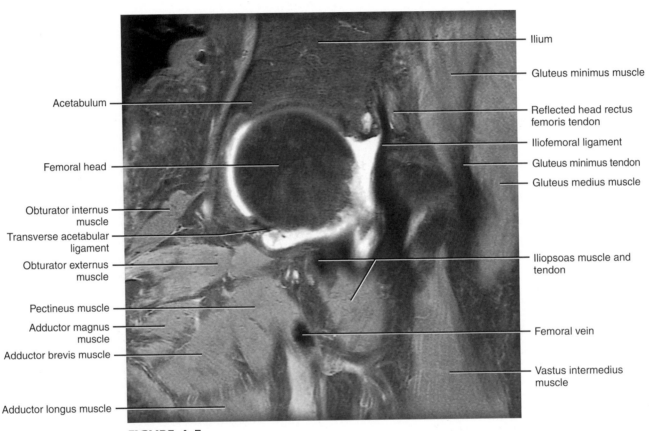

Acetabulum

Femoral head

Obturator internus
muscle

Transverse acetabular
ligament

Obturator externus
muscle

Pectineus muscle

Adductor magnus
muscle

Adductor brevis muscle

Adductor longus muscle

Ilium

Gluteus minimus muscle

Reflected head rectus
femoris tendon

Iliofemoral ligament

Gluteus minimus tendon

Gluteus medius muscle

Iliopsoas muscle and
tendon

Femoral vein

Vastus intermedius
muscle

FIGURE 4-5

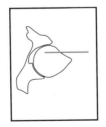

HIP: CORONAL

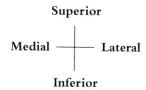

Superior

Medial — | — Lateral

Inferior

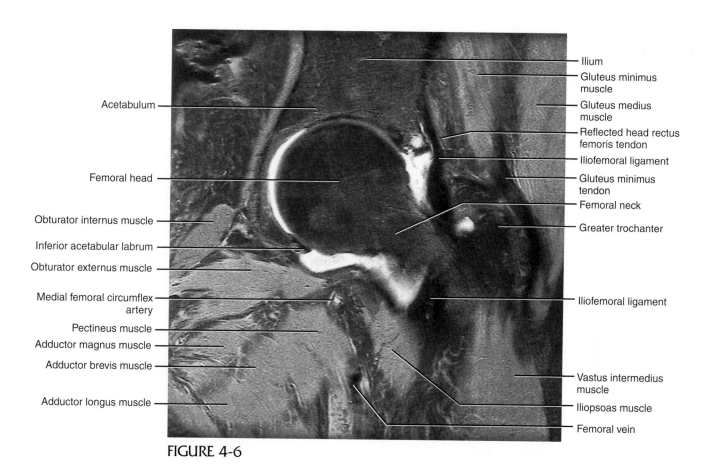

Ilium

Gluteus minimus muscle

Gluteus medius muscle

Reflected head rectus femoris tendon

Iliofemoral ligament

Gluteus minimus tendon

Femoral neck

Greater trochanter

Acetabulum

Femoral head

Obturator internus muscle

Inferior acetabular labrum

Obturator externus muscle

Medial femoral circumflex artery

Pectineus muscle

Adductor magnus muscle

Adductor brevis muscle

Adductor longus muscle

Iliofemoral ligament

Vastus intermedius muscle

Iliopsoas muscle

Femoral vein

FIGURE 4-6

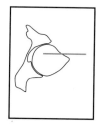

HIP: CORONAL

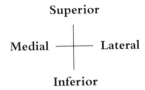

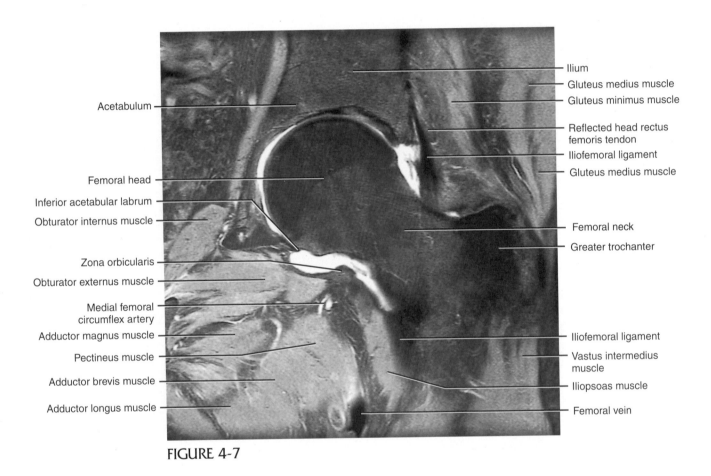

FIGURE 4-7

HIP: CORONAL

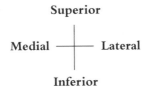

Superior

Medial ——|—— Lateral

Inferior

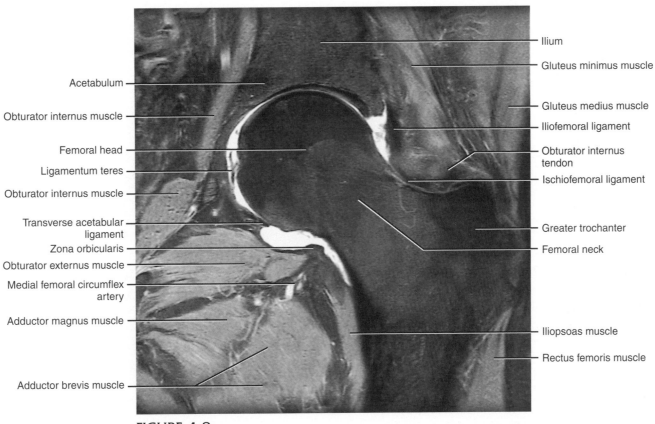

Acetabulum

Obturator internus muscle

Femoral head

Ligamentum teres

Obturator internus muscle

Transverse acetabular ligament

Zona orbicularis

Obturator externus muscle

Medial femoral circumflex artery

Adductor magnus muscle

Adductor brevis muscle

Ilium

Gluteus minimus muscle

Gluteus medius muscle

Iliofemoral ligament

Obturator internus tendon

Ischiofemoral ligament

Greater trochanter

Femoral neck

Iliopsoas muscle

Rectus femoris muscle

FIGURE 4-8

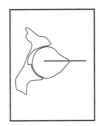

HIP: CORONAL

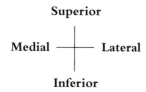

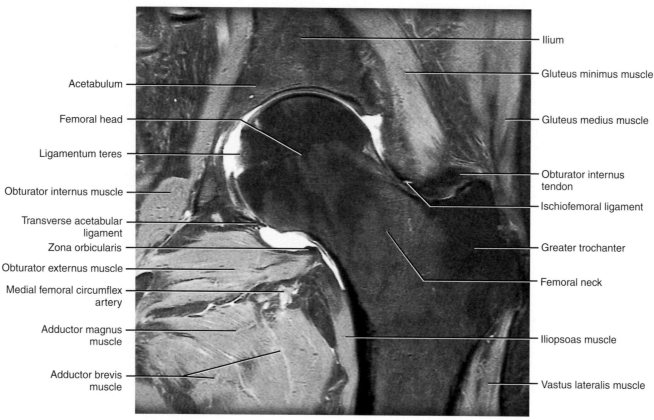

Acetabulum

Femoral head

Ligamentum teres

Obturator internus muscle

Transverse acetabular ligament

Zona orbicularis

Obturator externus muscle

Medial femoral circumflex artery

Adductor magnus muscle

Adductor brevis muscle

Ilium

Gluteus minimus muscle

Gluteus medius muscle

Obturator internus tendon

Ischiofemoral ligament

Greater trochanter

Femoral neck

Iliopsoas muscle

Vastus lateralis muscle

FIGURE 4-9

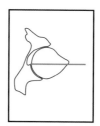

HIP: CORONAL

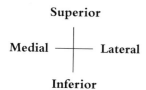

Superior

Medial ──┼── Lateral

Inferior

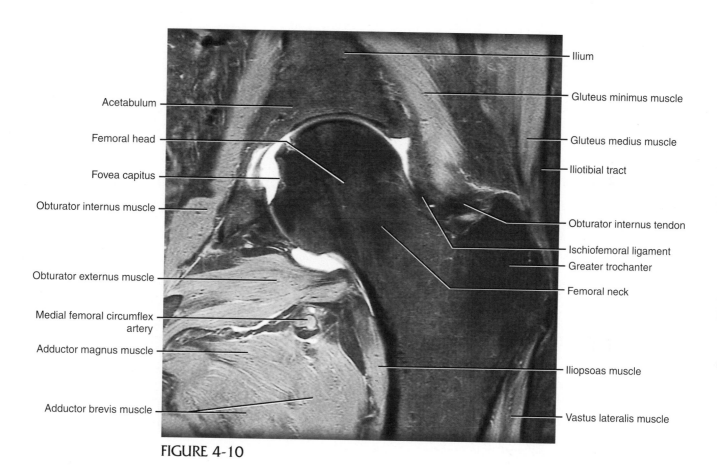

Acetabulum

Femoral head

Fovea capitus

Obturator internus muscle

Obturator externus muscle

Medial femoral circumflex artery

Adductor magnus muscle

Adductor brevis muscle

Ilium

Gluteus minimus muscle

Gluteus medius muscle

Iliotibial tract

Obturator internus tendon

Ischiofemoral ligament

Greater trochanter

Femoral neck

Iliopsoas muscle

Vastus lateralis muscle

FIGURE 4-10

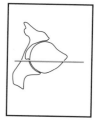

HIP: CORONAL

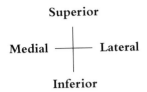

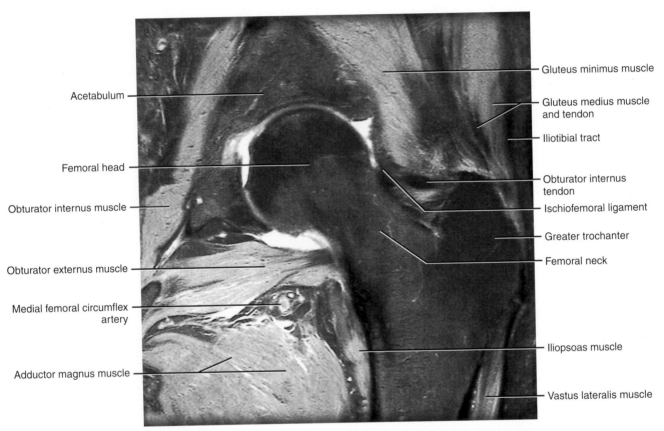

Acetabulum

Femoral head

Obturator internus muscle

Obturator externus muscle

Medial femoral circumflex artery

Adductor magnus muscle

Gluteus minimus muscle

Gluteus medius muscle and tendon

Iliotibial tract

Obturator internus tendon

Ischiofemoral ligament

Greater trochanter

Femoral neck

Iliopsoas muscle

Vastus lateralis muscle

FIGURE 4-11

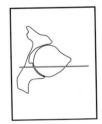

HIP: CORONAL

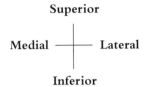

Superior

Medial ——|—— Lateral

Inferior

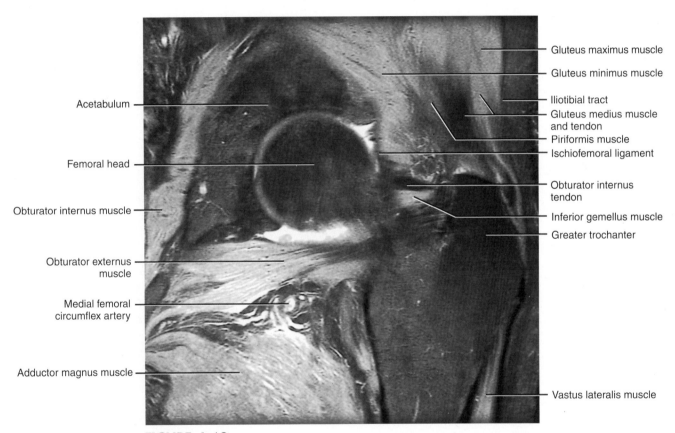

Gluteus maximus muscle

Gluteus minimus muscle

Iliotibial tract

Gluteus medius muscle
and tendon

Piriformis muscle

Ischiofemoral ligament

Obturator internus
tendon

Inferior gemellus muscle

Greater trochanter

Vastus lateralis muscle

Acetabulum

Femoral head

Obturator internus muscle

Obturator externus
muscle

Medial femoral
circumflex artery

Adductor magnus muscle

FIGURE 4-12

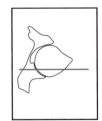

HIP: CORONAL

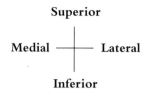

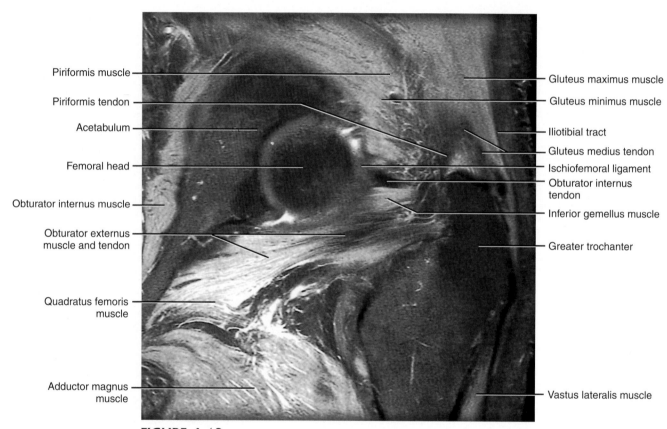

Piriformis muscle — Gluteus maximus muscle

Piriformis tendon — Gluteus minimus muscle

Acetabulum — Iliotibial tract

Femoral head — Gluteus medius tendon

Obturator internus muscle — Ischiofemoral ligament

Obturator externus muscle and tendon — Obturator internus tendon

Quadratus femoris muscle — Inferior gemellus muscle

Adductor magnus muscle — Greater trochanter

Vastus lateralis muscle

FIGURE 4-13

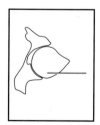

HIP: CORONAL

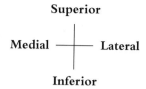

Superior

Medial —|— Lateral

Inferior

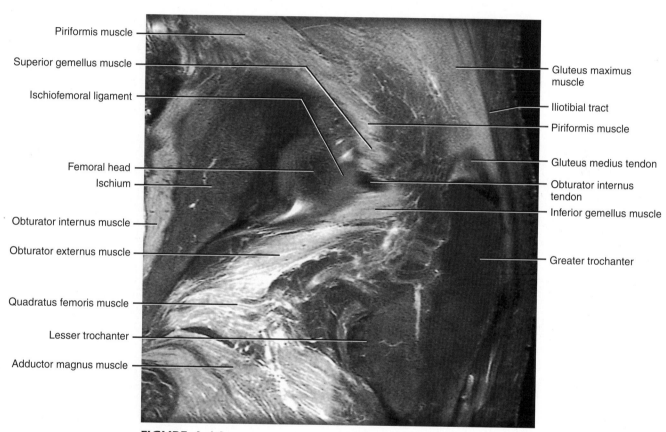

Piriformis muscle

Superior gemellus muscle

Ischiofemoral ligament

Femoral head

Ischium

Obturator internus muscle

Obturator externus muscle

Quadratus femoris muscle

Lesser trochanter

Adductor magnus muscle

Gluteus maximus muscle

Iliotibial tract

Piriformis muscle

Gluteus medius tendon

Obturator internus tendon

Inferior gemellus muscle

Greater trochanter

FIGURE 4-14

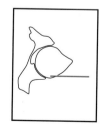

HIP: CORONAL

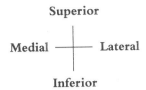

Superior

Medial ——|—— Lateral

Inferior

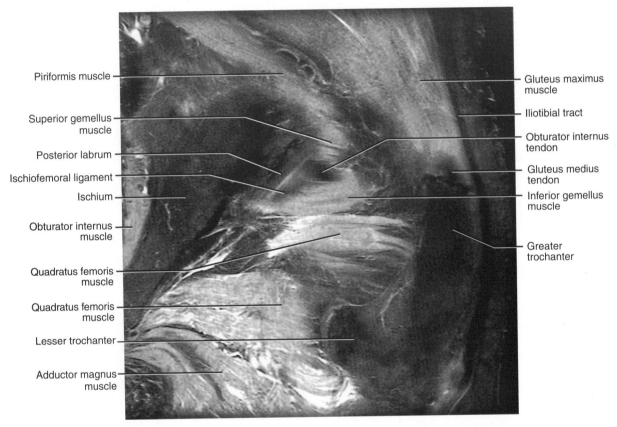

Piriformis muscle

Superior gemellus muscle

Posterior labrum

Ischiofemoral ligament

Ischium

Obturator internus muscle

Quadratus femoris muscle

Quadratus femoris muscle

Lesser trochanter

Adductor magnus muscle

Gluteus maximus muscle

Iliotibial tract

Obturator internus tendon

Gluteus medius tendon

Inferior gemellus muscle

Greater trochanter

FIGURE 4-15

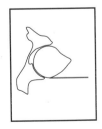

HIP: CORONAL

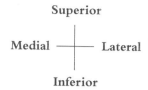

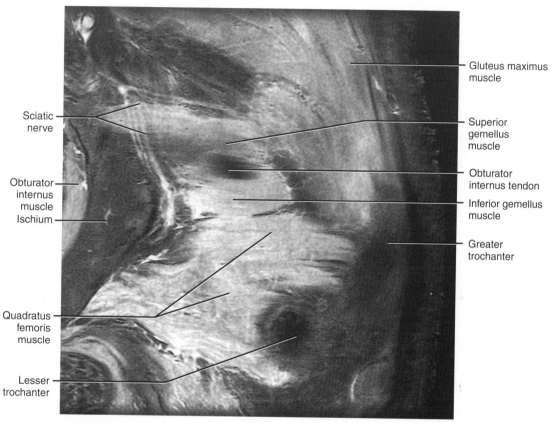

Gluteus maximus
muscle

Sciatic
nerve

Superior
gemellus
muscle

Obturator
internus tendon

Obturator
internus
muscle

Inferior gemellus
muscle

Ischium

Greater
trochanter

Quadratus
femoris
muscle

Lesser
trochanter

FIGURE 4-16

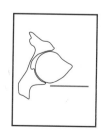

HIP: CORONAL

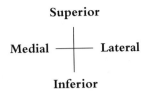

Superior

Medial —┼— Lateral

Inferior

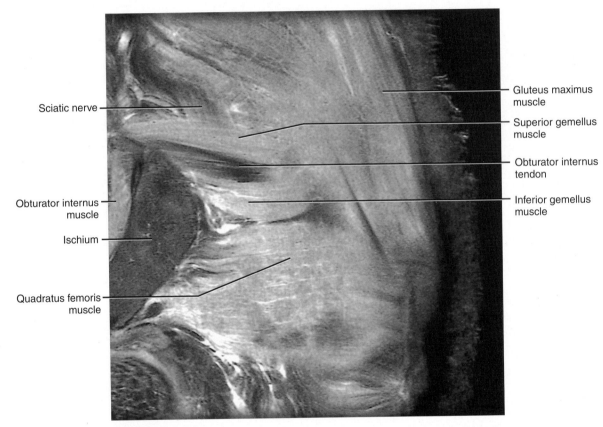

Sciatic nerve

Obturator internus muscle

Ischium

Quadratus femoris muscle

Gluteus maximus muscle

Superior gemellus muscle

Obturator internus tendon

Inferior gemellus muscle

FIGURE 4-17

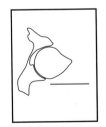

HIP: CORONAL

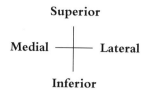

Superior

Medial ─┼─ Lateral

Inferior

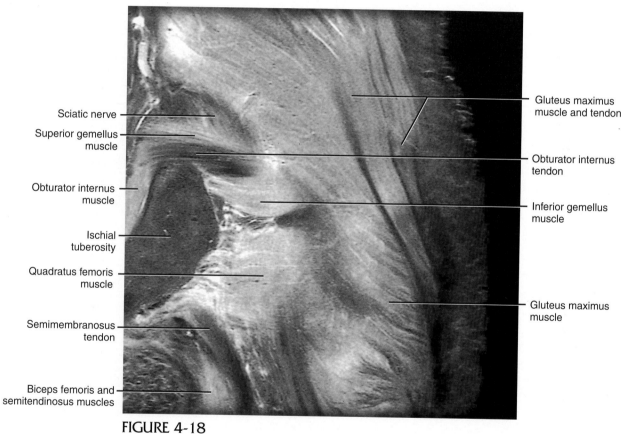

Sciatic nerve

Superior gemellus
muscle

Obturator internus
muscle

Ischial
tuberosity

Quadratus femoris
muscle

Semimembranosus
tendon

Biceps femoris and
semitendinosus muscles

Gluteus maximus
muscle and tendon

Obturator internus
tendon

Inferior gemellus
muscle

Gluteus maximus
muscle

FIGURE 4-18

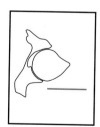

HIP: CORONAL

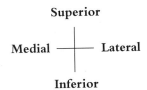

Superior

Medial —— Lateral

Inferior

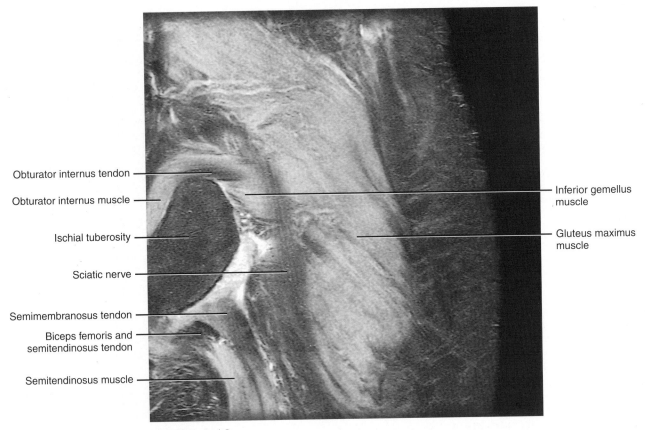

Obturator internus tendon ——

Inferior gemellus
muscle

Obturator internus muscle ——

Ischial tuberosity ——

Gluteus maximus
muscle

Sciatic nerve ——

Semimembranosus tendon ——

Biceps femoris and
semitendinosus tendon ——

Semitendinosus muscle ——

FIGURE 4-19

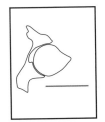

HIP: CORONAL

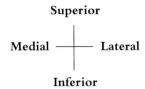

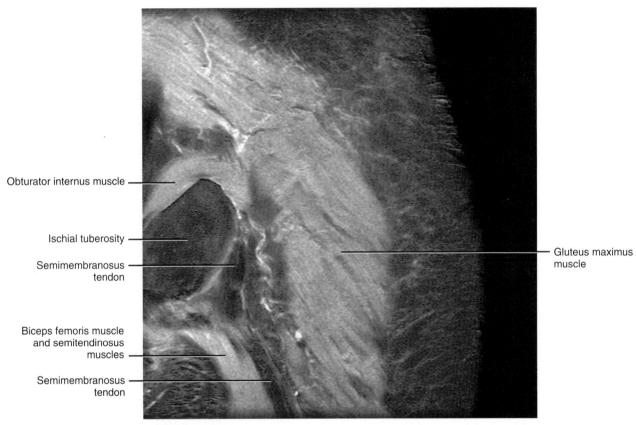

Obturator internus muscle

Ischial tuberosity

Semimembranosus tendon

Biceps femoris muscle and semitendinosus muscles

Semimembranosus tendon

Gluteus maximus muscle

FIGURE 4-20

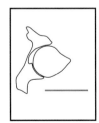

HIP: CORONAL

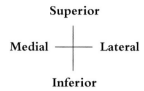

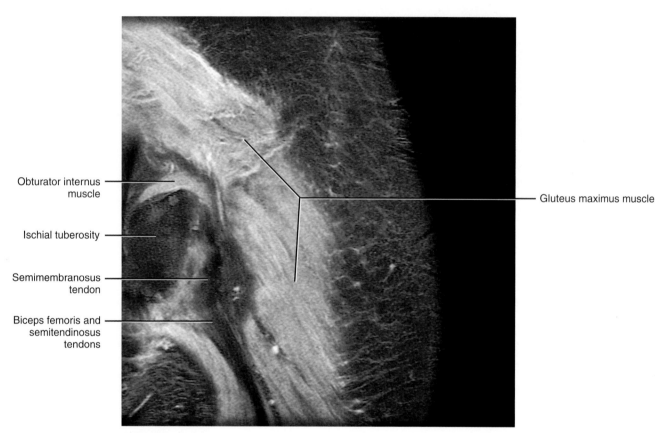

Obturator internus muscle

Ischial tuberosity

Semimembranosus tendon

Biceps femoris and semitendinosus tendons

Gluteus maximus muscle

FIGURE 4-21

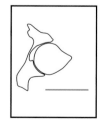

HIP: CORONAL

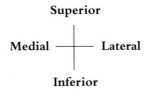

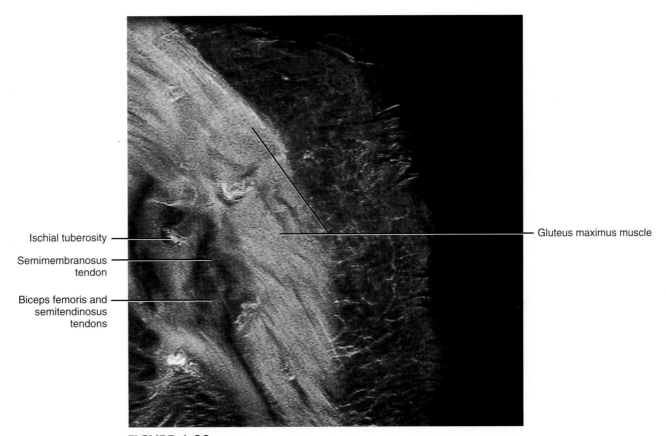

Ischial tuberosity

Semimembranosus tendon

Biceps femoris and semitendinosus tendons

Gluteus maximus muscle

FIGURE 4-22

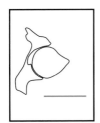

HIP: AXIAL

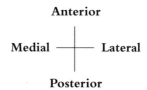

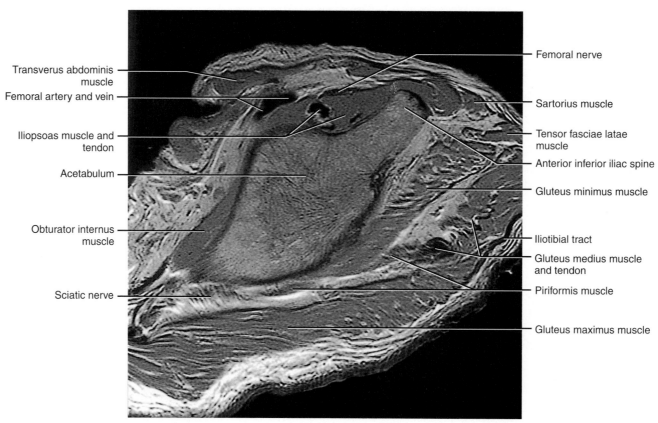

Transverus abdominis muscle

Femoral artery and vein

Iliopsoas muscle and tendon

Acetabulum

Obturator internus muscle

Sciatic nerve

Femoral nerve

Sartorius muscle

Tensor fasciae latae muscle

Anterior inferior iliac spine

Gluteus minimus muscle

Iliotibial tract

Gluteus medius muscle and tendon

Piriformis muscle

Gluteus maximus muscle

FIGURE 4-23

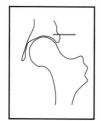

HIP: AXIAL

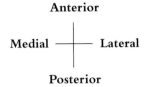

Anterior

Medial ——|—— Lateral

Posterior

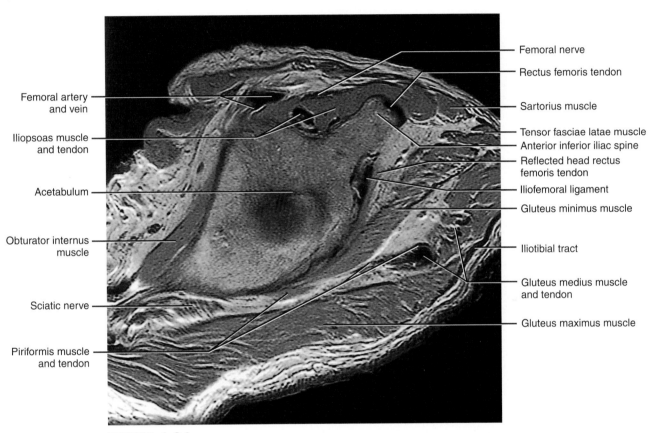

Femoral artery
and vein

Iliopsoas muscle
and tendon

Acetabulum

Obturator internus
muscle

Sciatic nerve

Piriformis muscle
and tendon

Femoral nerve

Rectus femoris tendon

Sartorius muscle

Tensor fasciae latae muscle

Anterior inferior iliac spine

Reflected head rectus
femoris tendon

Iliofemoral ligament

Gluteus minimus muscle

Iliotibial tract

Gluteus medius muscle
and tendon

Gluteus maximus muscle

FIGURE 4-24

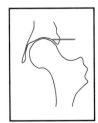

HIP: AXIAL

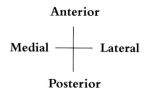

Anterior

Medial ——+—— Lateral

Posterior

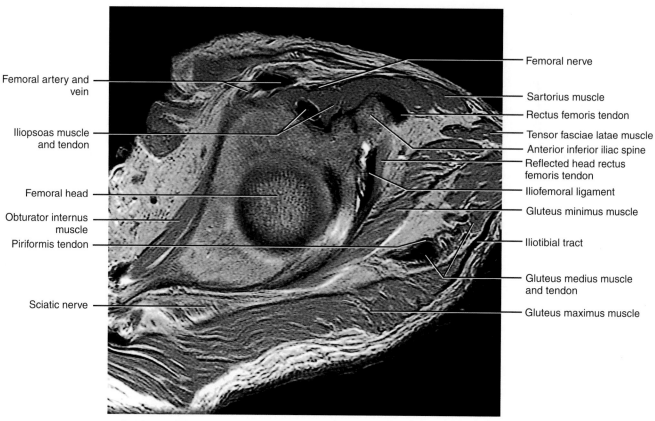

Femoral artery and vein

Iliopsoas muscle and tendon

Femoral head

Obturator internus muscle

Piriformis tendon

Sciatic nerve

Femoral nerve

Sartorius muscle

Rectus femoris tendon

Tensor fasciae latae muscle

Anterior inferior iliac spine

Reflected head rectus femoris tendon

Iliofemoral ligament

Gluteus minimus muscle

Iliotibial tract

Gluteus medius muscle and tendon

Gluteus maximus muscle

FIGURE 4-25

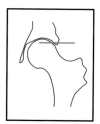

HIP: AXIAL

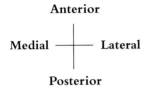

Anterior

Medial —|— Lateral

Posterior

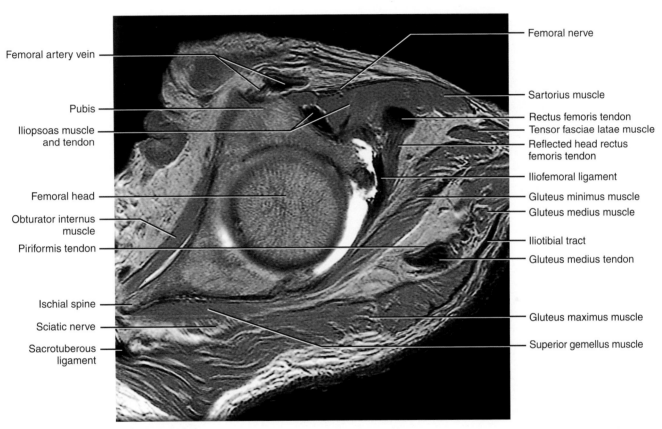

Femoral artery vein

Pubis

Iliopsoas muscle
and tendon

Femoral head

Obturator internus
muscle

Piriformis tendon

Ischial spine

Sciatic nerve

Sacrotuberous
ligament

Femoral nerve

Sartorius muscle

Rectus femoris tendon

Tensor fasciae latae muscle

Reflected head rectus
femoris tendon

Iliofemoral ligament

Gluteus minimus muscle

Gluteus medius muscle

Iliotibial tract

Gluteus medius tendon

Gluteus maximus muscle

Superior gemellus muscle

FIGURE 4-26

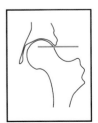

HIP: AXIAL

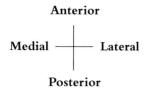

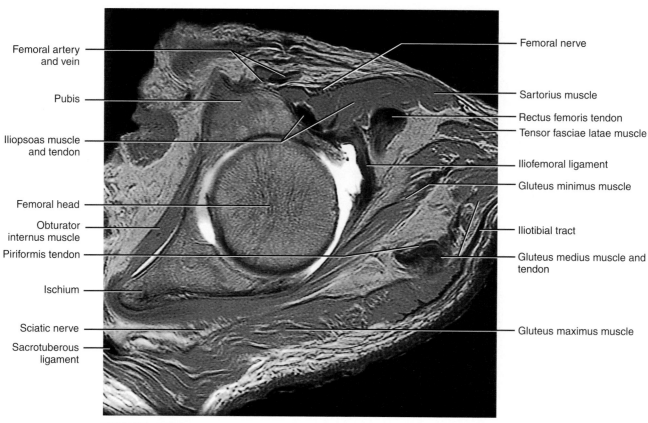

FIGURE 4-27

Femoral artery and vein

Pubis

Iliopsoas muscle and tendon

Femoral head

Obturator internus muscle

Piriformis tendon

Ischium

Sciatic nerve

Sacrotuberous ligament

Femoral nerve

Sartorius muscle

Rectus femoris tendon

Tensor fasciae latae muscle

Iliofemoral ligament

Gluteus minimus muscle

Iliotibial tract

Gluteus medius muscle and tendon

Gluteus maximus muscle

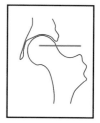

HIP: AXIAL

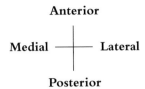

Anterior

Medial ── Lateral

Posterior

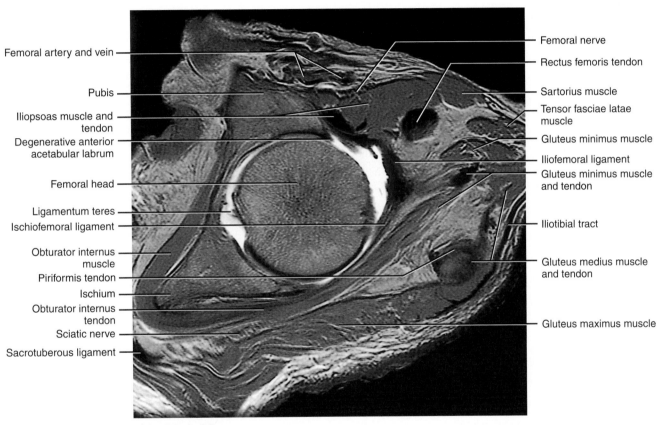

Femoral artery and vein

Pubis

Iliopsoas muscle and tendon

Degenerative anterior acetabular labrum

Femoral head

Ligamentum teres

Ischiofemoral ligament

Obturator internus muscle

Piriformis tendon

Ischium

Obturator internus tendon

Sciatic nerve

Sacrotuberous ligament

Femoral nerve

Rectus femoris tendon

Sartorius muscle

Tensor fasciae latae muscle

Gluteus minimus muscle

Iliofemoral ligament

Gluteus minimus muscle and tendon

Iliotibial tract

Gluteus medius muscle and tendon

Gluteus maximus muscle

FIGURE 4-28

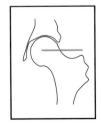

HIP: AXIAL

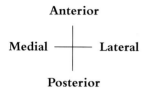

Anterior

Medial ─── Lateral

Posterior

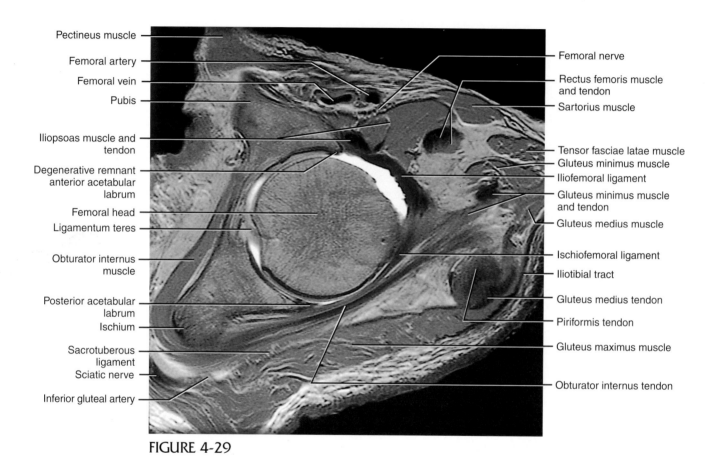

Pectineus muscle

Femoral artery

Femoral vein

Pubis

Iliopsoas muscle and tendon

Degenerative remnant anterior acetabular labrum

Femoral head

Ligamentum teres

Obturator internus muscle

Posterior acetabular labrum

Ischium

Sacrotuberous ligament

Sciatic nerve

Inferior gluteal artery

Femoral nerve

Rectus femoris muscle and tendon

Sartorius muscle

Tensor fasciae latae muscle

Gluteus minimus muscle

Iliofemoral ligament

Gluteus minimus muscle and tendon

Gluteus medius muscle

Ischiofemoral ligament

Iliotibial tract

Gluteus medius tendon

Piriformis tendon

Gluteus maximus muscle

Obturator internus tendon

FIGURE 4-29

HIP: AXIAL

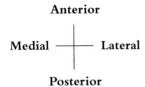

Anterior

Medial ——|—— **Lateral**

Posterior

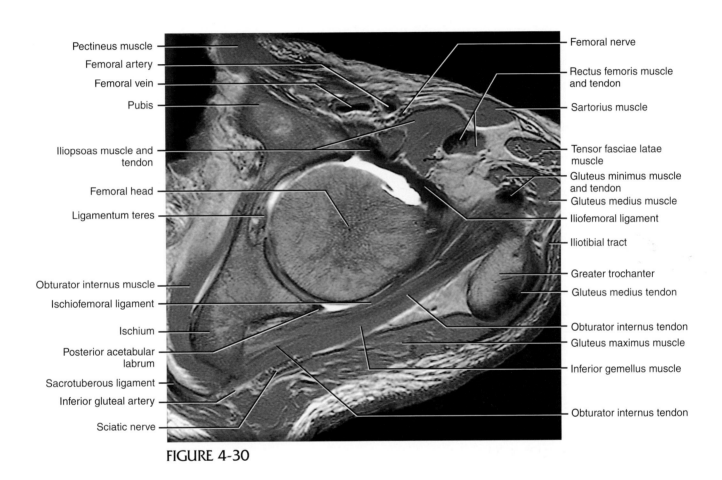

Pectineus muscle

Femoral artery

Femoral vein

Pubis

Iliopsoas muscle and tendon

Femoral head

Ligamentum teres

Obturator internus muscle

Ischiofemoral ligament

Ischium

Posterior acetabular labrum

Sacrotuberous ligament

Inferior gluteal artery

Sciatic nerve

Femoral nerve

Rectus femoris muscle and tendon

Sartorius muscle

Tensor fasciae latae muscle

Gluteus minimus muscle and tendon

Gluteus medius muscle

Iliofemoral ligament

Iliotibial tract

Greater trochanter

Gluteus medius tendon

Obturator internus tendon

Gluteus maximus muscle

Inferior gemellus muscle

Obturator internus tendon

FIGURE 4-30

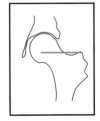

HIP: AXIAL

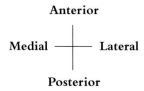

Anterior

Medial ——┼—— Lateral

Posterior

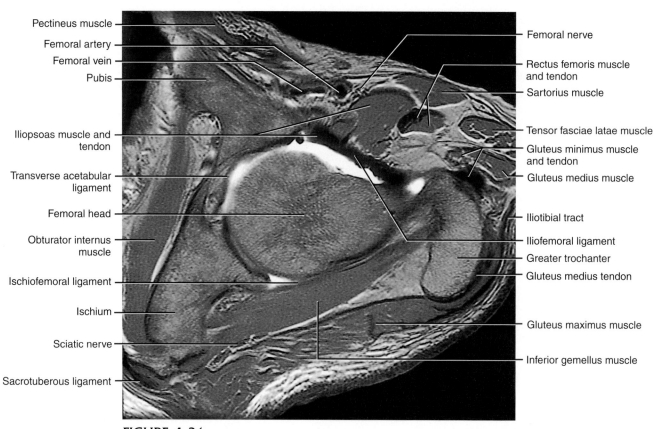

Pectineus muscle

Femoral artery

Femoral vein

Pubis

Iliopsoas muscle and tendon

Transverse acetabular ligament

Femoral head

Obturator internus muscle

Ischiofemoral ligament

Ischium

Sciatic nerve

Sacrotuberous ligament

Femoral nerve

Rectus femoris muscle and tendon

Sartorius muscle

Tensor fasciae latae muscle

Gluteus minimus muscle and tendon

Gluteus medius muscle

Iliotibial tract

Iliofemoral ligament

Greater trochanter

Gluteus medius tendon

Gluteus maximus muscle

Inferior gemellus muscle

FIGURE 4-31

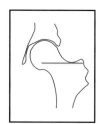

HIP: AXIAL

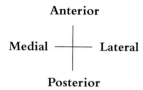

Anterior

Medial —|— Lateral

Posterior

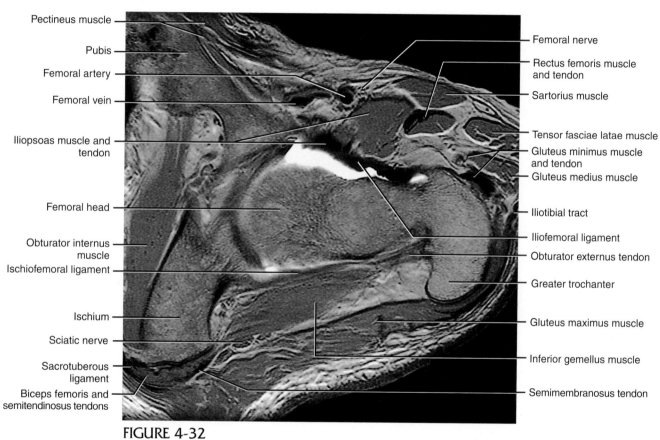

Pectineus muscle

Pubis

Femoral artery

Femoral vein

Iliopsoas muscle and tendon

Femoral head

Obturator internus muscle

Ischiofemoral ligament

Ischium

Sciatic nerve

Sacrotuberous ligament

Biceps femoris and semitendinosus tendons

Femoral nerve

Rectus femoris muscle and tendon

Sartorius muscle

Tensor fasciae latae muscle

Gluteus minimus muscle and tendon

Gluteus medius muscle

Iliotibial tract

Iliofemoral ligament

Obturator externus tendon

Greater trochanter

Gluteus maximus muscle

Inferior gemellus muscle

Semimembranosus tendon

FIGURE 4-32

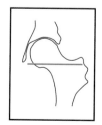

HIP: AXIAL

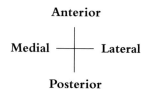

Anterior

Medial —|— Lateral

Posterior

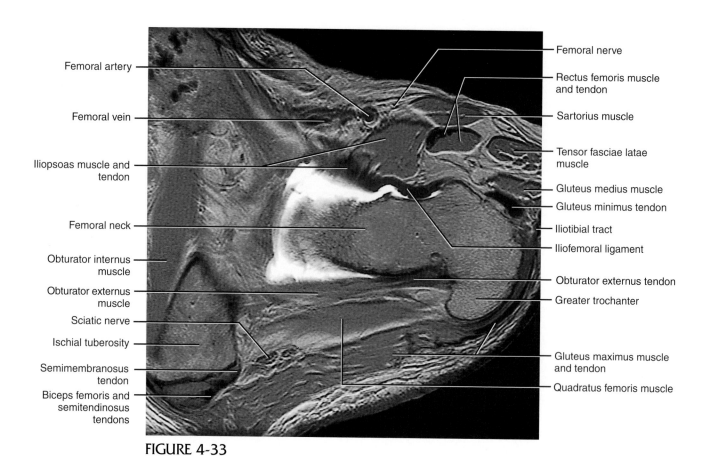

Femoral artery

Femoral vein

Iliopsoas muscle and tendon

Femoral neck

Obturator internus muscle

Obturator externus muscle

Sciatic nerve

Ischial tuberosity

Semimembranosus tendon

Biceps femoris and semitendinosus tendons

Femoral nerve

Rectus femoris muscle and tendon

Sartorius muscle

Tensor fasciae latae muscle

Gluteus medius muscle

Gluteus minimus tendon

Iliotibial tract

Iliofemoral ligament

Obturator externus tendon

Greater trochanter

Gluteus maximus muscle and tendon

Quadratus femoris muscle

FIGURE 4-33

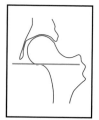

HIP: AXIAL

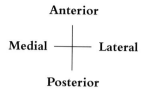

Anterior
Medial — Lateral
Posterior

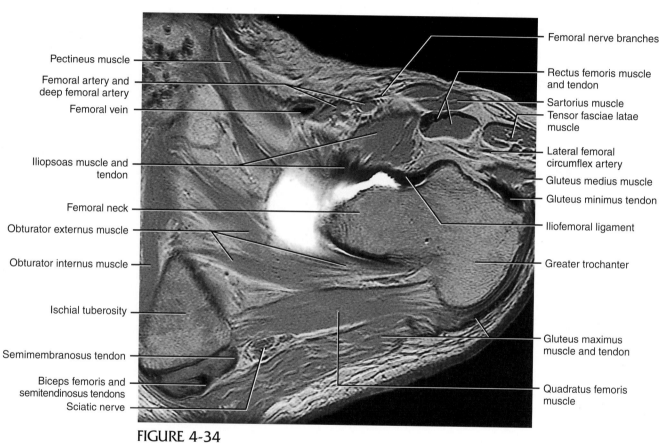

Pectineus muscle

Femoral artery and
deep femoral artery

Femoral vein

Iliopsoas muscle and
tendon

Femoral neck

Obturator externus muscle

Obturator internus muscle

Ischial tuberosity

Semimembranosus tendon

Biceps femoris and
semitendinosus tendons
Sciatic nerve

Femoral nerve branches

Rectus femoris muscle
and tendon

Sartorius muscle
Tensor fasciae latae
muscle

Lateral femoral
circumflex artery

Gluteus medius muscle

Gluteus minimus tendon

Iliofemoral ligament

Greater trochanter

Gluteus maximus
muscle and tendon

Quadratus femoris
muscle

FIGURE 4-34

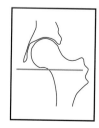

HIP: AXIAL

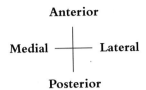

Anterior

Medial — Lateral

Posterior

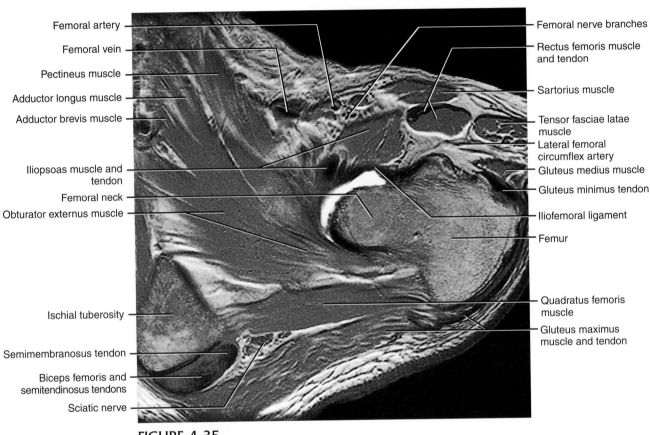

Femoral artery

Femoral vein

Pectineus muscle

Adductor longus muscle

Adductor brevis muscle

Iliopsoas muscle and tendon

Femoral neck

Obturator externus muscle

Ischial tuberosity

Semimembranosus tendon

Biceps femoris and semitendinosus tendons

Sciatic nerve

Femoral nerve branches

Rectus femoris muscle and tendon

Sartorius muscle

Tensor fasciae latae muscle

Lateral femoral circumflex artery

Gluteus medius muscle

Gluteus minimus tendon

Iliofemoral ligament

Femur

Quadratus femoris muscle

Gluteus maximus muscle and tendon

FIGURE 4-35

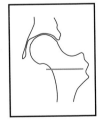

HIP: AXIAL

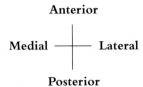

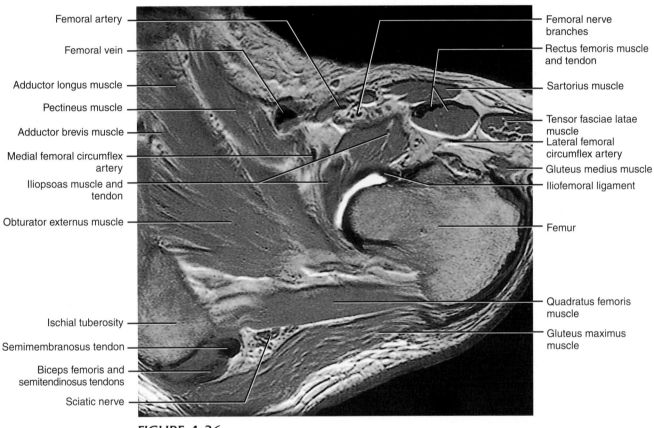

Label (left)		Label (right)

Femoral artery

Femoral vein

Adductor longus muscle

Pectineus muscle

Adductor brevis muscle

Medial femoral circumflex artery

Iliopsoas muscle and tendon

Obturator externus muscle

Ischial tuberosity

Semimembranosus tendon

Biceps femoris and semitendinosus tendons

Sciatic nerve

Femoral nerve branches

Rectus femoris muscle and tendon

Sartorius muscle

Tensor fasciae latae muscle

Lateral femoral circumflex artery

Gluteus medius muscle

Iliofemoral ligament

Femur

Quadratus femoris muscle

Gluteus maximus muscle

FIGURE 4-36

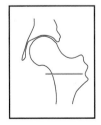

HIP: SAGITTAL

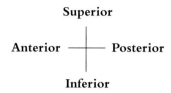

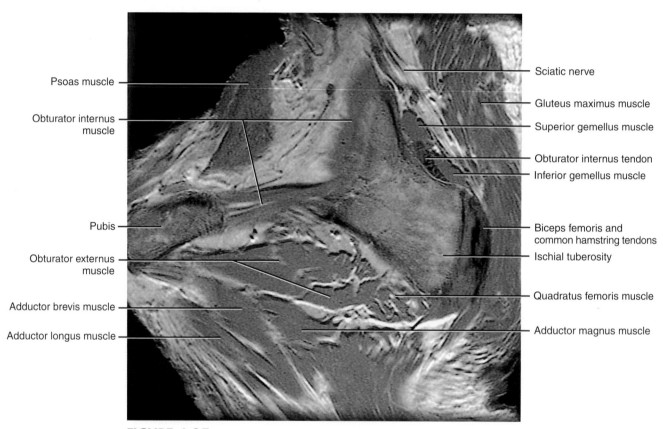

Psoas muscle

Obturator internus muscle

Pubis

Obturator externus muscle

Adductor brevis muscle

Adductor longus muscle

Sciatic nerve

Gluteus maximus muscle

Superior gemellus muscle

Obturator internus tendon

Inferior gemellus muscle

Biceps femoris and common hamstring tendons

Ischial tuberosity

Quadratus femoris muscle

Adductor magnus muscle

FIGURE 4-37

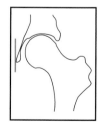

HIP: SAGITTAL

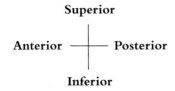

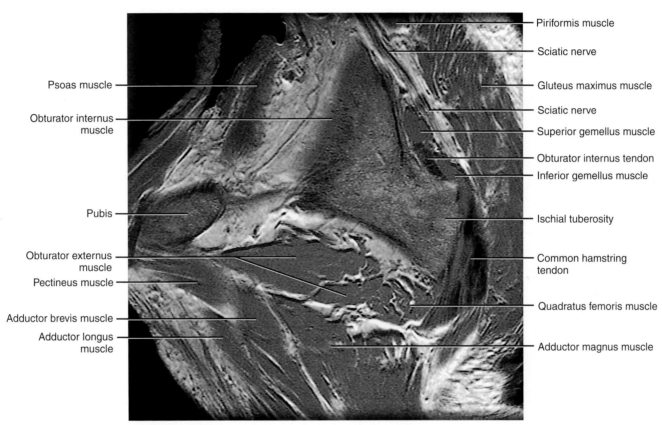

Piriformis muscle

Sciatic nerve

Psoas muscle

Gluteus maximus muscle

Sciatic nerve

Obturator internus
muscle

Superior gemellus muscle

Obturator internus tendon

Inferior gemellus muscle

Pubis

Ischial tuberosity

Obturator externus
muscle

Common hamstring
tendon

Pectineus muscle

Quadratus femoris muscle

Adductor brevis muscle

Adductor longus
muscle

Adductor magnus muscle

FIGURE 4-38

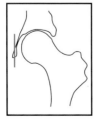

HIP: SAGITTAL

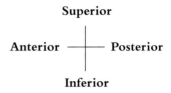

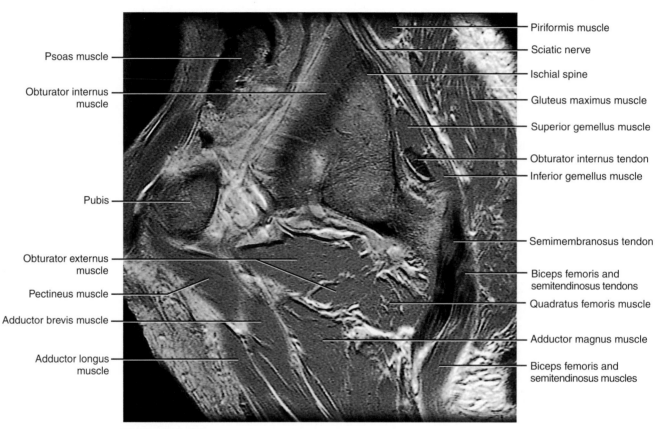

Psoas muscle

Obturator internus muscle

Pubis

Obturator externus muscle

Pectineus muscle

Adductor brevis muscle

Adductor longus muscle

Piriformis muscle

Sciatic nerve

Ischial spine

Gluteus maximus muscle

Superior gemellus muscle

Obturator internus tendon

Inferior gemellus muscle

Semimembranosus tendon

Biceps femoris and semitendinosus tendons

Quadratus femoris muscle

Adductor magnus muscle

Biceps femoris and semitendinosus muscles

FIGURE 4-39

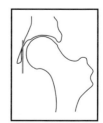

HIP: SAGITTAL

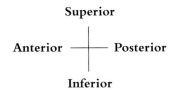

Superior

Anterior ——+—— Posterior

Inferior

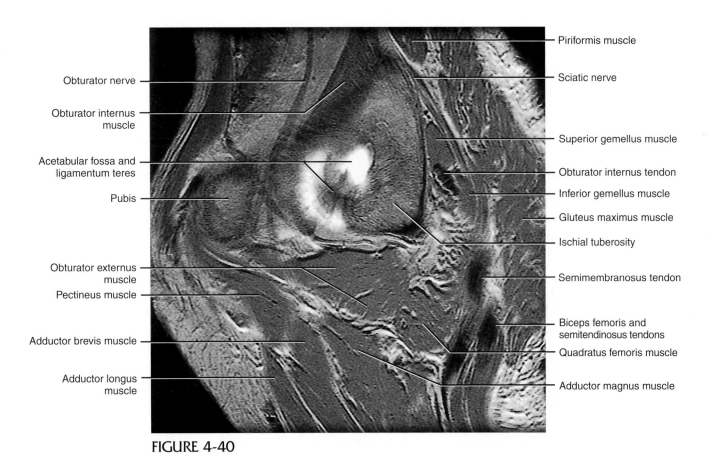

Obturator nerve

Obturator internus muscle

Acetabular fossa and ligamentum teres

Pubis

Obturator externus muscle

Pectineus muscle

Adductor brevis muscle

Adductor longus muscle

Piriformis muscle

Sciatic nerve

Superior gemellus muscle

Obturator internus tendon

Inferior gemellus muscle

Gluteus maximus muscle

Ischial tuberosity

Semimembranosus tendon

Biceps femoris and semitendinosus tendons

Quadratus femoris muscle

Adductor magnus muscle

FIGURE 4-40

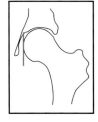

HIP: SAGITTAL

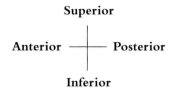

Superior

Anterior —— Posterior

Inferior

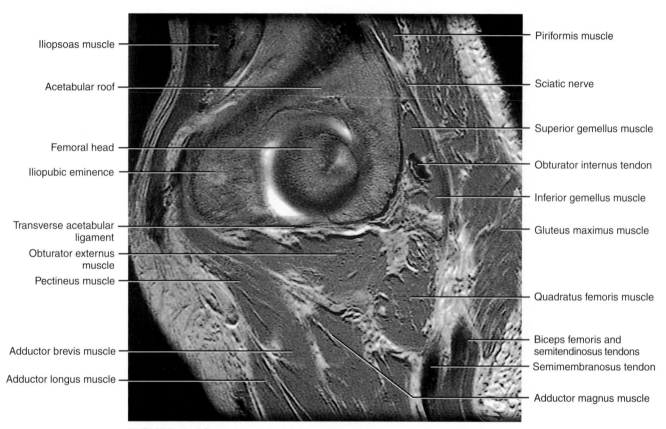

Iliopsoas muscle

Acetabular roof

Femoral head

Iliopubic eminence

Transverse acetabular ligament

Obturator externus muscle

Pectineus muscle

Adductor brevis muscle

Adductor longus muscle

Piriformis muscle

Sciatic nerve

Superior gemellus muscle

Obturator internus tendon

Inferior gemellus muscle

Gluteus maximus muscle

Quadratus femoris muscle

Biceps femoris and semitendinosus tendons

Semimembranosus tendon

Adductor magnus muscle

FIGURE 4-41

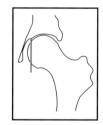

HIP: SAGITTAL

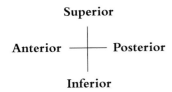

Superior

Anterior ——|—— Posterior

Inferior

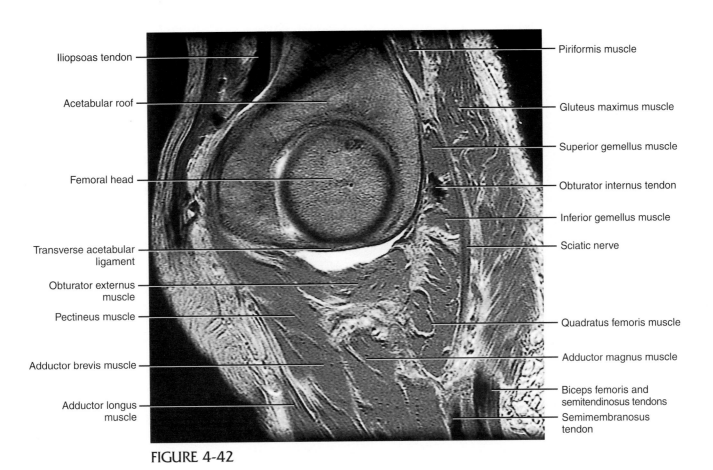

Iliopsoas tendon

Acetabular roof

Femoral head

Transverse acetabular ligament

Obturator externus muscle

Pectineus muscle

Adductor brevis muscle

Adductor longus muscle

Piriformis muscle

Gluteus maximus muscle

Superior gemellus muscle

Obturator internus tendon

Inferior gemellus muscle

Sciatic nerve

Quadratus femoris muscle

Adductor magnus muscle

Biceps femoris and semitendinosus tendons

Semimembranosus tendon

FIGURE 4-42

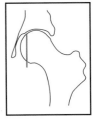

HIP: SAGITTAL

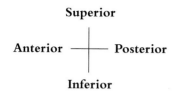

Superior

Anterior —|— Posterior

Inferior

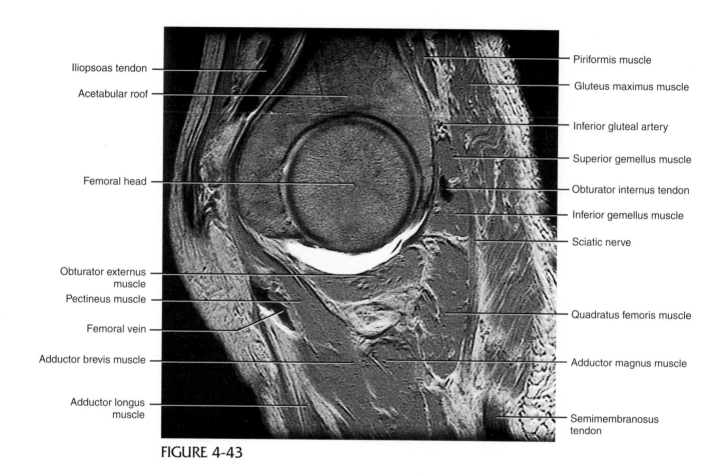

Iliopsoas tendon

Acetabular roof

Femoral head

Obturator externus muscle

Pectineus muscle

Femoral vein

Adductor brevis muscle

Adductor longus muscle

Piriformis muscle

Gluteus maximus muscle

Inferior gluteal artery

Superior gemellus muscle

Obturator internus tendon

Inferior gemellus muscle

Sciatic nerve

Quadratus femoris muscle

Adductor magnus muscle

Semimembranosus tendon

FIGURE 4-43

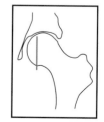

HIP: SAGITTAL

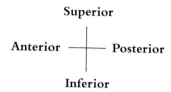

Superior

Anterior ——|—— Posterior

Inferior

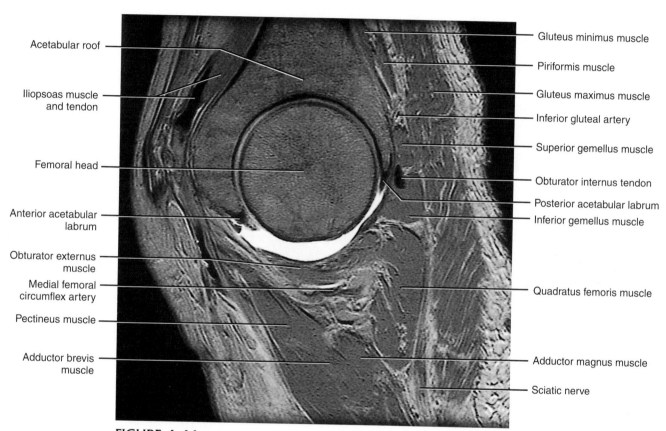

Acetabular roof

Iliopsoas muscle
and tendon

Femoral head

Anterior acetabular
labrum

Obturator externus
muscle

Medial femoral
circumflex artery

Pectineus muscle

Adductor brevis
muscle

Gluteus minimus muscle

Piriformis muscle

Gluteus maximus muscle

Inferior gluteal artery

Superior gemellus muscle

Obturator internus tendon

Posterior acetabular labrum

Inferior gemellus muscle

Quadratus femoris muscle

Adductor magnus muscle

Sciatic nerve

FIGURE 4-44

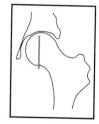

HIP: SAGITTAL

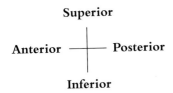

Iliopsoas muscle

Acetabular roof

Femoral head

Anterior acetabular labrum

Femoral nerve

Obturator externus tendon

Medial femoral circumflex artery

Deep femoral artery and vein

Pectineus muscle

Adductor brevis muscle

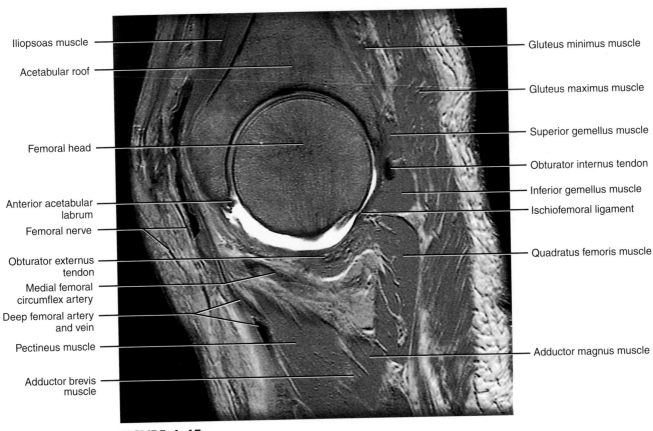

Gluteus minimus muscle

Gluteus maximus muscle

Superior gemellus muscle

Obturator internus tendon

Inferior gemellus muscle

Ischiofemoral ligament

Quadratus femoris muscle

Adductor magnus muscle

FIGURE 4-45

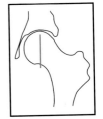

HIP: SAGITTAL

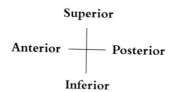

Superior

Anterior —|— Posterior

Inferior

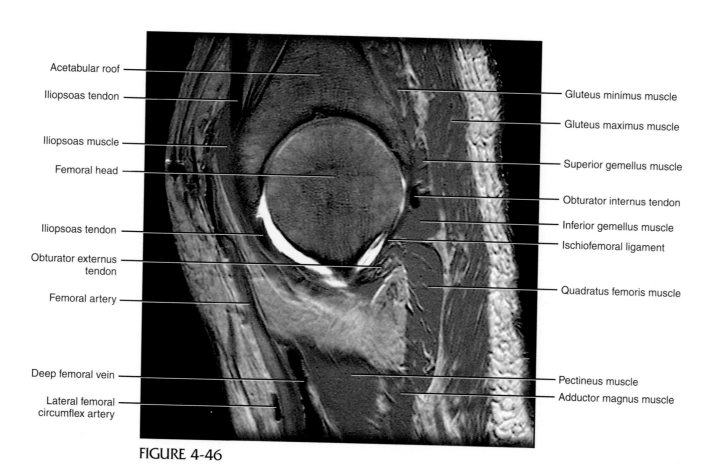

Acetabular roof

Iliopsoas tendon

Iliopsoas muscle

Femoral head

Iliopsoas tendon

Obturator externus tendon

Femoral artery

Deep femoral vein

Lateral femoral circumflex artery

Gluteus minimus muscle

Gluteus maximus muscle

Superior gemellus muscle

Obturator internus tendon

Inferior gemellus muscle

Ischiofemoral ligament

Quadratus femoris muscle

Pectineus muscle

Adductor magnus muscle

FIGURE 4-46

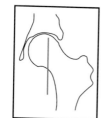

HIP: SAGITTAL

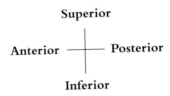

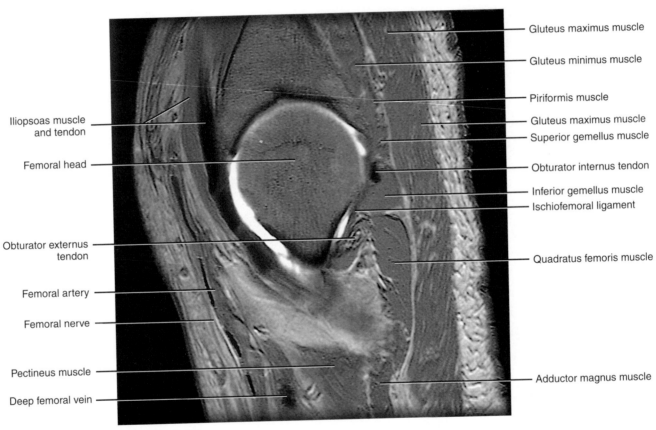

Iliopsoas muscle and tendon

Femoral head

Obturator externus tendon

Femoral artery

Femoral nerve

Pectineus muscle

Deep femoral vein

Gluteus maximus muscle

Gluteus minimus muscle

Piriformis muscle

Gluteus maximus muscle

Superior gemellus muscle

Obturator internus tendon

Inferior gemellus muscle

Ischiofemoral ligament

Quadratus femoris muscle

Adductor magnus muscle

FIGURE 4-47

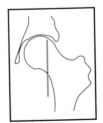

HIP: SAGITTAL

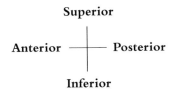

Superior

Anterior ——|—— Posterior

Inferior

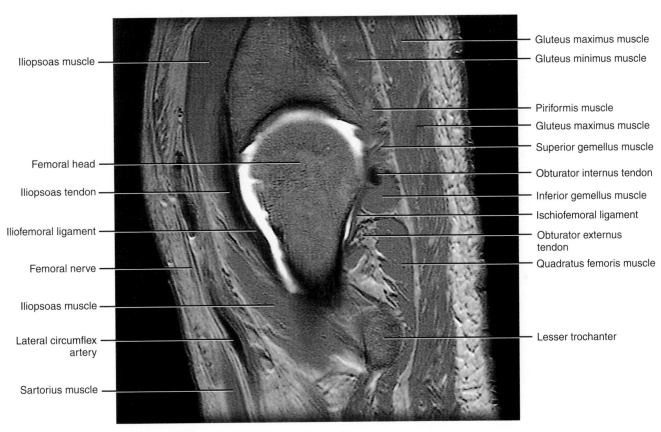

Iliopsoas muscle

Femoral head

Iliopsoas tendon

Iliofemoral ligament

Femoral nerve

Iliopsoas muscle

Lateral circumflex artery

Sartorius muscle

Gluteus maximus muscle

Gluteus minimus muscle

Piriformis muscle

Gluteus maximus muscle

Superior gemellus muscle

Obturator internus tendon

Inferior gemellus muscle

Ischiofemoral ligament

Obturator externus tendon

Quadratus femoris muscle

Lesser trochanter

FIGURE 4-48

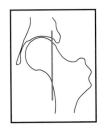

HIP: SAGITTAL

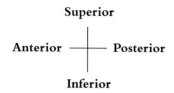

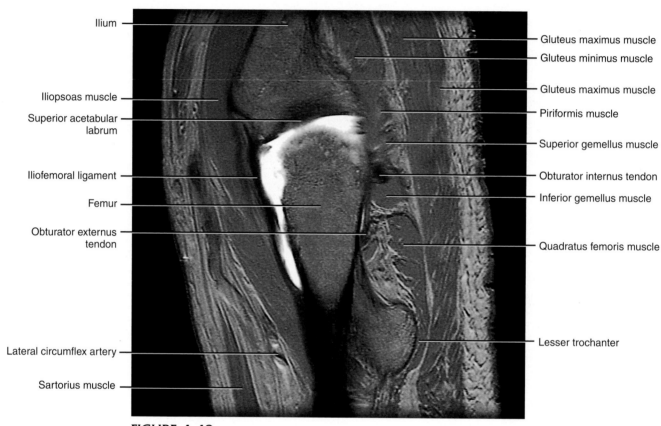

Ilium

Iliopsoas muscle

Superior acetabular labrum

Iliofemoral ligament

Femur

Obturator externus tendon

Lateral circumflex artery

Sartorius muscle

Gluteus maximus muscle

Gluteus minimus muscle

Gluteus maximus muscle

Piriformis muscle

Superior gemellus muscle

Obturator internus tendon

Inferior gemellus muscle

Quadratus femoris muscle

Lesser trochanter

FIGURE 4-49

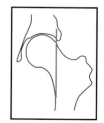

HIP: SAGITTAL

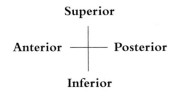

Superior

Anterior ——+—— Posterior

Inferior

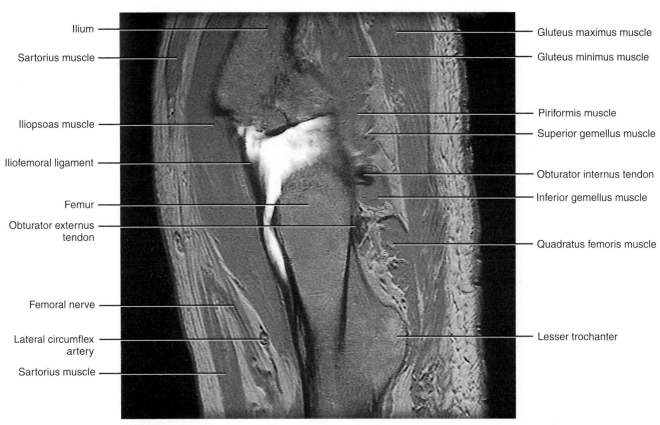

Ilium

Sartorius muscle

Iliopsoas muscle

Iliofemoral ligament

Femur

Obturator externus tendon

Femoral nerve

Lateral circumflex artery

Sartorius muscle

Gluteus maximus muscle

Gluteus minimus muscle

Piriformis muscle

Superior gemellus muscle

Obturator internus tendon

Inferior gemellus muscle

Quadratus femoris muscle

Lesser trochanter

FIGURE 4-50

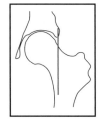

HIP: SAGITTAL

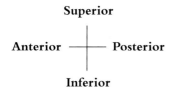

Superior

Anterior ——|—— Posterior

Inferior

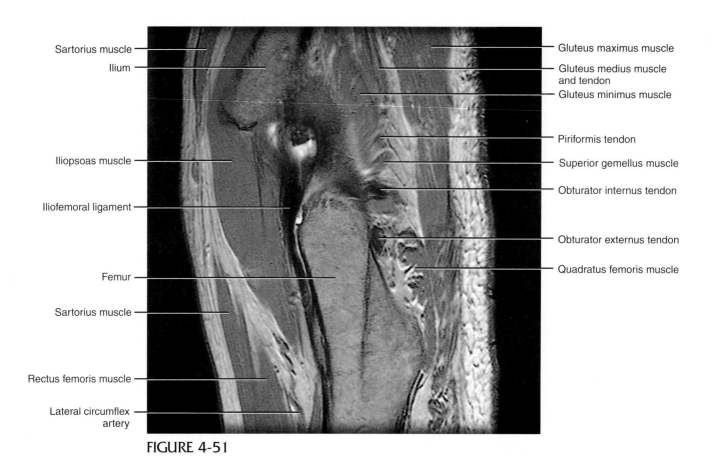

Sartorius muscle

Ilium

Iliopsoas muscle

Iliofemoral ligament

Femur

Sartorius muscle

Rectus femoris muscle

Lateral circumflex artery

Gluteus maximus muscle

Gluteus medius muscle and tendon

Gluteus minimus muscle

Piriformis tendon

Superior gemellus muscle

Obturator internus tendon

Obturator externus tendon

Quadratus femoris muscle

FIGURE 4-51

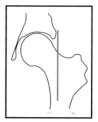

HIP: SAGITTAL

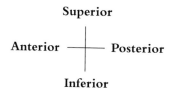

Superior

Anterior ——|—— Posterior

Inferior

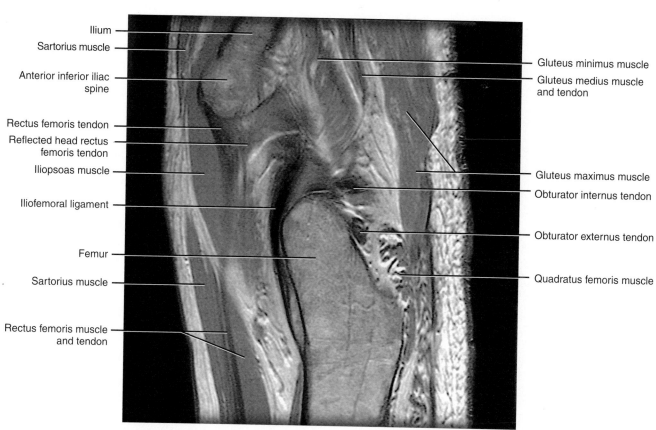

Ilium

Sartorius muscle

Anterior inferior iliac spine

Rectus femoris tendon

Reflected head rectus femoris tendon

Iliopsoas muscle

Iliofemoral ligament

Femur

Sartorius muscle

Rectus femoris muscle and tendon

Gluteus minimus muscle

Gluteus medius muscle and tendon

Gluteus maximus muscle

Obturator internus tendon

Obturator externus tendon

Quadratus femoris muscle

FIGURE 4-52

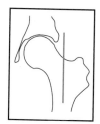

HIP: SAGITTAL

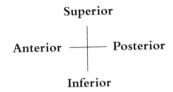

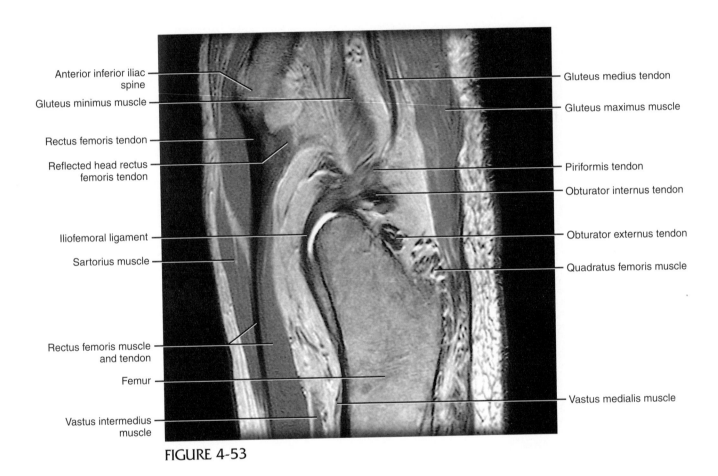

Anterior inferior iliac spine

Gluteus minimus muscle

Rectus femoris tendon

Reflected head rectus femoris tendon

Iliofemoral ligament

Sartorius muscle

Rectus femoris muscle and tendon

Femur

Vastus intermedius muscle

Gluteus medius tendon

Gluteus maximus muscle

Piriformis tendon

Obturator internus tendon

Obturator externus tendon

Quadratus femoris muscle

Vastus medialis muscle

FIGURE 4-53

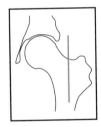

HIP: SAGITTAL

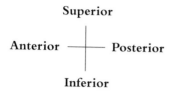

Superior

Anterior ——|—— Posterior

Inferior

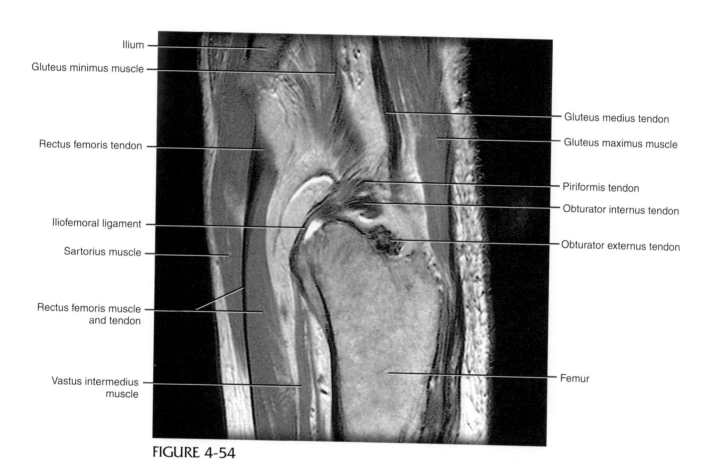

Ilium

Gluteus minimus muscle

Rectus femoris tendon

Iliofemoral ligament

Sartorius muscle

Rectus femoris muscle and tendon

Vastus intermedius muscle

Gluteus medius tendon

Gluteus maximus muscle

Piriformis tendon

Obturator internus tendon

Obturator externus tendon

Femur

FIGURE 4-54

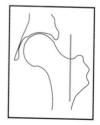

HIP: SAGITTAL

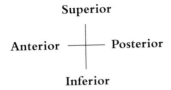

Superior

Anterior ——┼—— Posterior

Inferior

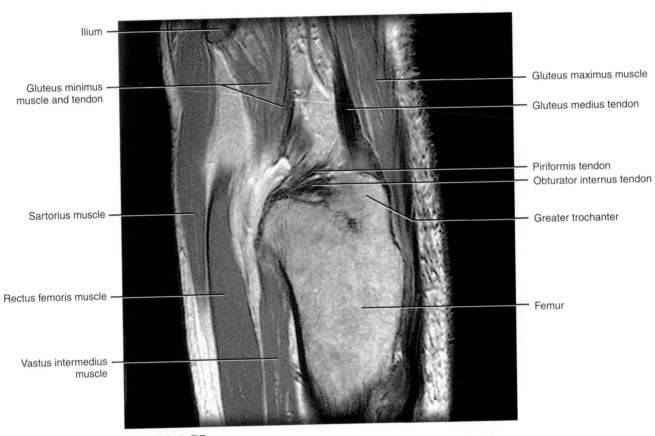

Ilium

Gluteus maximus muscle

Gluteus minimus muscle and tendon

Gluteus medius tendon

Piriformis tendon

Obturator internus tendon

Sartorius muscle

Greater trochanter

Rectus femoris muscle

Femur

Vastus intermedius muscle

FIGURE 4-55

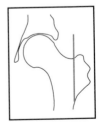

HIP: SAGITTAL

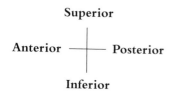

Superior

Anterior ——|—— Posterior

Inferior

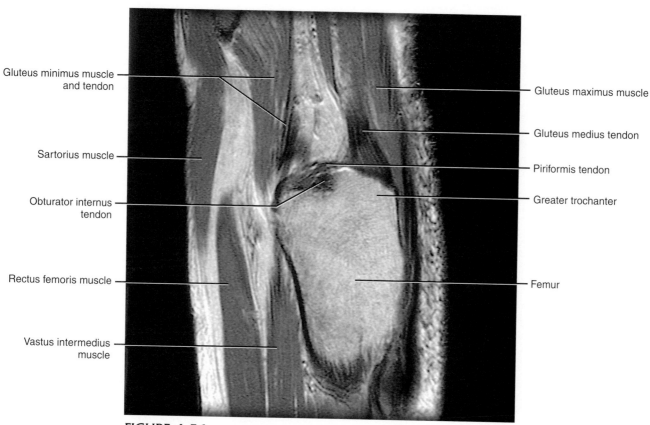

Gluteus minimus muscle and tendon

Sartorius muscle

Obturator internus tendon

Rectus femoris muscle

Vastus intermedius muscle

Gluteus maximus muscle

Gluteus medius tendon

Piriformis tendon

Greater trochanter

Femur

FIGURE 4-56

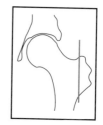

HIP: SAGITTAL

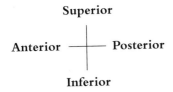

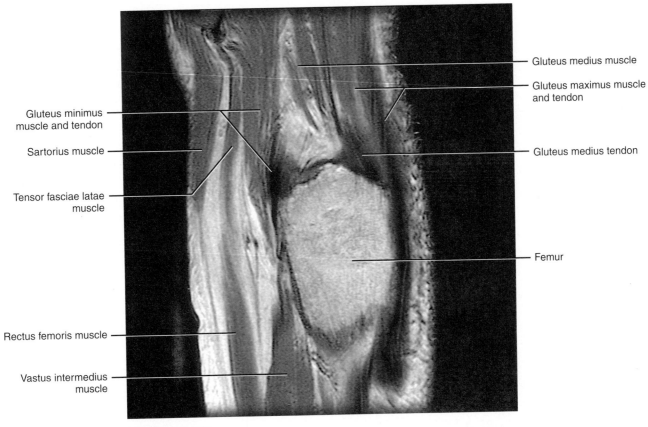

Gluteus minimus muscle and tendon

Sartorius muscle

Tensor fasciae latae muscle

Rectus femoris muscle

Vastus intermedius muscle

Gluteus medius muscle

Gluteus maximus muscle and tendon

Gluteus medius tendon

Femur

FIGURE 4-57

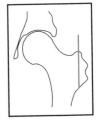

HIP: SAGITTAL

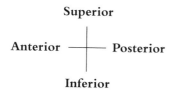

Superior

Anterior —┼— Posterior

Inferior

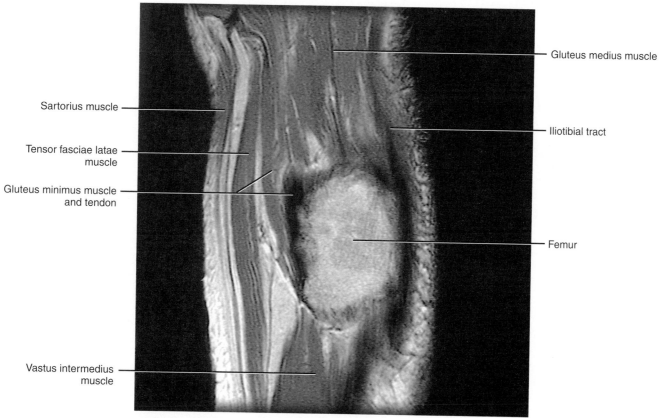

Gluteus medius muscle

Sartorius muscle

Iliotibial tract

Tensor fasciae latae muscle

Gluteus minimus muscle and tendon

Femur

Vastus intermedius muscle

FIGURE 4-58

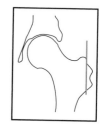

HIP: ANTERIOR VIEW

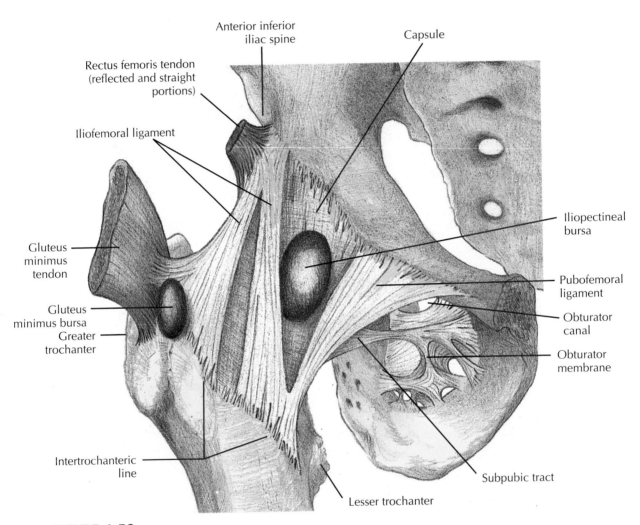

FIGURE 4-59

Anterior view of the hip capsule. The inelastic fibrous capsule of the hip joint is reinforced by the iliofemoral, pubofemoral, and ischiofemoral ligaments (thickenings of the hip capsule). The iliofemoral ligament, or ligament of Bigelow, is the strongest and thickest of the capsular ligaments and has an inverted Y shape anteriorly. The pubofemoral and ischiofemoral ligaments are less substantial. For related MR, arthroscopy, and surgical anatomy images see Figures 4-63, 4-64, and 4-66.

HIP: POSTERIOR VIEW

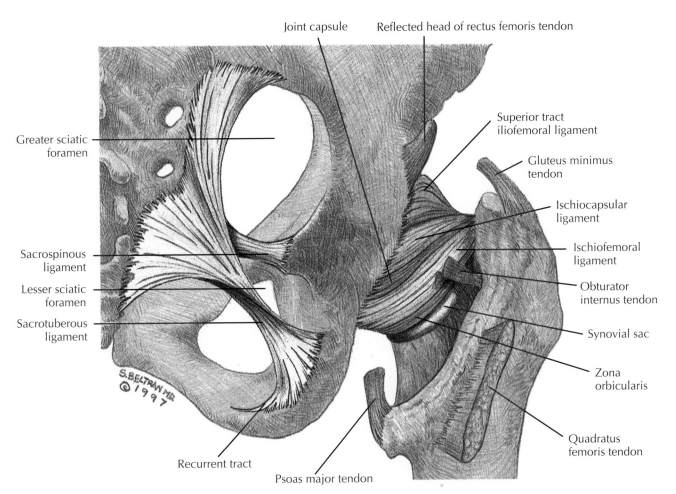

Joint capsule

Reflected head of rectus femoris tendon

Greater sciatic foramen

Superior tract iliofemoral ligament

Gluteus minimus tendon

Ischiocapsular ligament

Ischiofemoral ligament

Sacrospinous ligament

Obturator internus tendon

Lesser sciatic foramen

Sacrotuberous ligament

Synovial sac

Zona orbicularis

Quadratus femoris tendon

Recurrent tract

Psoas major tendon

FIGURE 4-60

Posterior view of the hip capsule. The ischiofemoral ligament is the weakest of the three capsular ligaments. Deep circular fibers from the ischiofemoral ligament form the zona orbicularis. Arthroscopically, the zona orbicularis may be mistaken for the acetabular labrum. The ischiocapsular ligament is part of the ischiofemoral ligament and more accurately describes the anatomy of this ligament. Only a few ischiofemoral fibers reach the femur. For related MR, arthroscopy, and surgical anatomy images see Figures 4-63 through 4-66.

HIP: JOINT OPENED, ANTEROLATERAL VIEW

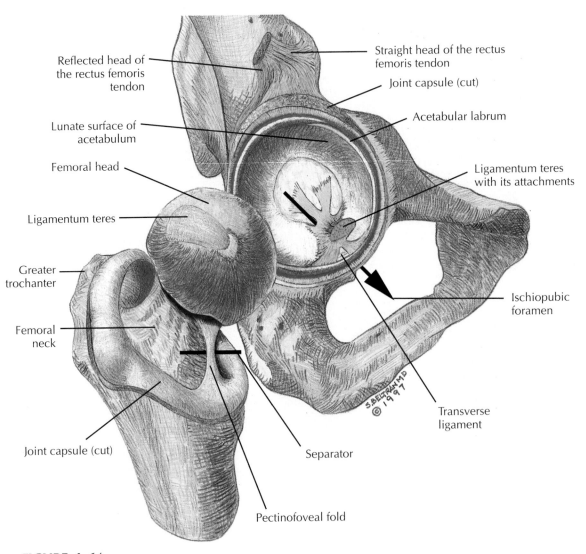

FIGURE 4-61

Anterolateral view of disarticulated hip joint. The acetabulum has a horseshoe-shaped lunate surface. The acetabular fossa lies in the inferomedial portion of the acetabulum and is occupied by the pulvinar (fat pad) and ligamentum teres. The transverse acetabular ligament bridges the notch at the inferolateral acetabulum and, together with the acetabular labrum, forms a complete ring around the acetabulum. The insertion of the ligamentum teres into the fovea capitis of the medial femoral head fills what has been referred to as a bare area. The reflected portion of the joint capsule maintains the nutrient arteries from the trochanteric anastomosis along the femoral neck, to supply the femoral head. For related MR, arthroscopy, and surgical anatomy images see Figures 4-67 through 4-72.

HIP: ACETABULUM, LATERAL VIEW

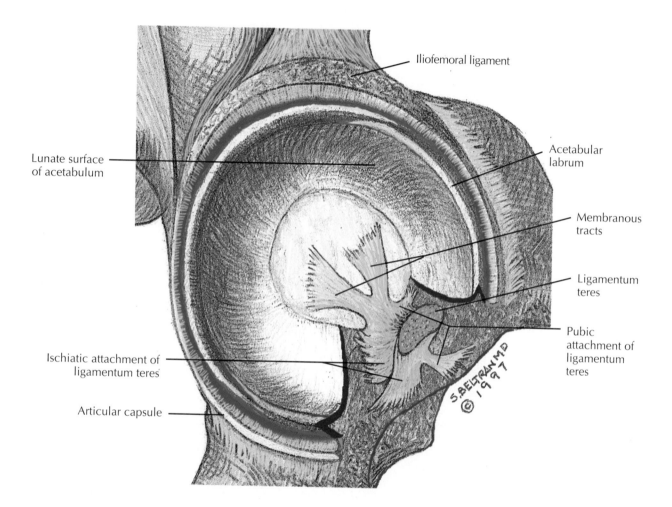

Iliofemoral ligament

Acetabular labrum

Membranous tracts

Ligamentum teres

Pubic attachment of ligamentum teres

Lunate surface of acetabulum

Ischiatic attachment of ligamentum teres

Articular capsule

FIGURE 4-62

The acetabular expansions of the ligamentum teres include membranous tracts and ischiatic and pubic attachments. The dense fibrocartilaginous labrum of the acetabulum increases the depth of the acetabulum. For related MR, arthroscopy, and surgical anatomy images see Figures 4-67, 4-68, 4-70, and 4-71.

HIP: ILIOPSOAS AND RECTUS FEMORIS

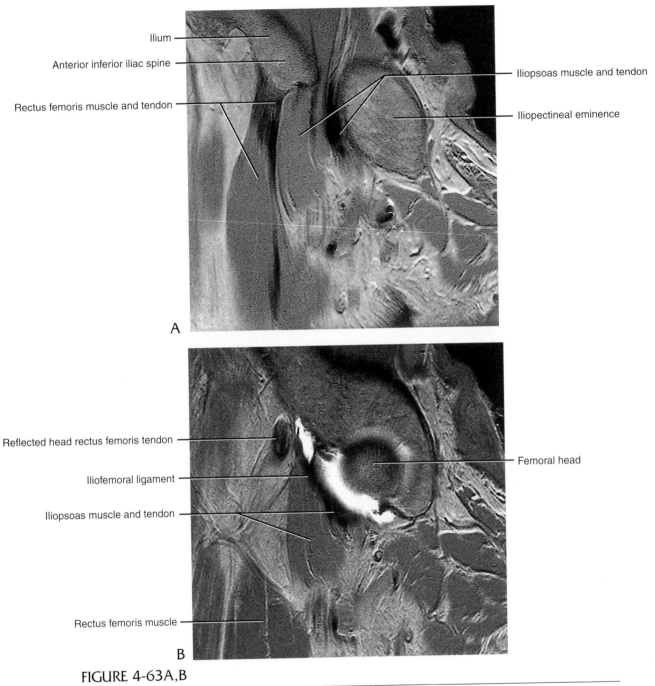

Ilium

Anterior inferior iliac spine

Rectus femoris muscle and tendon

Iliopsoas muscle and tendon

Iliopectineal eminence

A

Reflected head rectus femoris tendon

Iliofemoral ligament

Iliopsoas muscle and tendon

Femoral head

Rectus femoris muscle

B

FIGURE 4-63A,B

(**A** and **B**) T1-weighted coronal MR arthrograms showing the iliopsoas muscle and tendon and the rectus femoris muscle and tendon (**A**) and the iliofemoral ligament (**B**). The image in part **A** is more anterior than the image in part **B**.

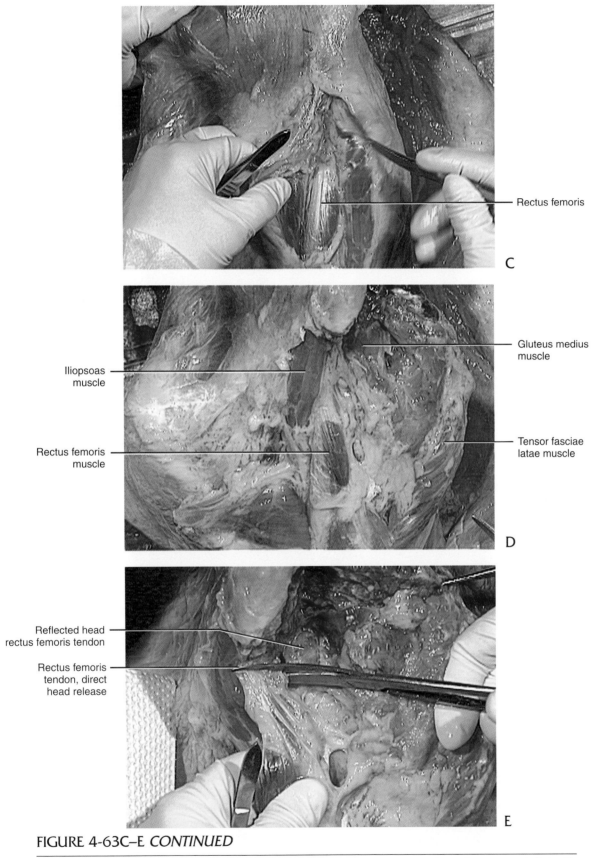

Rectus femoris

Gluteus medius
muscle

Iliopsoas
muscle

Tensor fasciae
latae muscle

Rectus femoris
muscle

C

D

Reflected head
rectus femoris tendon

Rectus femoris
tendon, direct
head release

E

FIGURE 4-63C–E *CONTINUED*

(**C, D,** and **E**) Corresponding dissections. (**C**) The rectus femoris with origin from the anterior inferior iliac spine and rim of acetabulum. (**D**) The iliopsoas muscle coursing to insert on the lesser trochanter. (**E**) The exposed direct and reflected head of the rectus femoris.

HIP: ILIOPSOAS AND RECTUS FEMORIS

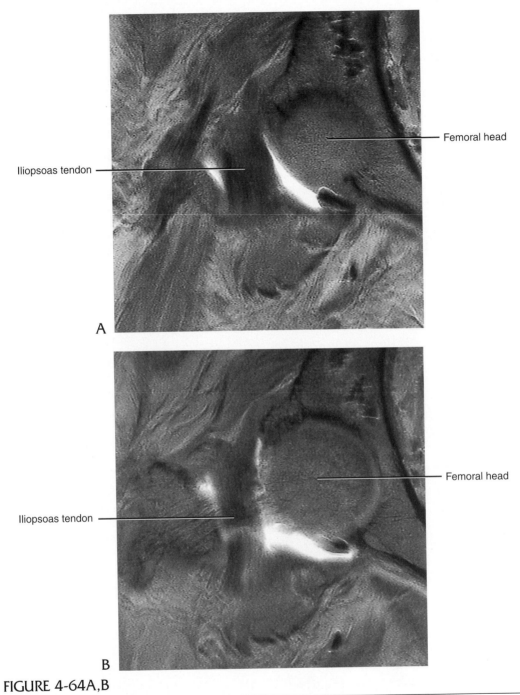

FIGURE 4-64A,B

(**A** and **B**) T1-weighted coronal MR arthrograms demonstrating the iliopsoas tendon (also correctly referred to as separate iliacus and psoas components) as it passes across the anterior aspect of the capsule of the hip joint. The image in part **A** is anterior to the image in part **B**.

HIP: ILIOPSOAS AND RECTUS FEMORIS

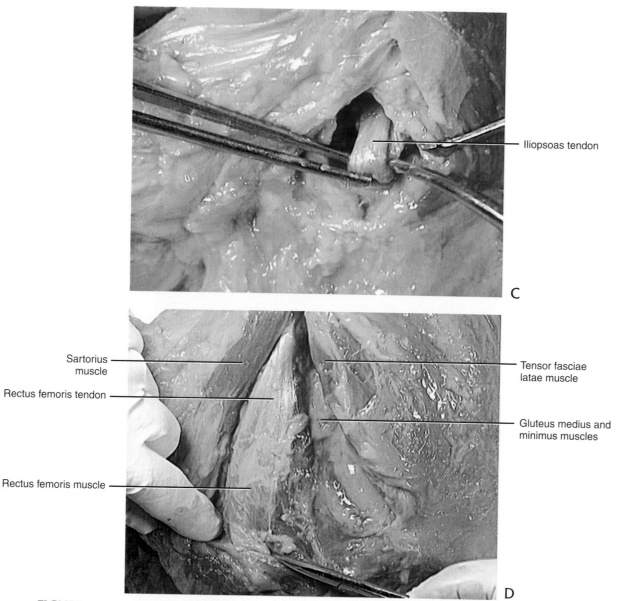

Iliopsoas tendon

Sartorius muscle

Rectus femoris tendon

Rectus femoris muscle

Tensor fasciae latae muscle

Gluteus medius and minimus muscles

C

D

FIGURE 4-64C,D *CONTINUED*

(C) The rounded tendon of the psoas is shown proximal to its insertion into the lesser trochanter. **(D)** The reflected head origin of the rectus femoris is superior to the acetabulum and the straight head origin is from the superior half of the anterior inferior iliac spine above the iliofemoral ligament. The gross dissection shows the spindle-shaped (bipenniform) morphology of the muscle.

HIP: SCIATIC NERVE

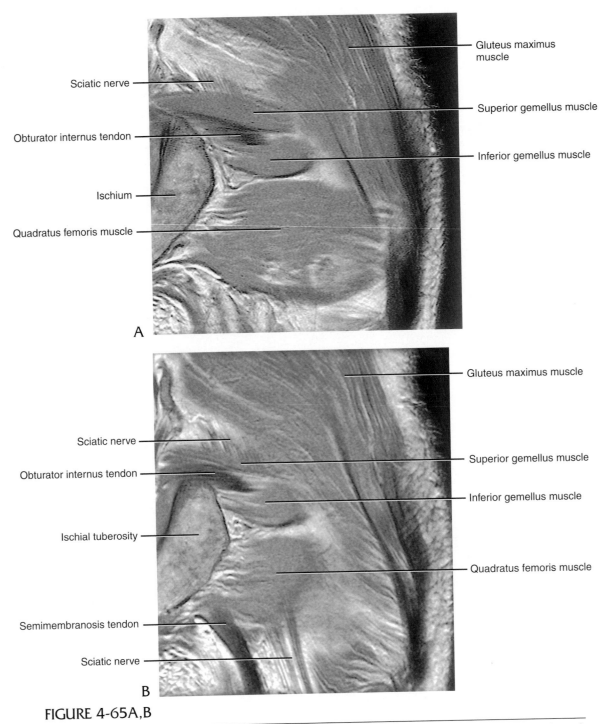

FIGURE 4-65A,B

(A and B) T1-weighted posterior coronal images illustrating the sciatic nerve as it leaves the pelvis through the greater sciatic foramen below the piriformis muscle. The gemelli insert into the obturator internus tendon. The image in part A is anterior to the image in part B.

HIP: SCIATIC NERVE

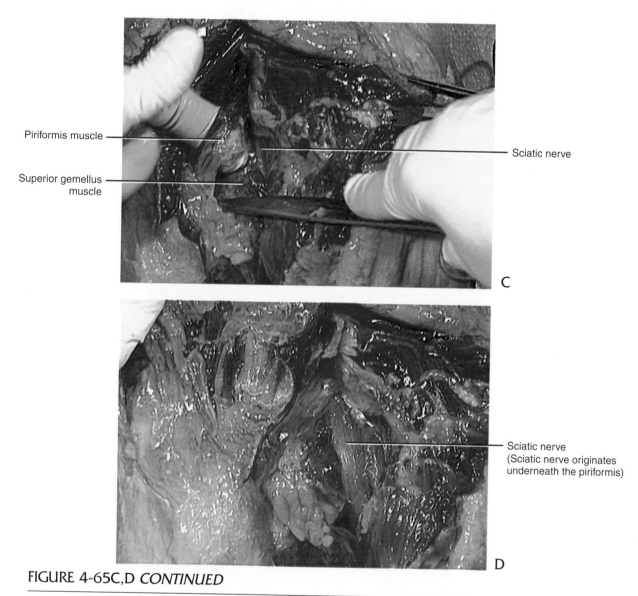

Piriformis muscle

Superior gemellus muscle

Sciatic nerve

Sciatic nerve
(Sciatic nerve originates underneath the piriformis)

C

D

FIGURE 4-65C,D *CONTINUED*

(**C** and **D**) Corresponding dissections showing the piriformis (**C**) and sciatic nerve (**D**).

HIP: CAPSULE

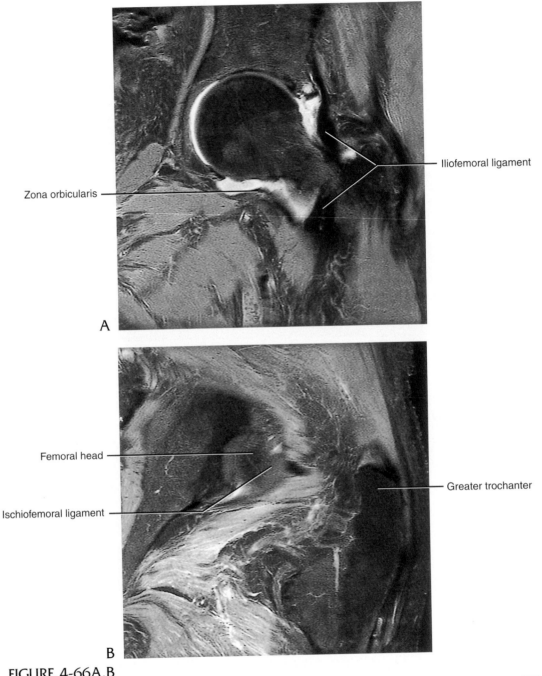

FIGURE 4-66A,B

(**A** and **B**) Fat-suppressed T2-weighted fast spin–echo coronal images showing the iliofemoral ligament (Y ligament of Bigelow) on an anterior coronal image (**A**) and the ischiofemoral ligament on a posterior coronal image (**B**). The zona orbicularis represents a condensed collar of deep circular fibers from the ischiofemoral ligament. These fibers are best visualized along the posterior inferior aspect of the ischiofemoral ligament.

HIP: CAPSULE

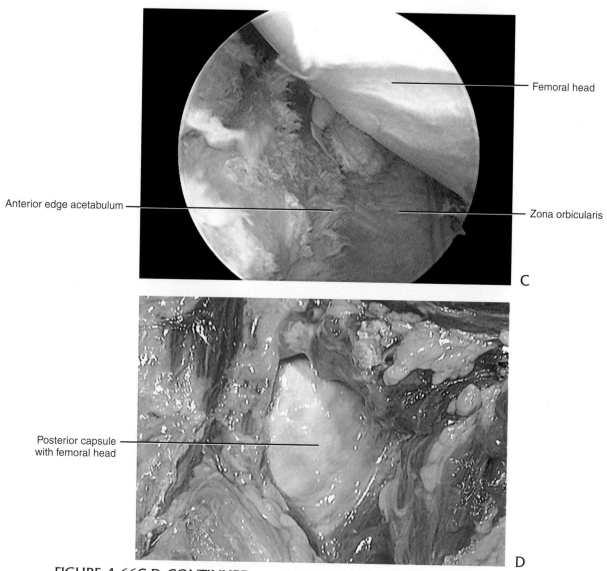

Femoral head

Anterior edge acetabulum

Zona orbicularis

C

Posterior capsule
with femoral head

D

FIGURE 4-66C,D *CONTINUED*

(C) Arthroscopic view of the capsular condensation of the zona orbicularis. **(D)** Posterior view of the fibrous hip capsule.

HIP: LIGAMENTUM TERES

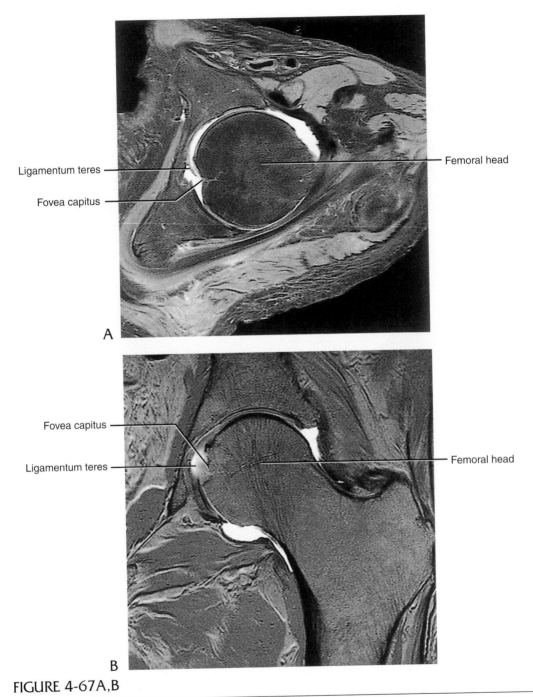

FIGURE 4-67A,B

(**A** and **B**) A fat-suppressed T2-weighted axial MR arthrogram (**A**) and a T1-weighted coronal MR arthrogram (**B**) illustrating the ligamentum teres attachment to the non-articulating fovea of the femoral head.

HIP: LIGAMENTUM TERES

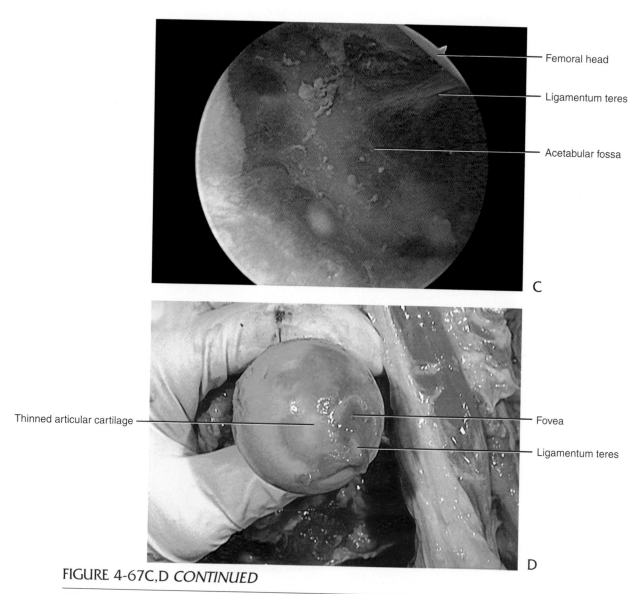

Femoral head

Ligamentum teres

Acetabular fossa

C

Thinned articular cartilage

Fovea

Ligamentum teres

D

FIGURE 4-67C,D *CONTINUED*

(C) Corresponding arthroscopic view of the ligamentum teres. (D) Dislocated femoral head.

HIP: ACETABULUM AND FEMORAL HEAD

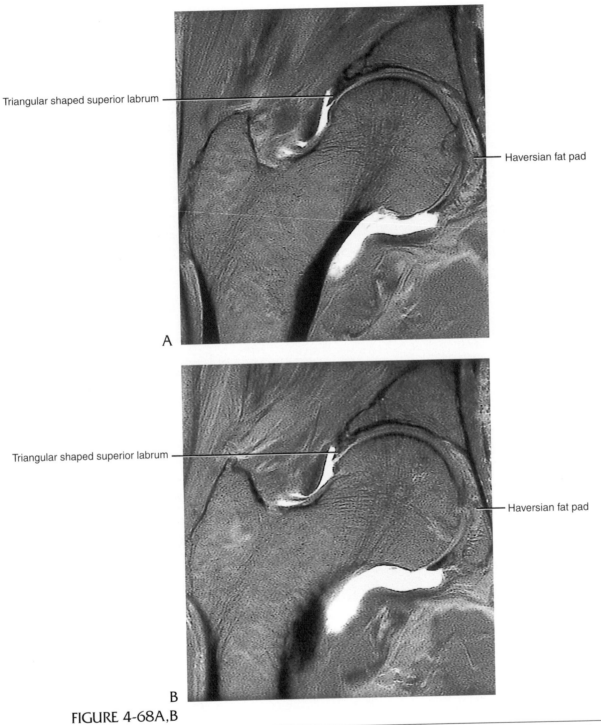

Triangular shaped superior labrum

Haversian fat pad

A

Triangular shaped superior labrum

Haversian fat pad

B

FIGURE 4-68A,B

(**A** and **B**) T1-weighted coronal MR arthrograms illustrating the haversian fat pad (intraarticular and extrasynovial), which occupies the central non-articular acetabular fossa. This fat pad slides underneath the transverse ligament to the obturator area during extension and remains within the acetabular notch during flexion.

HIP: ACETABULUM AND FEMORAL HEAD

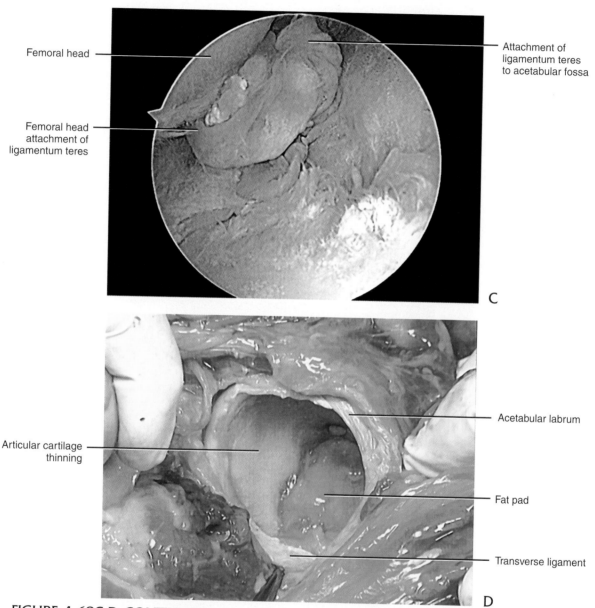

Femoral head

Attachment of
ligamentum teres
to acetabular fossa

Femoral head
attachment of
ligamentum teres

C

Articular cartilage
thinning

Acetabular labrum

Fat pad

Transverse ligament

D

FIGURE 4-68C,D *CONTINUED*

(C) Arthroscopic view showing the ligamentum teres arising from the posteroinferior aspect of the acetabular fossa and inserting on the femoral head. **(D)** The fat pad, labrum, and lunate surface of the acetabulum are demonstrated on this lateral view of the acetabulum.

HIP: TRANSVERSE LIGAMENT

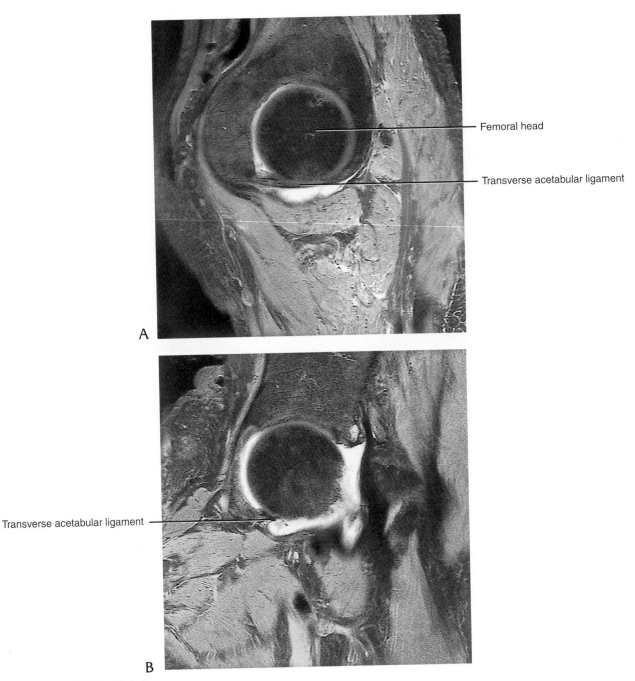

— Femoral head

— Transverse acetabular ligament

Transverse acetabular ligament —

FIGURE 4-69A,B

(**A** and **B**) A fat-suppressed T2-weighted sagittal MR arthrogram (**A**) and a fat-suppressed T2-weighted coronal MR arthrogram (**B**) showing the transverse ligament, which connects the anterior and posterior labrum across the acetabular notch.

HIP: TRANSVERSE LIGAMENT

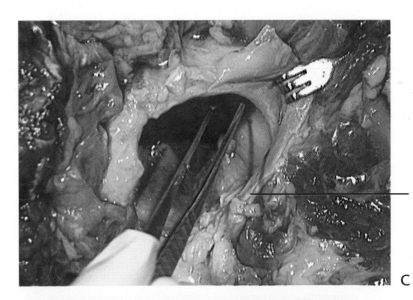

Transverse ligament
forms floor of acetabular
fossa and connects anterior
and posterior labrum

C

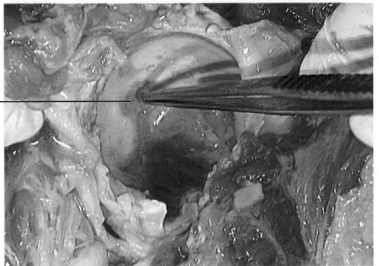

Articular cartilage loss on
acetabular lunate surface

D

FIGURE 4-69C,D *CONTINUED*

(C) Corresponding gross specimen showing the transverse ligament forming the floor of the acetabular fossa. The transverse ligament also provides attachment for the ligamentum teres. (D) The lunate surface of the acetabulum (peripheral articular margin) is absent inferiorly. The probe indicates a chondral lesion of the articular surface.

HIP: ACETABULAR SURFACE AND LABRUM

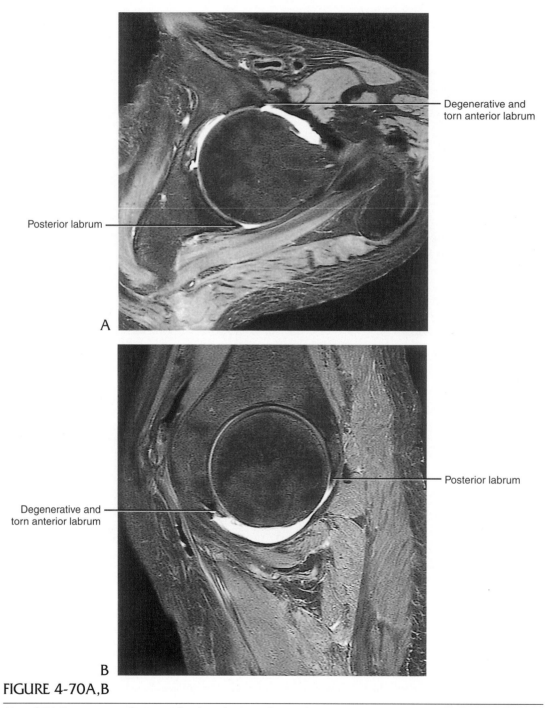

FIGURE 4-70A,B

(**A** and **B**) Fat-suppressed T2-weighted axial (**A**) and sagittal (**B**) MR arthrograms illustrating a degenerative anterior labrum. The posterior labrum has normal morphology.

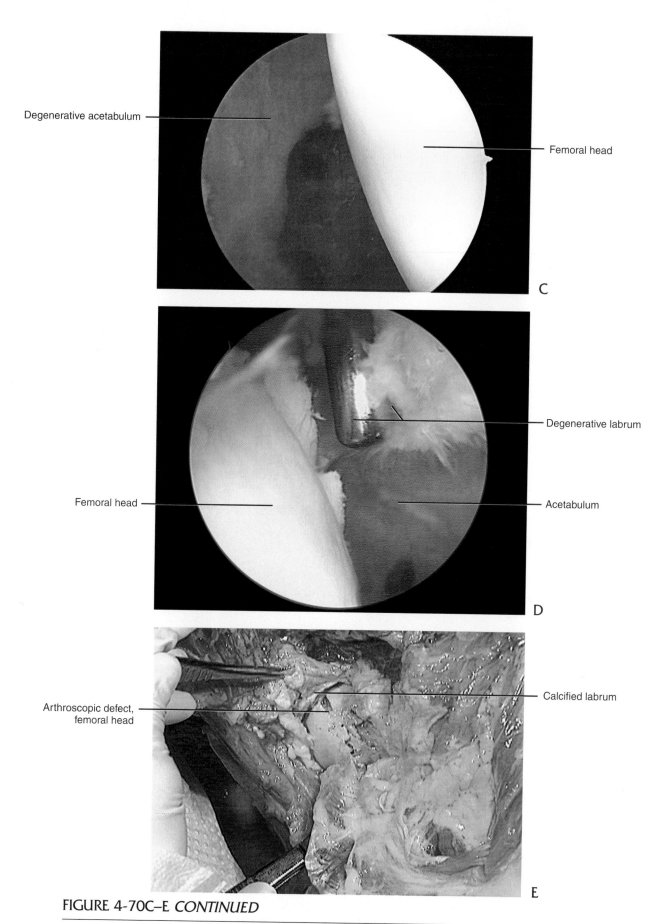

Degenerative acetabulum

Femoral head

C

Degenerative labrum

Femoral head

Acetabulum

D

Calcified labrum

Arthroscopic defect, femoral head

E

FIGURE 4-70C–E *CONTINUED*

(**C** and **D**) Arthroscopic views of the degenerative articular surface of the acetabulum (**C**) and the degenerative labrum (**D**). (**E**) The corresponding labrum is calcified in this degenerative specimen.

HIP: LABRUM

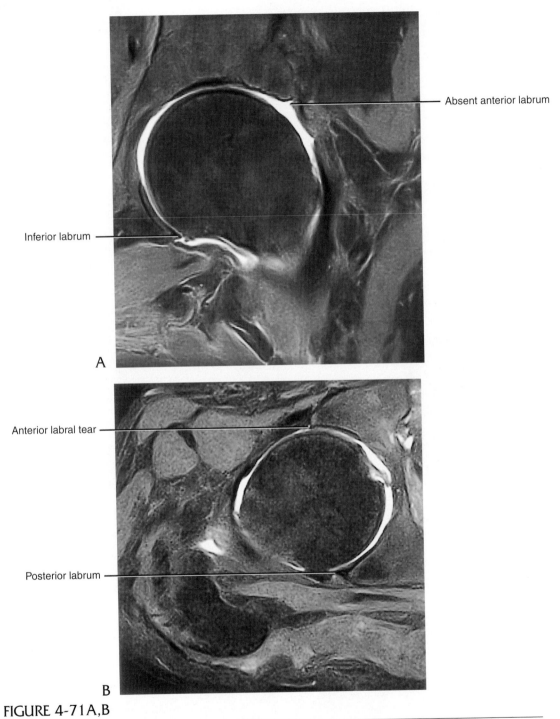

Absent anterior labrum

Inferior labrum

A

Anterior labral tear

Posterior labrum

B

FIGURE 4-71A,B

(A) A fat-suppressed T1-weighted coronal MR arthrogram showing a torn anterior labrum. (B) A fat-suppressed T1-weighted axial MR arthrogram showing an intact posterior labrum. (C and D) Corresponding arthroscopic views of the torn anterosuperior labrum (C) and normal posterior labrum (D). (E) Acetabular dissection demonstrates complete absence of the anterior labrum.

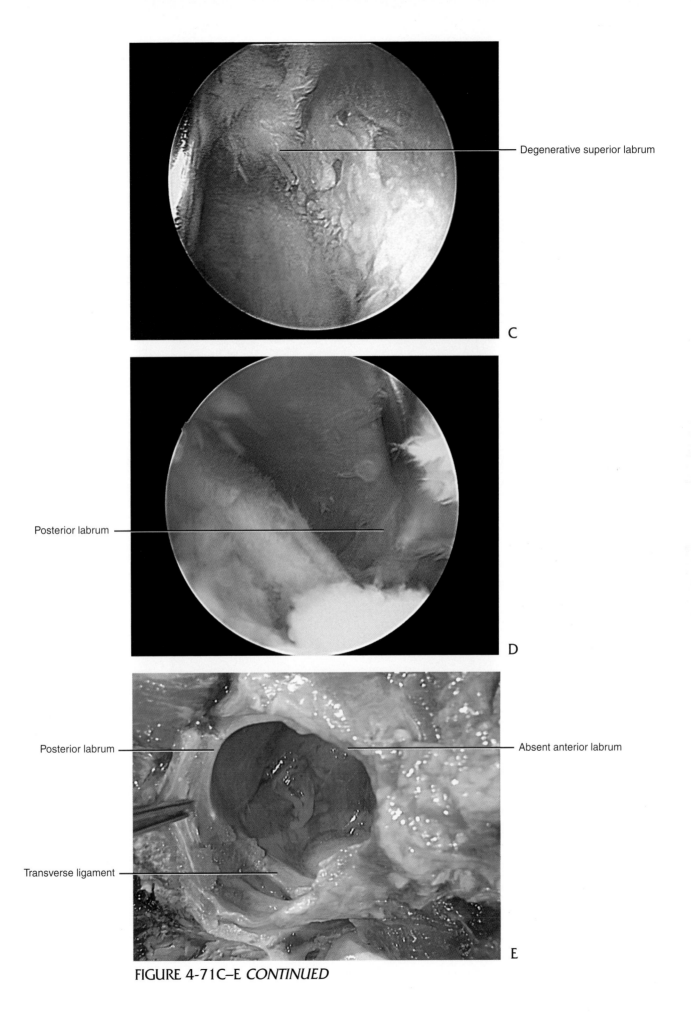

Degenerative superior labrum

C

Posterior labrum

D

Posterior labrum

Absent anterior labrum

Transverse ligament

E

FIGURE 4-71C–E *CONTINUED*

HIP: FEMORAL HEAD

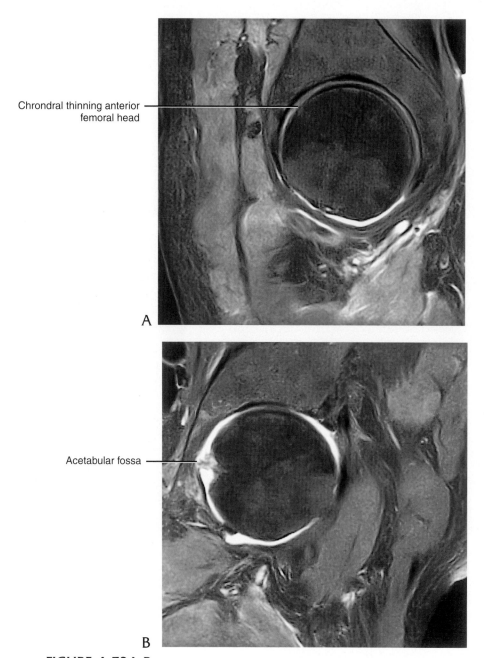

Chrondral thinning anterior femoral head

Acetabular fossa

A

B

FIGURE 4-72A,B

(A) Chondral thinning seen anteriorly on a fat-suppressed T1-weighted sagittal image. (B) Note the normal absence of articular cartilage in the acetabular fossa as seen on a fat-suppressed T1-weighted coronal MR arthrogram.

HIP: FEMORAL HEAD

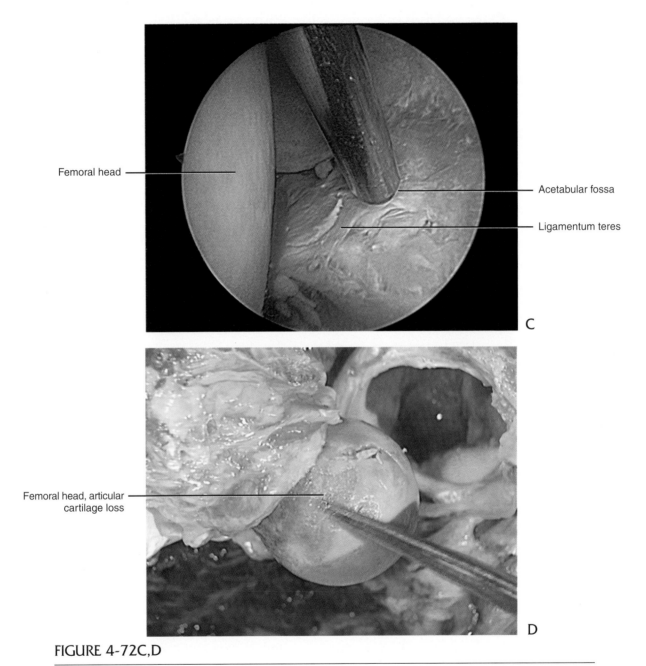

Femoral head ———

Acetabular fossa

Ligamentum teres

C

Femoral head, articular
cartilage loss ———

D

FIGURE 4-72C,D

(C and D) Corresponding arthroscopic view of the acetabular fossa (C) and a gross specimen of the degenerative femoral head (D).

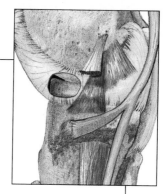

C H A P T E R 5

THE KNEE

David W. Stoller
W. Dilworth Cannon, Jr.
Scott Dye
Salvador Beltran
Charles P. Ho

KNEE ARTHROSCOPY AND DISSECTION
MR NORMAL ANATOMY

COLOR ANATOMIC ILLUSTRATIONS
MR, ARTHROSCOPY, AND SURGICAL CORRELATION

———— KNEE ARTHROSCOPY ————

THE OPTIMAL AND CONVENTIONAL PORTAL FOR KNEE ARTHRO-SCOPY is an anterolateral portal. An anteromedial portal is used for both instrument introduction and probing, and is also used as an alternative arthroscopic portal. Additional alternative portals include a central portal, which requires a transpatellar approach, and a midpatellar lateral portal, which is used to visualize the anterior aspect of the knee joint. A superolateral portal is used for placement of the pressure-sensing cannula for the pump. A superolateral or superomedial portal is used for arthroscopic assessment of the congruency of the patellofemoral joint through the range of motion from extension to flexion. The posteromedial and posterolateral portals are primarily surgical portals, but may also be used for visualization.

Evaluation of the knee begins by moving the arthroscope into the lateral recess of the anterolateral portal and performing a sweep of the lateral gutter down to the popliteus hiatus. The superior and inferior fasciculi of the lateral meniscus are visualized from the hiatus. The meniscosynovial junction of the middle third of the lateral meniscus is viewed up to the anterolateral corner of the knee. The anterior horn of the lateral meniscus and the anterior cruciate ligament (ACL) within the intercondylar notch can be seen with the knee in partial flexion and applied varus force.

The arthroscope is then moved to the medial recess and proximally into the suprapatellar pouch. A normal suprapatellar plica is seen in 80% to 89% of knees. The suprapatellar plica may cross the suprapatellar pouch to the lateral sidewall and, rarely, may compartmentalize the suprapatellar pouch.

With the knee in extension, the arthroscope is placed between the patella and medial parapatellar plica. A medial parapatellar plica is present in 50% to 60% of normal individuals, and there is enlargement or thickening in 19%. A thickened medial parapatellar plica may overlap the medial femoral condyle and impinge on the articular surface of the medial patellar facet.

The patellofemoral joint, including the medial and lateral facets, is inspected with the upward orientation of the arthroscope. The articular cartilage of the trochlear groove is inspected from a lateral to medial direction. The medial side of the trochlear groove and the medial patellar facet of the patella normally articulate between 45° and 55° of flexion, otherwise lateral subluxation occurs.

The arthroscope is next moved into the medial compartment, looking in a posterior direction. Opening of the medial compartment is facilitated by placing the knee in 15° to 20° of flexion with an applied valgus load. The posterior horn origin of the medial meniscus is inspected, and a sweep to the anterior horn is then performed. The articular cartilage of the medial femoral condyle and medial tibial plateau is assessed by gradually flexing the knee through an arc of 90°. The articular cartilage is followed from the medial edge of the intercondylar notch upward and over the ligamentum mucosum, which attaches at the top of the intercondylar notch.

The arthroscope is then oriented downward, on the lateral side of the notch, prior to inspection of the ACL within the notch. For inspection of the lateral compartment a probe is placed through the anteromedial portal and directed to the posterior horn of the lateral meniscus. The posterior horn origin and both superior and inferior surfaces of the lateral meniscus are inspected. Pulling the anterior horn anteriorly generates circumferential hoop stresses, helpful in identifying radial split tears of the middle third of the lateral meniscus. The ACL is then probed. The probe is introduced into the medial compartment through a separate synovial puncture with the knee in partial flexion and an applied valgus load. The medial meniscus, including its posterior horn origin, is then probed.

Next, the arthroscope is passed through the intercondylar notch to the posteromedial compartment, medial to the posterior cruciate ligament, which is also visualized. Arthroscopic visualization of the posterolateral compartment through the anteromedial portal is used to view the posterolateral structures. The posterior horn of the lateral meniscus can be further palpated by a probe introduced anterolaterally. Indications for arthroscopy include loose bodies, meniscal tears, soft tissue impingement, osteochondral lesions, cruciate ligament endoscopic reconstruction, tibial plateau fracture reduction, lateral retinacular release, and other patellar disorders as well as synovial pathology.

SURGICAL DISSECTION
OF THE KNEE

Anterior Dissection

There are three potential bursal spaces anterior to the patella. The prepatellar bursa, the most superficial of the three, is located between the skin and
arciform fascia. The arciform fascia consists of transverse fibers, which partially originate from the iliotibial tract and extend over the patellar tendon.
There is an intermediate oblique layer between the more superficial arciform layer and the deeper longitudinal fibers of the rectus femoris. Distally,
the intermediate oblique layer attenuates and becomes more delicate. Bursal
spaces lie between the arciform layer and the intermediate oblique layer and
the intermediate oblique layer and the deep fibers of the rectus femoris. The
longitudinal fibers of the rectus femoris continue over the top of the patella
and become the patellar tendon. A vascular ring between the rectus femoris
and the intermediate oblique layer provides blood supply to the patella.

Medial Dissection

Circumferential transverse fibers form the investing fascia, which covers the
vastus medialis obliquus muscle (VMO). The sartorial fascia, bound to the
sartorius muscle, is a suspensory system that inserts into fascia superficially
(superficial to the VMO and gastrocnemius) and to the proximal portion of
the pes anserinus. The anterior and superior borders of the pes anserinus are
formed by the sartorius muscle. The infrapatellar branch of the saphenous
nerve penetrates the sartorius muscle and is potentially at risk during
arthroscopy. The main sensory branch of the infrapatellar nerve exits below
the inferior border of the sartorius. The undersurface of the sartorius is
"spot-welded" to the fascia that extends to the posterior aspect of the calf.
Longitudinal and vertical fibers of the sartorial fascia produce flexibility and
dampening capabilities in this interlaced, or mesh-like, system. The tendon
of the gracilis is dissected deep to the condensation of sartorial fascia at the
insertion of the sartorius muscle. Fibrous and elastin suspensory ligaments
connect the gracilis to the femur. The sartorius is superficial to both the gracilis and semitendinosus. These three structures constitute the pes anserinus
or "goose's foot." The gracilis and semitendinosus are "spot-welded" to one
another at their pes insertion. The broad insertion of the semitendinosus is
associated with juncturi that need to be cut in order to harvest the pes tendons. The superficial medial collateral ligament (MCL) is deep to the pes
anserinus. The adductor tubercle is the point of insertion of the adductor
magnus. The superficial MCL originates from the medial epicondyle. The
MCL is asymmetric with respect to the length of fibers above and below
the medial joint line (in a ratio of 2:7, above and below the joint line, respectively). The posterior oblique ligament is contiguous with the MCL. In
flexion the posterior oblique ligament is lax, whereas the MCL remains relatively taut. This helps to define the posterior border of the MCL. With the
knee in full extension, the posterior oblique ligament becomes indistin-

guishable from the MCL. The posterior oblique ligament covers the semi-membranosus tendon, which has five separate insertions including:

1. An attachment to the tibial tubercle
2. An anterior branch (underneath the posterior oblique ligament and superficial MCL)
3. A medial collateral ligament branch blending with the posterior border of the MCL
4. An attachment to the posterior horn of the medial meniscus
5. An oblique popliteal ligament branch

The insertion of the semimembranosus is below the level of the joint line.

Lateral Dissection

The iliotibial band inserts into Gerdy's tubercle. The inferior border of the iliotibial band demarcates the lateral intermuscular septum, which gives attachment to the short head fibers of the biceps femoris. The lateral collateral ligament (LCL), or fibular collateral ligament, is partially lax in flexion and difficult to define as a separate structure. The long head fibers of the biceps femoris continue superficially over the LCL and blend in posteriorly and inferiorly. There is no separate free border to the LCL. The short head fibers of the biceps femoris also blend in with the posterior inferior border of the LCL. There is a bursa between the long tract fibers of the biceps femoris and the LCL. The peroneal nerve enters the lateral compartment below the termination of the distal fibers of the LCL. There is an osseous ridge on the fibula, which demarcates the distal LCL fibers from the peroneal nerve. The peroneal nerve arborizes into the lateral and anterior compartments and is located 2 to 3 cm below the joint line. The insertion of the popliteus tendon onto the popliteus fossa of the lateral femoral condyle is distal and anterior to the proximal LCL (the popliteus tendon crosses deep to the LCL). The popliteal hiatus is at the level of the lateral joint line. The superior fasciculus defines the posterior aspect of the hiatus. The popliteofibular ligament, the arcuate ligament, and the fabellofibular ligament reinforce the posterolateral corner of the knee. Posterolateral instability is usually associated with a posterior cruciate ligament tear but may also be associated with an anterior cruciate ligament tear. The popliteofibular ligament should be reconstructed during posterolateral corner surgery. Acute ACL injuries are associated with edema of the popliteus muscle and fluid posterior to the popliteus tendon. Osseous impaction occurs at the sulcus terminalis and posterolateral tibial plateau with twisting flexion ACL injuries in a "pivot shift." Osseous contusions may occur at the sulcus terminalis and anterior lateral tibial plateau with hyperextension ACL and PCL injuries. In full knee extension, the anterior horn of the lateral meniscus is located in the sulcus terminalis of the lateral femoral condyle. The popliteal artery is located just posterior to the origin of the posterior horn of the lateral meniscus and can be damaged during lateral meniscal repair. The popliteal artery sends geniculate branches medially and laterally, and a middle geniculate artery enters the intercondylar notch to supply the cruciate ligaments.

Posterior Dissection

The neurovascular structures are reflected to view the posterior aspect of the joint. The posterior cruciate ligament (PCL) is composed of a larger and stronger anterolateral bundle (ALB) and a smaller posteromedial bundle (PMB). The ALB is the more important bundle addressed during ligament reconstruction. The PCL lies 1 to 1.5 cm below the joint line, and drill holes need to be made below the joint line during arthroscopic reconstruction. The PMB of the posterior cruciate ligament is tight in extension and lax in flexion. The ALB is tight in flexion but lax in extension. The average diameter of the PCL is 11 mm at its midsection and 13 mm at its tibial insertion. It expands to a 32 mm insertion at its femoral origin (at 12 o'clock on the intercondylar notch when looking down medially). The PCL can also be reconstructed posteriorly, by making a trough in the posterior femur and inserting a bone-patellar tendon-bone autograft. In 80% of knees, there is either a meniscofemoral ligament of Wrisberg, ligament of Humphrey, or both. The meniscofemoral ligaments may contribute approximately 15% of the functional strength of the PCL. The ligament of Wrisberg originates from the posterior horn of the lateral meniscus, courses posterior to the PCL, and attaches to the medial femoral condyle. In the Wrisberg-type of discoid lateral meniscus, the capsular attachment to the posterior horn of the lateral meniscus is deficient.

The posterior origin of the ACL is visualized after reflecting the PCL posteriorly. In an over-the-top procedure for ACL reconstruction, a lateral femoral condylar trough is created for the graft, approximating the true isometric position of the ACL. The ACL is composed of an anteromedial bundle (AMB) and posterolateral bundle (PLB). The AMB is tight in flexion. and the PLB is tight in extension. If the femoral drill holes for an ACL reconstruction are placed too far anteriorly in the lateral femoral condyle, there will be a lack of isometry and the graft will become loose or stretch. The suprapatellar bursa (pouch) extends 4 to 5 cm superior to the superior pole of the patella. If the PCL remains intact, the knee is stable in full extension (to varus and valgus stress), even if other ligamentous structures are sectioned.

The medial meniscus is C-shaped with a broader posterior horn. The more O-shaped lateral meniscus is symmetrically rounded. In a gorilla, the lateral meniscus forms a complete torus, allowing greater rotational mobility. The lateral meniscus has 24 mm of mobility (compared to 10 to 11 mm for the medial meniscus), accounting for its greater rollback on the lateral tibial plateau. The medial meniscus is more constrained, which helps to explain its greater susceptibility to tearing in an ACL deficient knee. The posterior border of the lateral tibial plateau slopes inferiorly, to allow for this greater motion (rollback).

KNEE: CORONAL

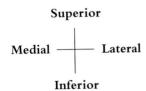

Superior

Medial ⎯⟊⎯ Lateral

Inferior

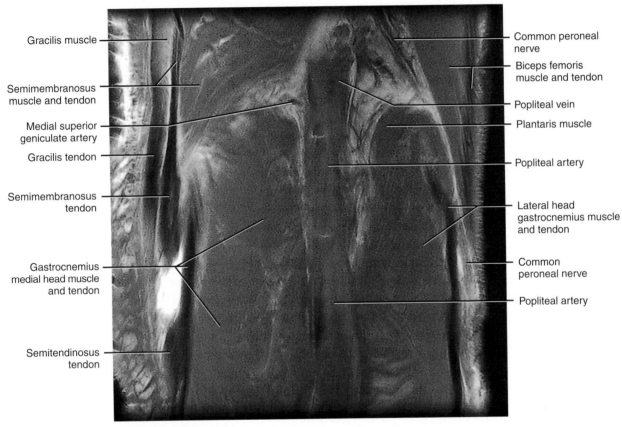

Gracilis muscle

Semimembranosus muscle and tendon

Medial superior geniculate artery

Gracilis tendon

Semimembranosus tendon

Gastrocnemius medial head muscle and tendon

Semitendinosus tendon

Common peroneal nerve

Biceps femoris muscle and tendon

Popliteal vein

Plantaris muscle

Popliteal artery

Lateral head gastrocnemius muscle and tendon

Common peroneal nerve

Popliteal artery

FIGURE 5-1

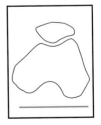

KNEE: CORONAL

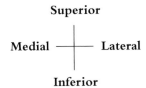

Superior

Medial ——|—— Lateral

Inferior

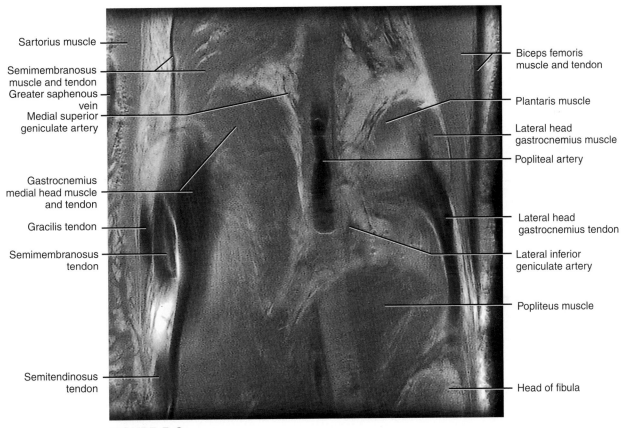

Sartorius muscle

Semimembranosus muscle and tendon

Greater saphenous vein

Medial superior geniculate artery

Gastrocnemius medial head muscle and tendon

Gracilis tendon

Semimembranosus tendon

Semitendinosus tendon

Biceps femoris muscle and tendon

Plantaris muscle

Lateral head gastrocnemius muscle

Popliteal artery

Lateral head gastrocnemius tendon

Lateral inferior geniculate artery

Popliteus muscle

Head of fibula

FIGURE 5-2

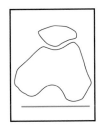

KNEE: CORONAL

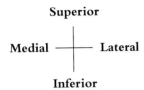

Superior

Medial ——|—— Lateral

Inferior

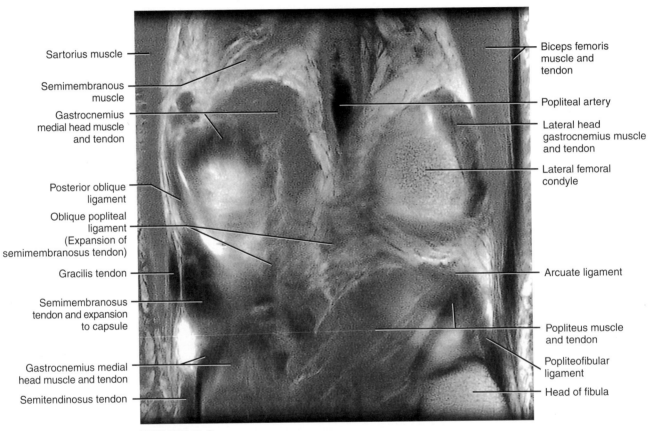

Sartorius muscle

Semimembranous muscle

Gastrocnemius medial head muscle and tendon

Posterior oblique ligament

Oblique popliteal ligament (Expansion of semimembranosus tendon)

Gracilis tendon

Semimembranosus tendon and expansion to capsule

Gastrocnemius medial head muscle and tendon

Semitendinosus tendon

Biceps femoris muscle and tendon

Popliteal artery

Lateral head gastrocnemius muscle and tendon

Lateral femoral condyle

Arcuate ligament

Popliteus muscle and tendon

Popliteofibular ligament

Head of fibula

FIGURE 5-3

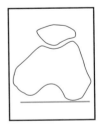

KNEE: CORONAL

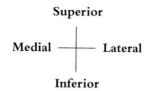

Superior

Medial ──┼── Lateral

Inferior

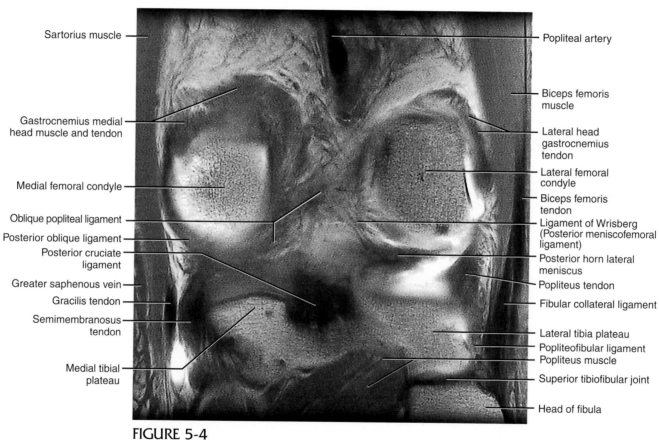

Sartorius muscle

Popliteal artery

Biceps femoris muscle

Gastrocnemius medial head muscle and tendon

Lateral head gastrocnemius tendon

Medial femoral condyle

Lateral femoral condyle

Biceps femoris tendon

Oblique popliteal ligament

Ligament of Wrisberg (Posterior meniscofemoral ligament)

Posterior oblique ligament

Posterior cruciate ligament

Posterior horn lateral meniscus

Greater saphenous vein

Popliteus tendon

Gracilis tendon

Fibular collateral ligament

Semimembranosus tendon

Lateral tibia plateau

Popliteofibular ligament

Popliteus muscle

Medial tibial plateau

Superior tibiofibular joint

Head of fibula

FIGURE 5-4

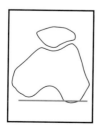

KNEE: CORONAL

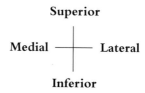

Sartorius muscle

Gastrocnemius
medial head muscle
and tendon

Medial femoral
condyle

Posterior oblique
ligament

Posterior cruciate
ligament

Sartorius muscle

Medial meniscus,
posterior horn

Semimembranosus
tendon

Gracilis tendon

Posterior tibia

Popliteus muscle

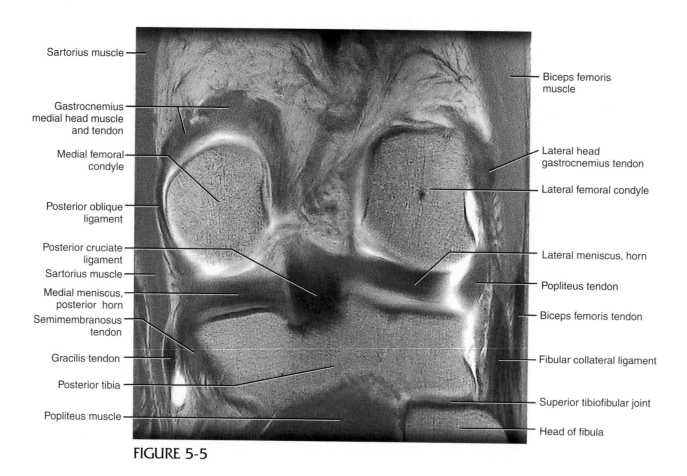

Biceps femoris
muscle

Lateral head
gastrocnemius tendon

Lateral femoral condyle

Lateral meniscus, horn

Popliteus tendon

Biceps femoris tendon

Fibular collateral ligament

Superior tibiofibular joint

Head of fibula

FIGURE 5-5

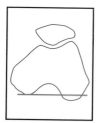

KNEE: CORONAL

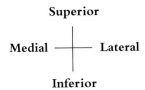

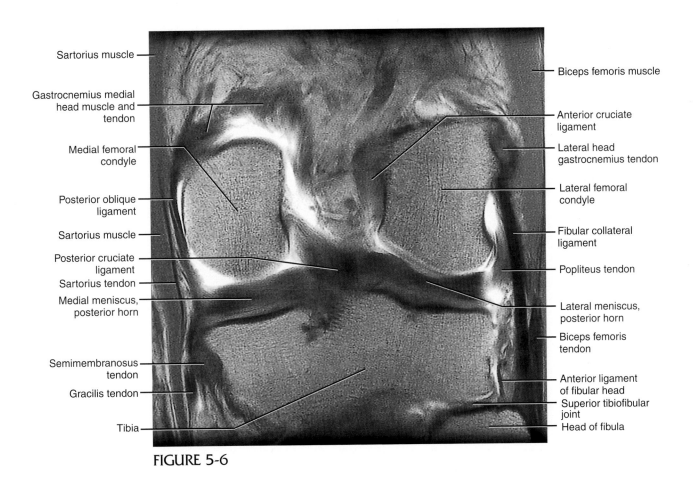

Sartorius muscle

Gastrocnemius medial head muscle and tendon

Medial femoral condyle

Posterior oblique ligament

Sartorius muscle

Posterior cruciate ligament

Sartorius tendon

Medial meniscus, posterior horn

Semimembranosus tendon

Gracilis tendon

Tibia

Biceps femoris muscle

Anterior cruciate ligament

Lateral head gastrocnemius tendon

Lateral femoral condyle

Fibular collateral ligament

Popliteus tendon

Lateral meniscus, posterior horn

Biceps femoris tendon

Anterior ligament of fibular head

Superior tibiofibular joint

Head of fibula

FIGURE 5-6

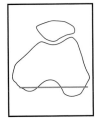

KNEE: CORONAL

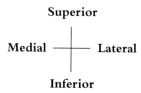

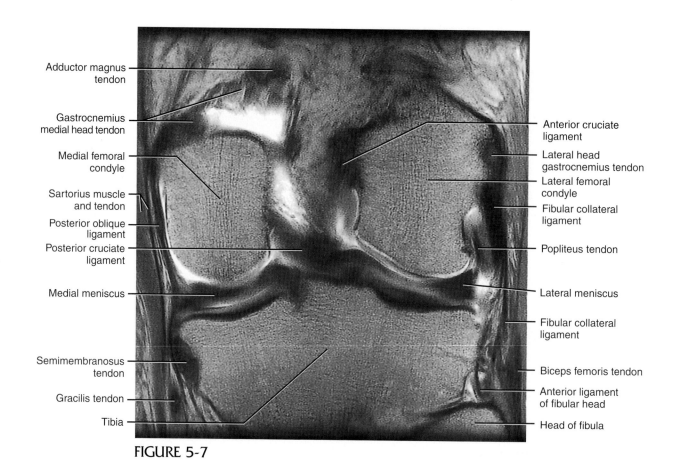

Adductor magnus tendon

Gastrocnemius medial head tendon

Medial femoral condyle

Sartorius muscle and tendon

Posterior oblique ligament

Posterior cruciate ligament

Medial meniscus

Semimembranosus tendon

Gracilis tendon

Tibia

Anterior cruciate ligament

Lateral head gastrocnemius tendon

Lateral femoral condyle

Fibular collateral ligament

Popliteus tendon

Lateral meniscus

Fibular collateral ligament

Biceps femoris tendon

Anterior ligament of fibular head

Head of fibula

FIGURE 5-7

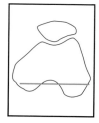

KNEE: CORONAL

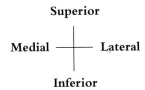

Superior

Medial ——┼—— Lateral

Inferior

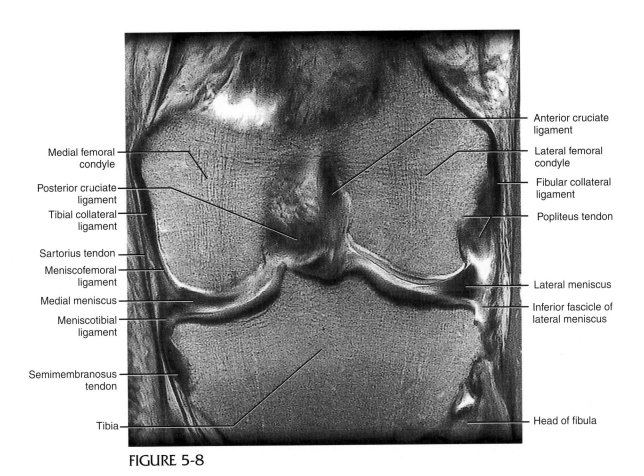

Medial femoral condyle

Posterior cruciate ligament

Tibial collateral ligament

Sartorius tendon

Meniscofemoral ligament

Medial meniscus

Meniscotibial ligament

Semimembranosus tendon

Tibia

Anterior cruciate ligament

Lateral femoral condyle

Fibular collateral ligament

Popliteus tendon

Lateral meniscus

Inferior fascicle of lateral meniscus

Head of fibula

FIGURE 5-8

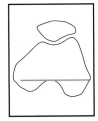

KNEE: CORONAL

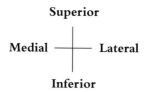

Superior

Medial ── ── Lateral

Inferior

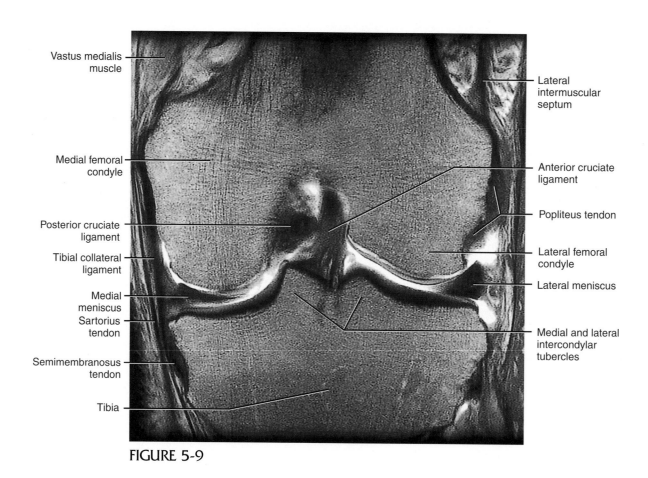

Vastus medialis
muscle

Lateral
intermuscular
septum

Medial femoral
condyle

Anterior cruciate
ligament

Popliteus tendon

Posterior cruciate
ligament

Lateral femoral
condyle

Tibial collateral
ligament

Lateral meniscus

Medial
meniscus

Sartorius
tendon

Medial and lateral
intercondylar
tubercles

Semimembranosus
tendon

Tibia

FIGURE 5-9

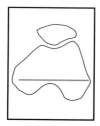

KNEE: CORONAL

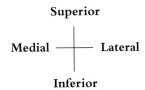

Superior

Medial ——|—— Lateral

Inferior

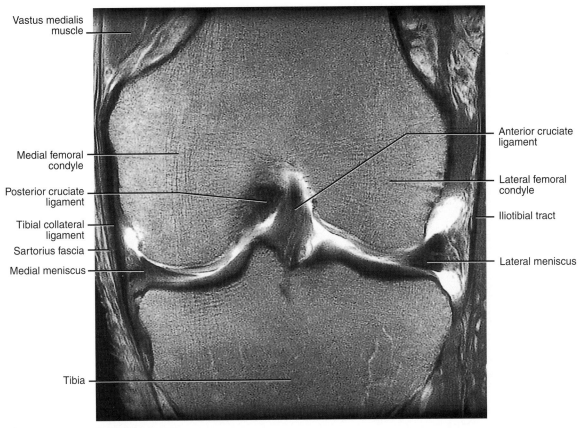

Vastus medialis muscle

Medial femoral condyle

Posterior cruciate ligament

Tibial collateral ligament

Sartorius fascia

Medial meniscus

Tibia

Anterior cruciate ligament

Lateral femoral condyle

Iliotibial tract

Lateral meniscus

FIGURE 5-10

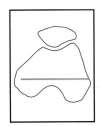

KNEE: CORONAL

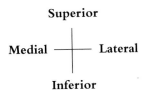

Superior

Medial — Lateral

Inferior

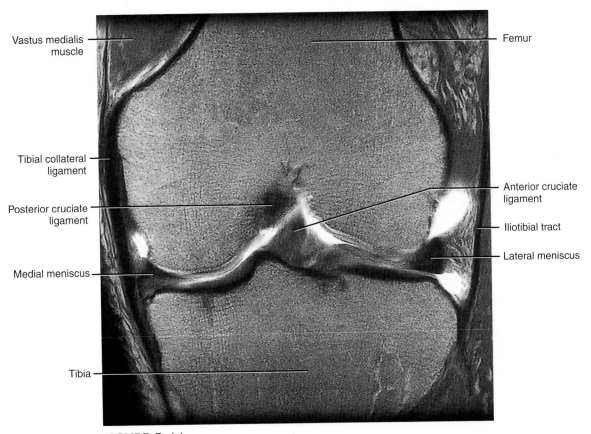

Vastus medialis
muscle

Femur

Tibial collateral
ligament

Anterior cruciate
ligament

Posterior cruciate
ligament

Iliotibial tract

Lateral meniscus

Medial meniscus

Tibia

FIGURE 5-11

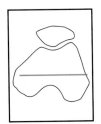

KNEE: CORONAL

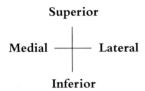

Superior

Medial ——|—— Lateral

Inferior

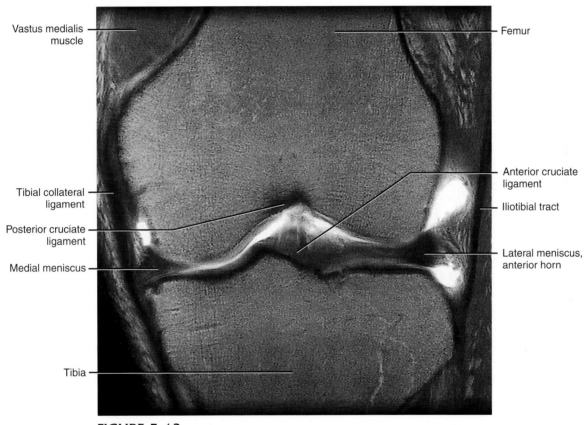

Vastus medialis muscle

Femur

Tibial collateral ligament

Anterior cruciate ligament

Iliotibial tract

Posterior cruciate ligament

Medial meniscus

Lateral meniscus, anterior horn

Tibia

FIGURE 5-12

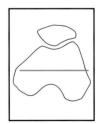

KNEE: CORONAL

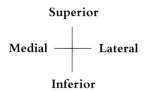

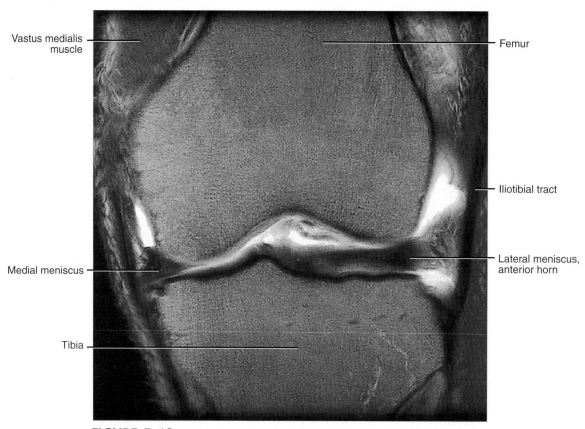

Vastus medialis muscle

Femur

Iliotibial tract

Medial meniscus

Lateral meniscus, anterior horn

Tibia

FIGURE 5-13

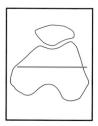

KNEE: CORONAL

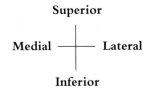

Superior

Medial ——|—— Lateral

Inferior

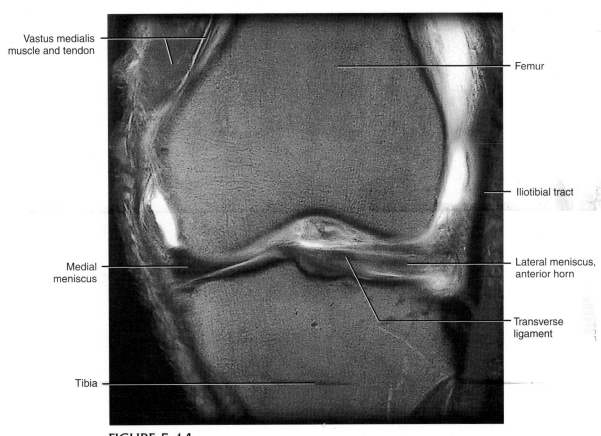

Vastus medialis
muscle and tendon

Femur

Iliotibial tract

Medial
meniscus

Lateral meniscus,
anterior horn

Transverse
ligament

Tibia

FIGURE 5-14

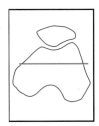

KNEE: CORONAL

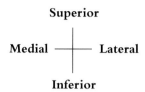

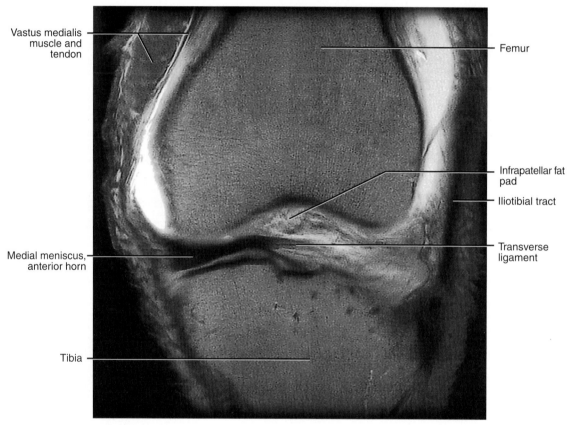

Vastus medialis muscle and tendon

Femur

Infrapatellar fat pad

Iliotibial tract

Medial meniscus, anterior horn

Transverse ligament

Tibia

FIGURE 5-15

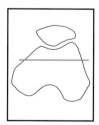

KNEE: CORONAL

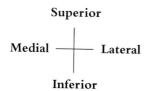

Superior

Medial — Lateral

Inferior

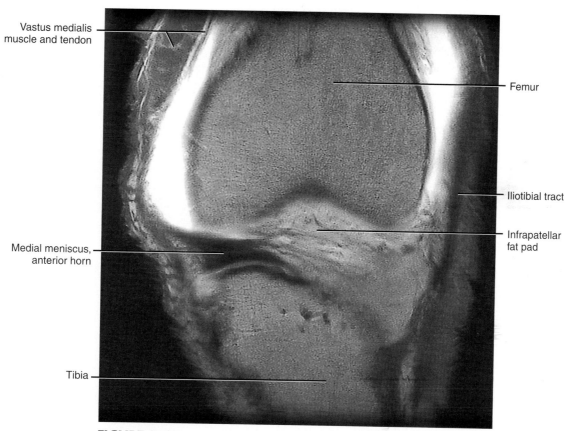

Vastus medialis
muscle and tendon

Femur

Iliotibial tract

Infrapatellar
fat pad

Medial meniscus,
anterior horn

Tibia

FIGURE 5-16

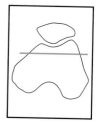

KNEE: CORONAL

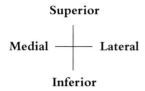

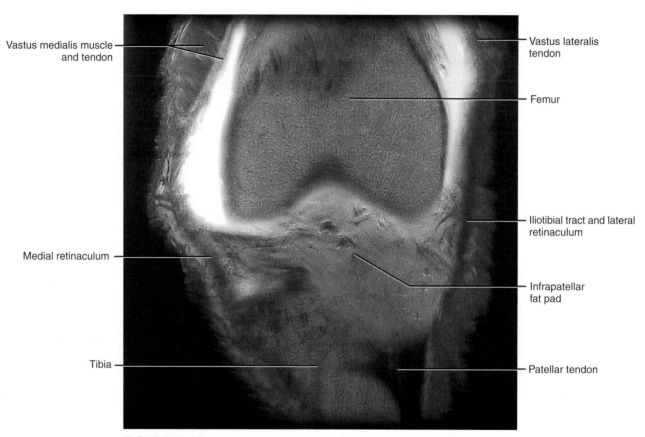

Vastus medialis muscle and tendon

Vastus lateralis tendon

Femur

Medial retinaculum

Iliotibial tract and lateral retinaculum

Infrapatellar fat pad

Tibia

Patellar tendon

FIGURE 5-17

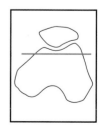

KNEE: CORONAL

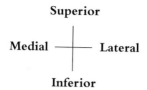

Superior

Medial — Lateral

Inferior

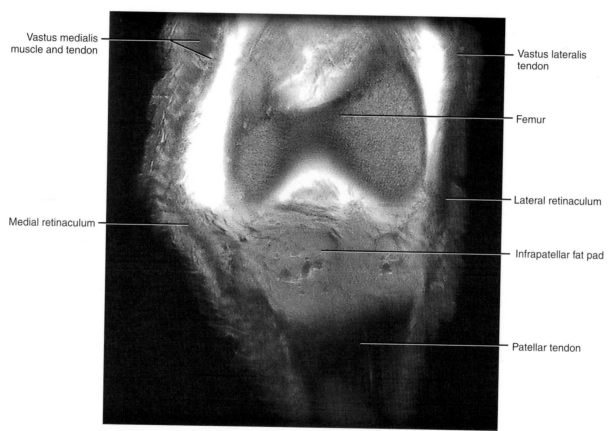

Vastus medialis muscle and tendon

Vastus lateralis tendon

Femur

Lateral retinaculum

Medial retinaculum

Infrapatellar fat pad

Patellar tendon

FIGURE 5-18

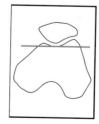

KNEE: CORONAL

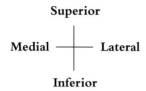

Superior

Medial ——|—— Lateral

Inferior

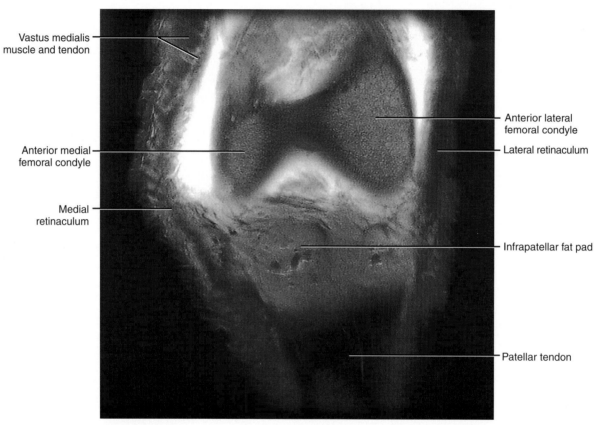

Vastus medialis
muscle and tendon

Anterior lateral
femoral condyle

Anterior medial
femoral condyle

Lateral retinaculum

Medial
retinaculum

Infrapatellar fat pad

Patellar tendon

FIGURE 5-19

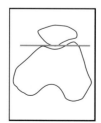

KNEE: CORONAL

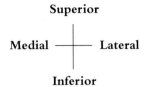

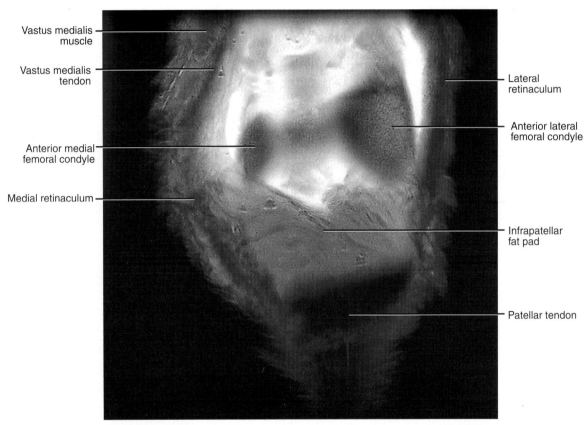

Vastus medialis muscle

Vastus medialis tendon

Anterior medial femoral condyle

Medial retinaculum

Lateral retinaculum

Anterior lateral femoral condyle

Infrapatellar fat pad

Patellar tendon

FIGURE 5-20

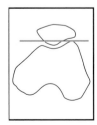

KNEE: CORONAL

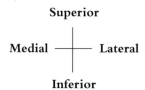

Vastus medialis tendon

Medial patellar facet

Medial retinaculum

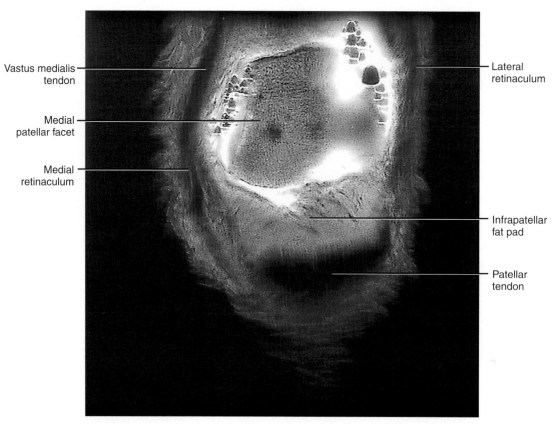

Lateral retinaculum

Infrapatellar fat pad

Patellar tendon

FIGURE 5-21

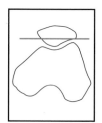

KNEE: CORONAL

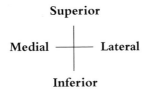

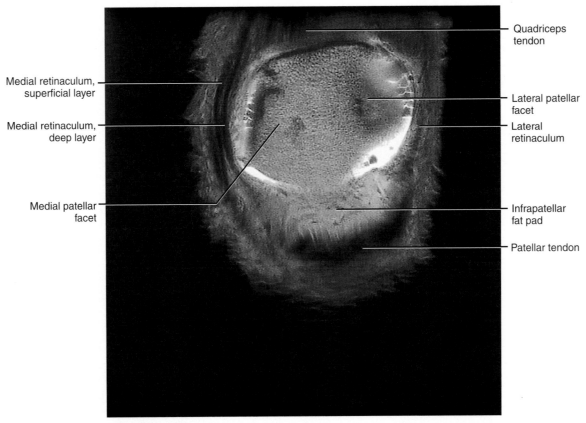

Quadriceps tendon

Medial retinaculum, superficial layer

Lateral patellar facet

Medial retinaculum, deep layer

Lateral retinaculum

Medial patellar facet

Infrapatellar fat pad

Patellar tendon

FIGURE 5-22

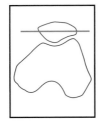

KNEE: CORONAL

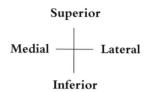

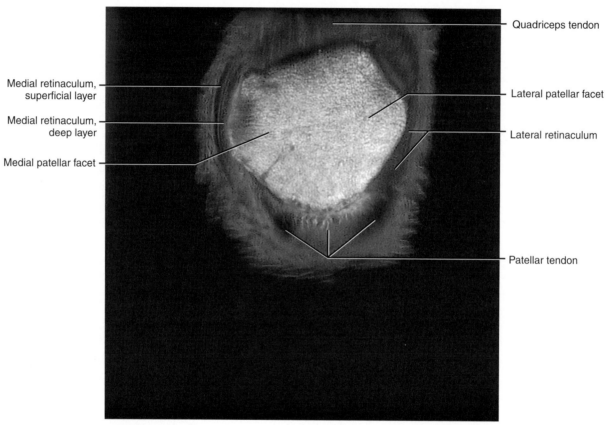

Quadriceps tendon

Medial retinaculum, superficial layer

Lateral patellar facet

Medial retinaculum, deep layer

Lateral retinaculum

Medial patellar facet

Patellar tendon

FIGURE 5-23

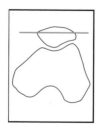

KNEE: CORONAL

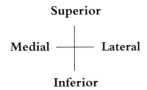

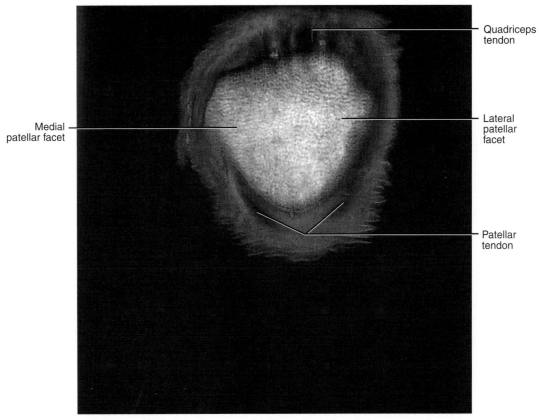

Medial
patellar facet

Quadriceps
tendon

Lateral
patellar
facet

Patellar
tendon

FIGURE 5-24

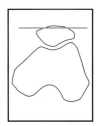

KNEE: AXIAL

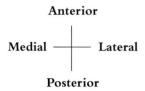

Anterior

Medial —— Lateral

Posterior

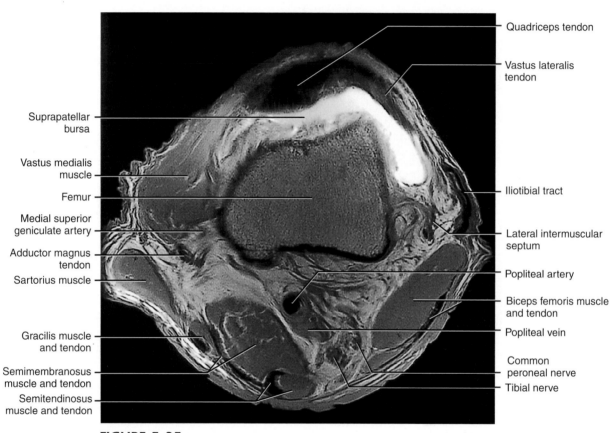

Quadriceps tendon

Vastus lateralis tendon

Suprapatellar bursa

Vastus medialis muscle

Femur

Medial superior geniculate artery

Adductor magnus tendon

Sartorius muscle

Iliotibial tract

Lateral intermuscular septum

Popliteal artery

Biceps femoris muscle and tendon

Gracilis muscle and tendon

Popliteal vein

Semimembranosus muscle and tendon

Common peroneal nerve

Tibial nerve

Semitendinosus muscle and tendon

FIGURE 5-25

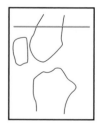

KNEE: AXIAL

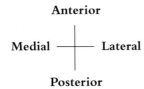

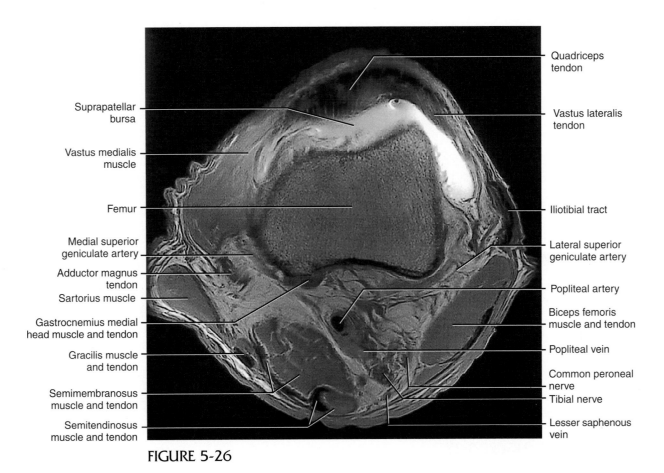

FIGURE 5-26

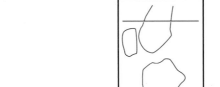

KNEE: AXIAL

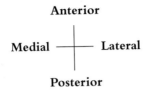

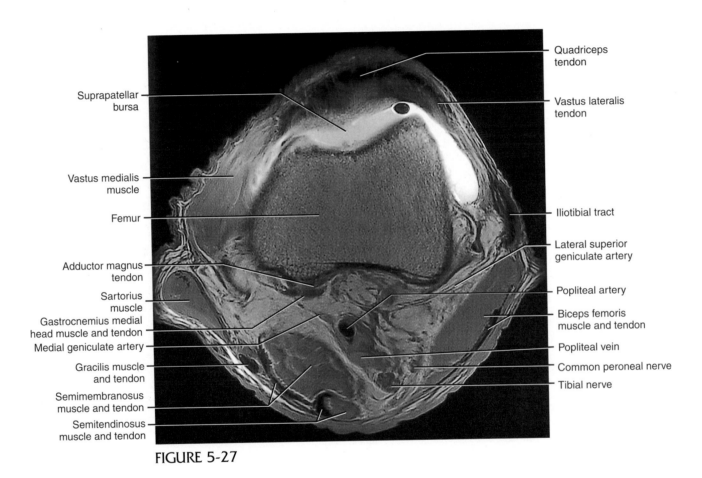

Quadriceps tendon

Suprapatellar bursa

Vastus lateralis tendon

Vastus medialis muscle

Femur

Iliotibial tract

Adductor magnus tendon

Lateral superior geniculate artery

Sartorius muscle

Popliteal artery

Gastrocnemius medial head muscle and tendon

Biceps femoris muscle and tendon

Medial geniculate artery

Popliteal vein

Gracilis muscle and tendon

Common peroneal nerve

Semimembranosus muscle and tendon

Tibial nerve

Semitendinosus muscle and tendon

FIGURE 5-27

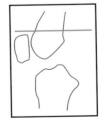

KNEE: AXIAL

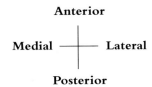

Anterior

Medial ——|—— Lateral

Posterior

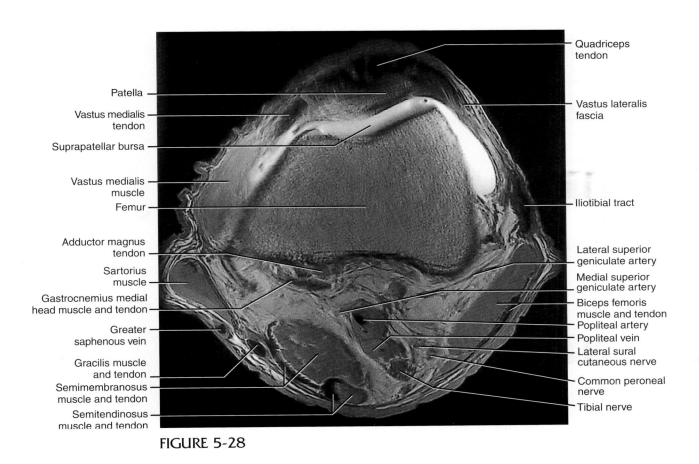

Quadriceps tendon

Patella

Vastus medialis tendon

Suprapatellar bursa

Vastus medialis muscle

Femur

Adductor magnus tendon

Sartorius muscle

Gastrocnemius medial head muscle and tendon

Greater saphenous vein

Gracilis muscle and tendon

Semimembranosus muscle and tendon

Semitendinosus muscle and tendon

Vastus lateralis fascia

Iliotibial tract

Lateral superior geniculate artery

Medial superior geniculate artery

Biceps femoris muscle and tendon

Popliteal artery

Popliteal vein

Lateral sural cutaneous nerve

Common peroneal nerve

Tibial nerve

FIGURE 5-28

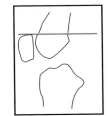

KNEE: AXIAL

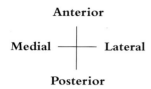

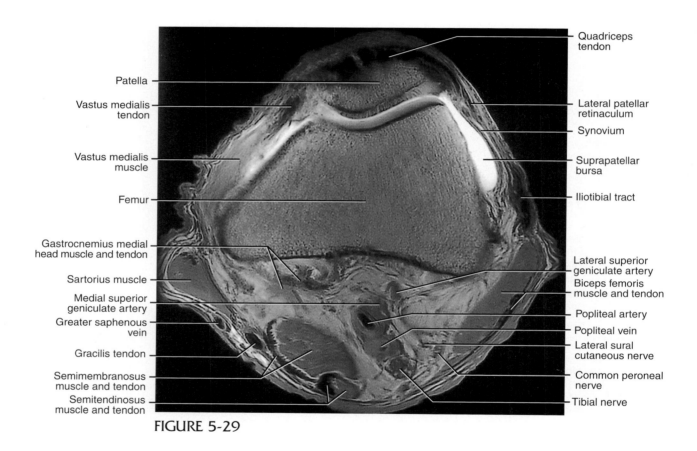

Quadriceps tendon

Patella

Vastus medialis tendon

Lateral patellar retinaculum

Synovium

Vastus medialis muscle

Suprapatellar bursa

Femur

Iliotibial tract

Gastrocnemius medial head muscle and tendon

Sartorius muscle

Lateral superior geniculate artery

Medial superior geniculate artery

Biceps femoris muscle and tendon

Greater saphenous vein

Popliteal artery

Gracilis tendon

Popliteal vein

Lateral sural cutaneous nerve

Semimembranosus muscle and tendon

Common peroneal nerve

Semitendinosus muscle and tendon

Tibial nerve

FIGURE 5-29

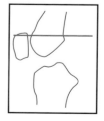

KNEE: AXIAL

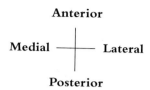

Anterior

Medial —|— Lateral

Posterior

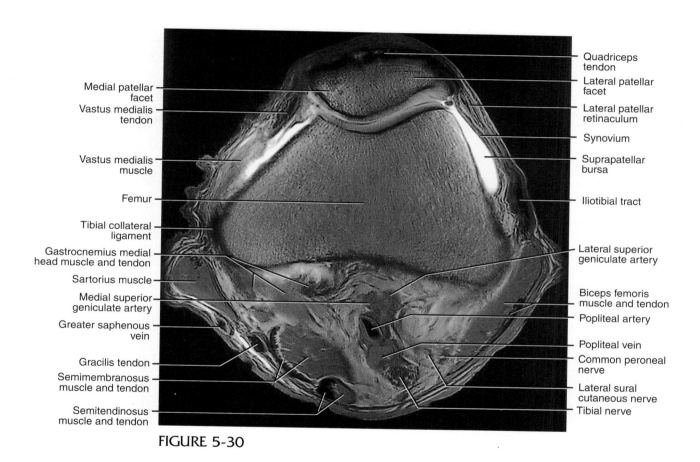

Medial patellar facet

Vastus medialis tendon

Vastus medialis muscle

Femur

Tibial collateral ligament

Gastrocnemius medial head muscle and tendon

Sartorius muscle

Medial superior geniculate artery

Greater saphenous vein

Gracilis tendon

Semimembranosus muscle and tendon

Semitendinosus muscle and tendon

Quadriceps tendon

Lateral patellar facet

Lateral patellar retinaculum

Synovium

Suprapatellar bursa

Iliotibial tract

Lateral superior geniculate artery

Biceps femoris muscle and tendon

Popliteal artery

Popliteal vein

Common peroneal nerve

Lateral sural cutaneous nerve

Tibial nerve

FIGURE 5-30

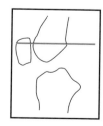

KNEE: AXIAL

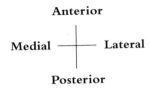

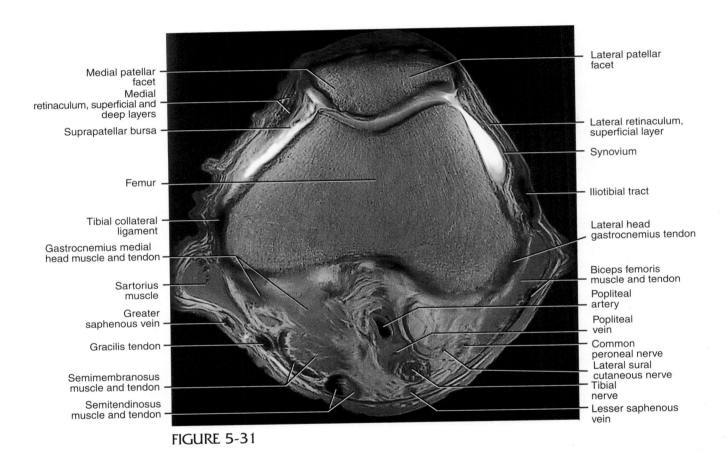

Medial patellar facet

Medial retinaculum, superficial and deep layers

Suprapatellar bursa

Femur

Tibial collateral ligament

Gastrocnemius medial head muscle and tendon

Sartorius muscle

Greater saphenous vein

Gracilis tendon

Semimembranosus muscle and tendon

Semitendinosus muscle and tendon

Lateral patellar facet

Lateral retinaculum, superficial layer

Synovium

Iliotibial tract

Lateral head gastrocnemius tendon

Biceps femoris muscle and tendon

Popliteal artery

Popliteal vein

Common peroneal nerve

Lateral sural cutaneous nerve

Tibial nerve

Lesser saphenous vein

FIGURE 5-31

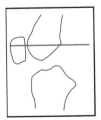

KNEE: AXIAL

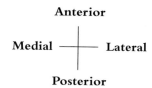

Anterior

Medial ── Lateral

Posterior

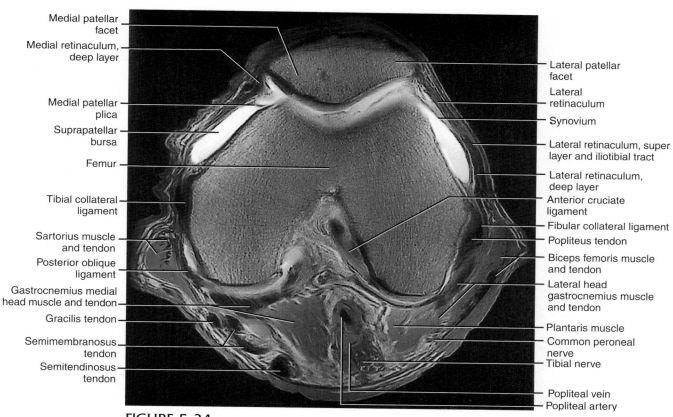

Medial patellar facet

Medial retinaculum, deep layer

Medial patellar plica

Suprapatellar bursa

Femur

Tibial collateral ligament

Sartorius muscle and tendon

Posterior oblique ligament

Gastrocnemius medial head muscle and tendon

Gracilis tendon

Semimembranosus tendon

Semitendinosus tendon

Lateral patellar facet

Lateral retinaculum

Synovium

Lateral retinaculum, super layer and iliotibial tract

Lateral retinaculum, deep layer

Anterior cruciate ligament

Fibular collateral ligament

Popliteus tendon

Biceps femoris muscle and tendon

Lateral head gastrocnemius muscle and tendon

Plantaris muscle

Common peroneal nerve

Tibial nerve

Popliteal vein

Popliteal artery

FIGURE 5-34

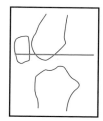

KNEE: AXIAL

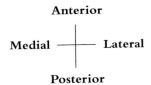

Anterior

Medial —|— Lateral

Posterior

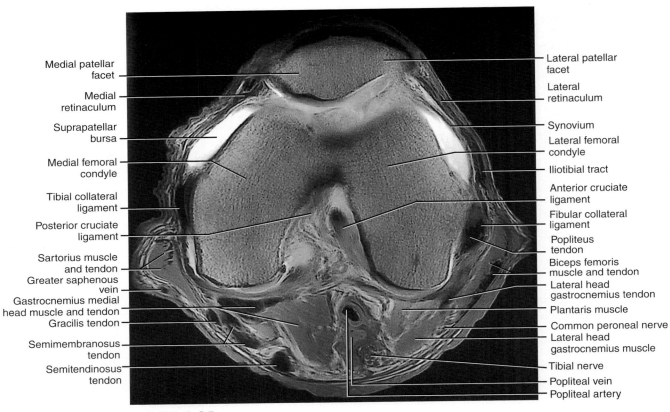

Medial patellar facet

Medial retinaculum

Suprapatellar bursa

Medial femoral condyle

Tibial collateral ligament

Posterior cruciate ligament

Sartorius muscle and tendon

Greater saphenous vein

Gastrocnemius medial head muscle and tendon

Gracilis tendon

Semimembranosus tendon

Semitendinosus tendon

Lateral patellar facet

Lateral retinaculum

Synovium

Lateral femoral condyle

Iliotibial tract

Anterior cruciate ligament

Fibular collateral ligament

Popliteus tendon

Biceps femoris muscle and tendon

Lateral head gastrocnemius tendon

Plantaris muscle

Common peroneal nerve

Lateral head gastrocnemius muscle

Tibial nerve

Popliteal vein

Popliteal artery

FIGURE 5-35

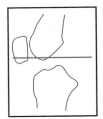

KNEE: AXIAL

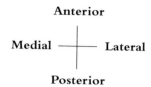

Anterior

Medial ——|—— Lateral

Posterior

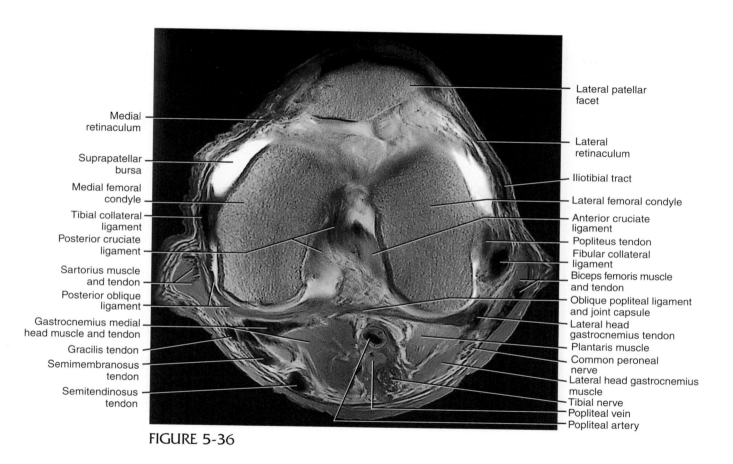

Medial retinaculum

Suprapatellar bursa

Medial femoral condyle

Tibial collateral ligament

Posterior cruciate ligament

Sartorius muscle and tendon

Posterior oblique ligament

Gastrocnemius medial head muscle and tendon

Gracilis tendon

Semimembranosus tendon

Semitendinosus tendon

Lateral patellar facet

Lateral retinaculum

Iliotibial tract

Lateral femoral condyle

Anterior cruciate ligament

Popliteus tendon

Fibular collateral ligament

Biceps femoris muscle and tendon

Oblique popliteal ligament and joint capsule

Lateral head gastrocnemius tendon

Plantaris muscle

Common peroneal nerve

Lateral head gastrocnemius muscle

Tibial nerve

Popliteal vein

Popliteal artery

FIGURE 5-36

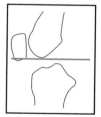

KNEE: AXIAL

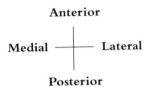

Anterior

Medial —— Lateral

Posterior

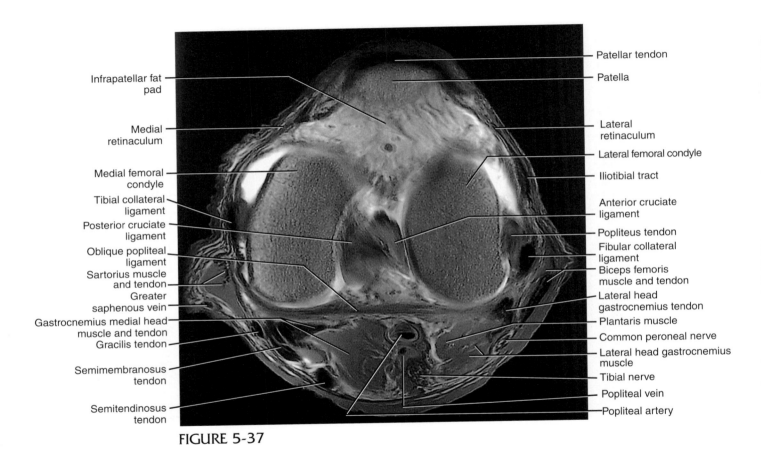

Infrapatellar fat pad

Medial retinaculum

Medial femoral condyle

Tibial collateral ligament

Posterior cruciate ligament

Oblique popliteal ligament

Sartorius muscle and tendon

Greater saphenous vein

Gastrocnemius medial head muscle and tendon

Gracilis tendon

Semimembranosus tendon

Semitendinosus tendon

Patellar tendon

Patella

Lateral retinaculum

Lateral femoral condyle

Iliotibial tract

Anterior cruciate ligament

Popliteus tendon

Fibular collateral ligament

Biceps femoris muscle and tendon

Lateral head gastrocnemius tendon

Plantaris muscle

Common peroneal nerve

Lateral head gastrocnemius muscle

Tibial nerve

Popliteal vein

Popliteal artery

FIGURE 5-37

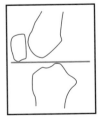

KNEE: AXIAL

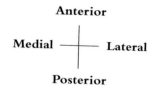

Anterior

Medial ——|—— Lateral

Posterior

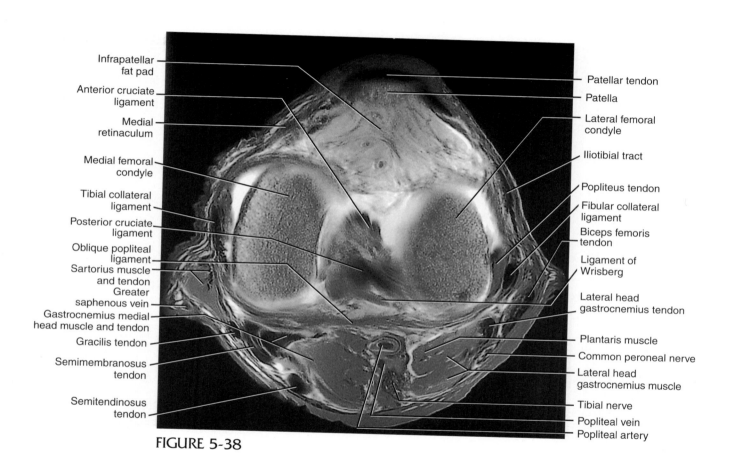

Infrapatellar fat pad

Anterior cruciate ligament

Medial retinaculum

Medial femoral condyle

Tibial collateral ligament

Posterior cruciate ligament

Oblique popliteal ligament

Sartorius muscle and tendon

Greater saphenous vein

Gastrocnemius medial head muscle and tendon

Gracilis tendon

Semimembranosus tendon

Semitendinosus tendon

Patellar tendon

Patella

Lateral femoral condyle

Iliotibial tract

Popliteus tendon

Fibular collateral ligament

Biceps femoris tendon

Ligament of Wrisberg

Lateral head gastrocnemius tendon

Plantaris muscle

Common peroneal nerve

Lateral head gastrocnemius muscle

Tibial nerve

Popliteal vein

Popliteal artery

FIGURE 5-38

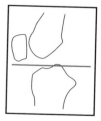

KNEE: AXIAL

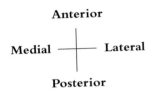

Anterior

Medial —— Lateral

Posterior

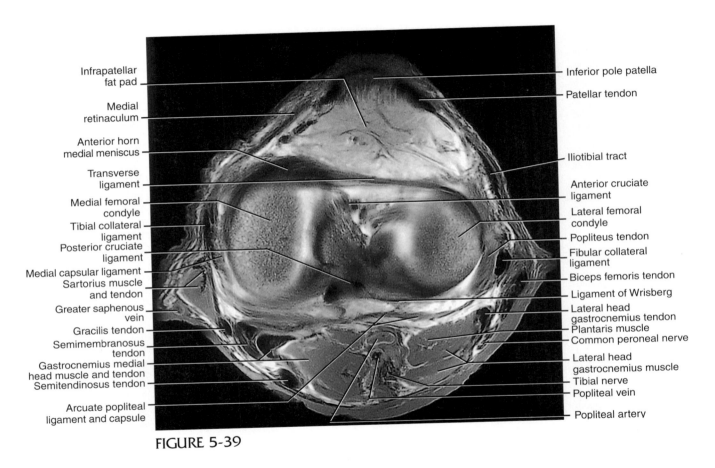

Infrapatellar fat pad

Medial retinaculum

Anterior horn medial meniscus

Transverse ligament

Medial femoral condyle

Tibial collateral ligament

Posterior cruciate ligament

Medial capsular ligament

Sartorius muscle and tendon

Greater saphenous vein

Gracilis tendon

Semimembranosus tendon

Gastrocnemius medial head muscle and tendon

Semitendinosus tendon

Arcuate popliteal ligament and capsule

Inferior pole patella

Patellar tendon

Iliotibial tract

Anterior cruciate ligament

Lateral femoral condyle

Popliteus tendon

Fibular collateral ligament

Biceps femoris tendon

Ligament of Wrisberg

Lateral head gastrocnemius tendon

Plantaris muscle

Common peroneal nerve

Lateral head gastrocnemius muscle

Tibial nerve

Popliteal vein

Popliteal artery

FIGURE 5-39

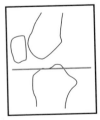

KNEE: AXIAL

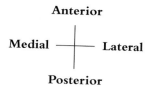

Anterior

Medial —|— Lateral

Posterior

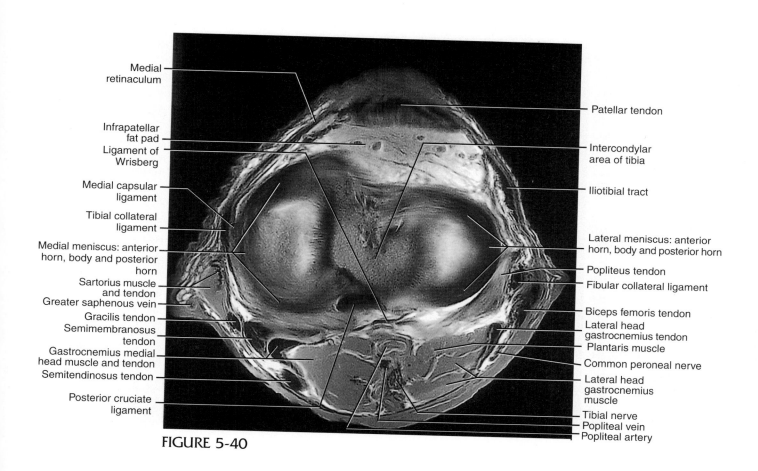

Medial retinaculum

Infrapatellar fat pad

Ligament of Wrisberg

Medial capsular ligament

Tibial collateral ligament

Medial meniscus: anterior horn, body and posterior horn

Sartorius muscle and tendon

Greater saphenous vein

Gracilis tendon

Semimembranosus tendon

Gastrocnemius medial head muscle and tendon

Semitendinosus tendon

Posterior cruciate ligament

Patellar tendon

Intercondylar area of tibia

Iliotibial tract

Lateral meniscus: anterior horn, body and posterior horn

Popliteus tendon

Fibular collateral ligament

Biceps femoris tendon

Lateral head gastrocnemius tendon

Plantaris muscle

Common peroneal nerve

Lateral head gastrocnemius muscle

Tibial nerve

Popliteal vein

Popliteal artery

FIGURE 5-40

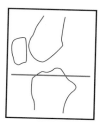

KNEE: AXIAL

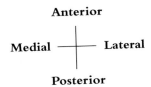

Anterior

Medial —|— Lateral

Posterior

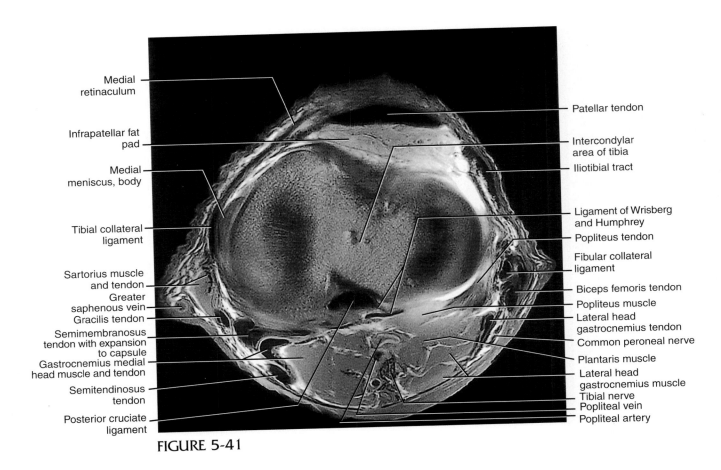

Medial
retinaculum

Infrapatellar fat
pad

Medial
meniscus, body

Tibial collateral
ligament

Sartorius muscle
and tendon

Greater
saphenous vein

Gracilis tendon

Semimembranosus
tendon with expansion
to capsule

Gastrocnemius medial
head muscle and tendon

Semitendinosus
tendon

Posterior cruciate
ligament

Patellar tendon

Intercondylar
area of tibia

Iliotibial tract

Ligament of Wrisberg
and Humphrey

Popliteus tendon

Fibular collateral
ligament

Biceps femoris tendon

Popliteus muscle

Lateral head
gastrocnemius tendon

Common peroneal nerve

Plantaris muscle

Lateral head
gastrocnemius muscle

Tibial nerve

Popliteal vein

Popliteal artery

FIGURE 5-41

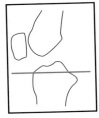

KNEE: AXIAL

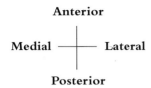

Anterior

Medial ——+—— Lateral

Posterior

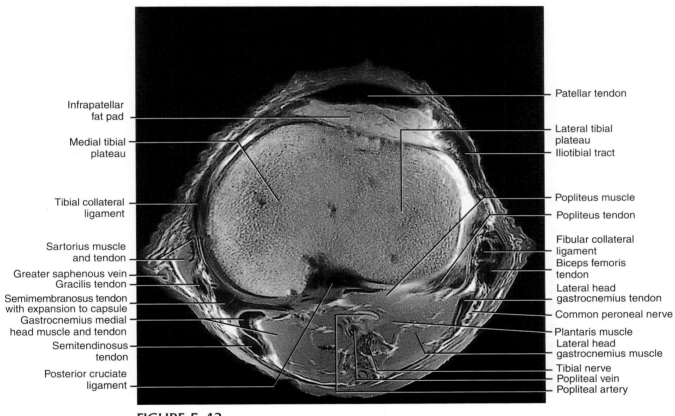

Infrapatellar
fat pad

Medial tibial
plateau

Tibial collateral
ligament

Sartorius muscle
and tendon

Greater saphenous vein
Gracilis tendon

Semimembranosus tendon
with expansion to capsule
Gastrocnemius medial
head muscle and tendon

Semitendinosus
tendon

Posterior cruciate
ligament

Patellar tendon

Lateral tibial
plateau
Iliotibial tract

Popliteus muscle
Popliteus tendon

Fibular collateral
ligament
Biceps femoris
tendon

Lateral head
gastrocnemius tendon

Common peroneal nerve

Plantaris muscle
Lateral head
gastrocnemius muscle

Tibial nerve
Popliteal vein
Popliteal artery

FIGURE 5-42

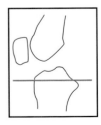

KNEE: AXIAL

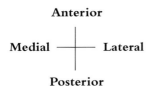

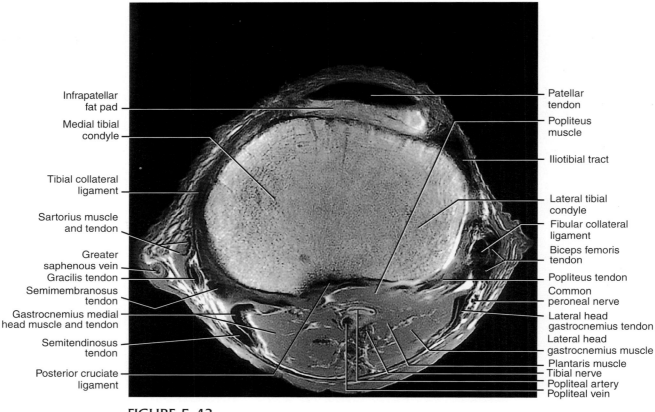

Infrapatellar fat pad

Medial tibial condyle

Tibial collateral ligament

Sartorius muscle and tendon

Greater saphenous vein

Gracilis tendon

Semimembranosus tendon

Gastrocnemius medial head muscle and tendon

Semitendinosus tendon

Posterior cruciate ligament

Patellar tendon

Popliteus muscle

Iliotibial tract

Lateral tibial condyle

Fibular collateral ligament

Biceps femoris tendon

Popliteus tendon

Common peroneal nerve

Lateral head gastrocnemius tendon

Lateral head gastrocnemius muscle

Plantaris muscle

Tibial nerve

Popliteal artery

Popliteal vein

FIGURE 5-43

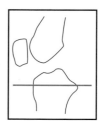

KNEE: AXIAL

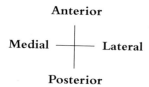

Anterior

Medial ——|—— Lateral

Posterior

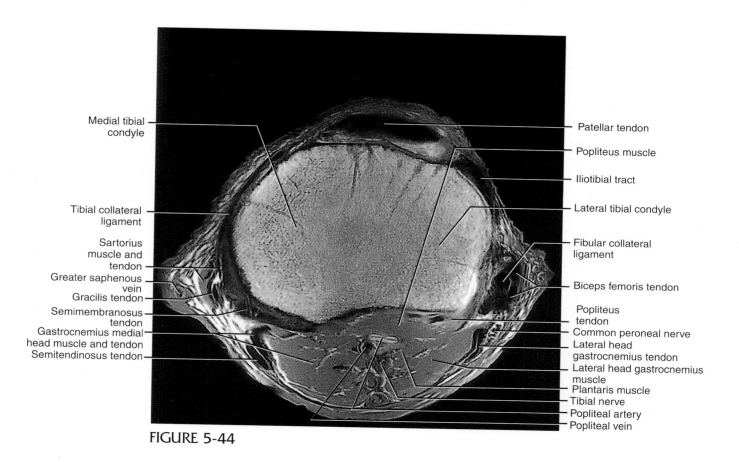

Medial tibial condyle

Tibial collateral ligament

Sartorius muscle and tendon

Greater saphenous vein

Gracilis tendon

Semimembranosus tendon

Gastrocnemius medial head muscle and tendon

Semitendinosus tendon

Patellar tendon

Popliteus muscle

Iliotibial tract

Lateral tibial condyle

Fibular collateral ligament

Biceps femoris tendon

Popliteus tendon

Common peroneal nerve

Lateral head gastrocnemius tendon

Lateral head gastrocnemius muscle

Plantaris muscle

Tibial nerve

Popliteal artery

Popliteal vein

FIGURE 5-44

KNEE: AXIAL

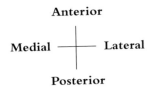

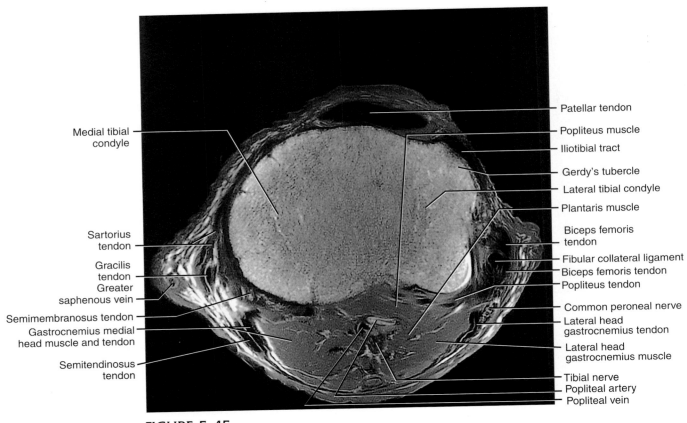

Medial tibial condyle

Patellar tendon

Popliteus muscle

Iliotibial tract

Gerdy's tubercle

Lateral tibial condyle

Plantaris muscle

Biceps femoris tendon

Sartorius tendon

Gracilis tendon

Greater saphenous vein

Fibular collateral ligament

Biceps femoris tendon

Popliteus tendon

Semimembranosus tendon

Gastrocnemius medial head muscle and tendon

Common peroneal nerve

Lateral head gastrocnemius tendon

Semitendinosus tendon

Lateral head gastrocnemius muscle

Tibial nerve

Popliteal artery

Popliteal vein

FIGURE 5-45

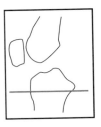

KNEE: AXIAL

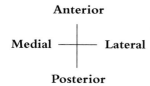

Anterior

Medial —— Lateral

Posterior

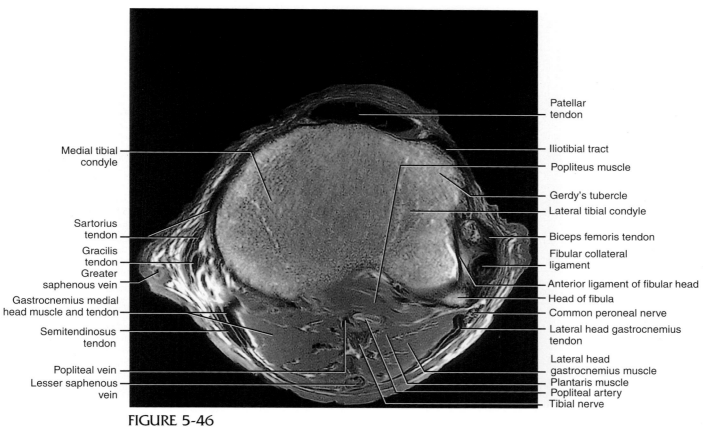

Medial tibial condyle

Sartorius tendon

Gracilis tendon

Greater saphenous vein

Gastrocnemius medial head muscle and tendon

Semitendinosus tendon

Popliteal vein

Lesser saphenous vein

Patellar tendon

Iliotibial tract

Popliteus muscle

Gerdy's tubercle

Lateral tibial condyle

Biceps femoris tendon

Fibular collateral ligament

Anterior ligament of fibular head

Head of fibula

Common peroneal nerve

Lateral head gastrocnemius tendon

Lateral head gastrocnemius muscle

Plantaris muscle

Popliteal artery

Tibial nerve

FIGURE 5-46

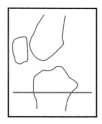

KNEE: AXIAL

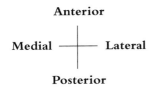

Anterior

Medial ——— Lateral

Posterior

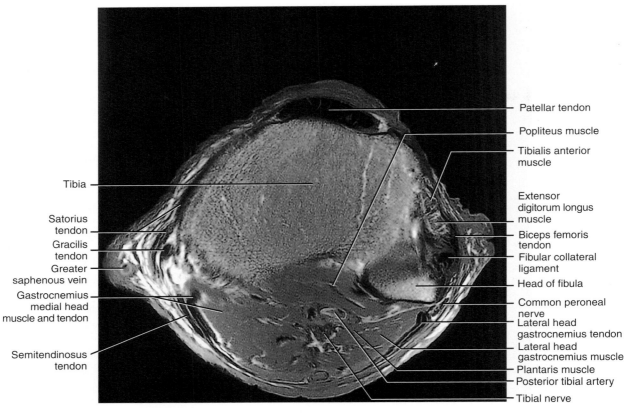

Tibia

Satorius tendon

Gracilis tendon

Greater saphenous vein

Gastrocnemius medial head muscle and tendon

Semitendinosus tendon

Patellar tendon

Popliteus muscle

Tibialis anterior muscle

Extensor digitorum longus muscle

Biceps femoris tendon

Fibular collateral ligament

Head of fibula

Common peroneal nerve

Lateral head gastrocnemius tendon

Lateral head gastrocnemius muscle

Plantaris muscle

Posterior tibial artery

Tibial nerve

FIGURE 5-47

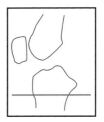

KNEE: AXIAL

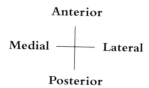

Anterior

Medial ── Lateral

Posterior

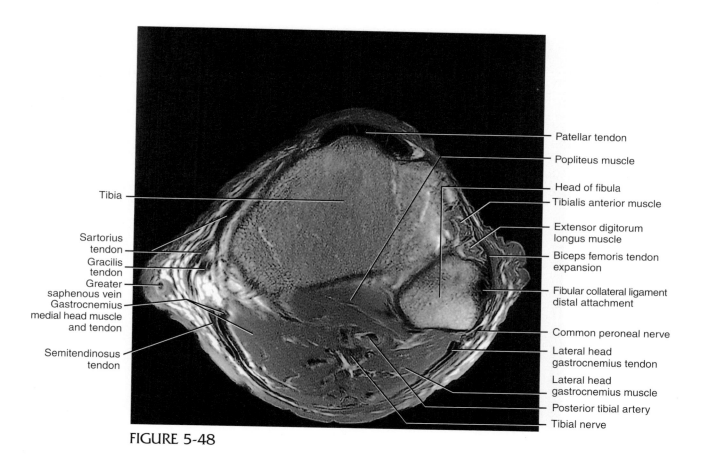

Tibia

Sartorius tendon

Gracilis tendon

Greater saphenous vein

Gastrocnemius medial head muscle and tendon

Semitendinosus tendon

Patellar tendon

Popliteus muscle

Head of fibula

Tibialis anterior muscle

Extensor digitorum longus muscle

Biceps femoris tendon expansion

Fibular collateral ligament distal attachment

Common peroneal nerve

Lateral head gastrocnemius tendon

Lateral head gastrocnemius muscle

Posterior tibial artery

Tibial nerve

FIGURE 5-48

KNEE: SAGITTAL

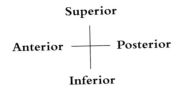

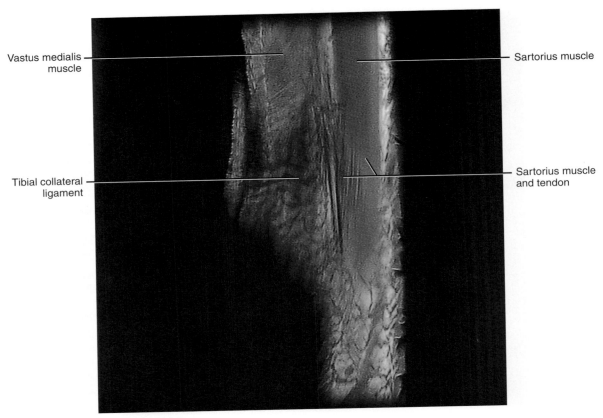

Vastus medialis
muscle

Sartorius muscle

Tibial collateral
ligament

Sartorius muscle
and tendon

FIGURE 5-49

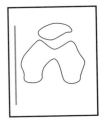

KNEE: SAGITTAL

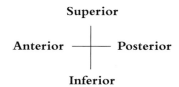

Superior

Anterior — Posterior

Inferior

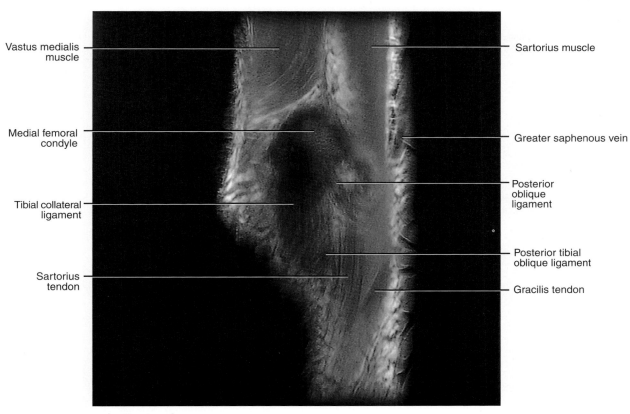

Vastus medialis muscle

Sartorius muscle

Medial femoral condyle

Greater saphenous vein

Posterior oblique ligament

Tibial collateral ligament

Posterior tibial oblique ligament

Sartorius tendon

Gracilis tendon

FIGURE 5-50

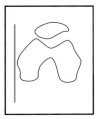

KNEE: SAGITTAL

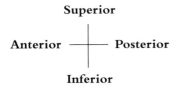

Superior

Anterior —|— Posterior

Inferior

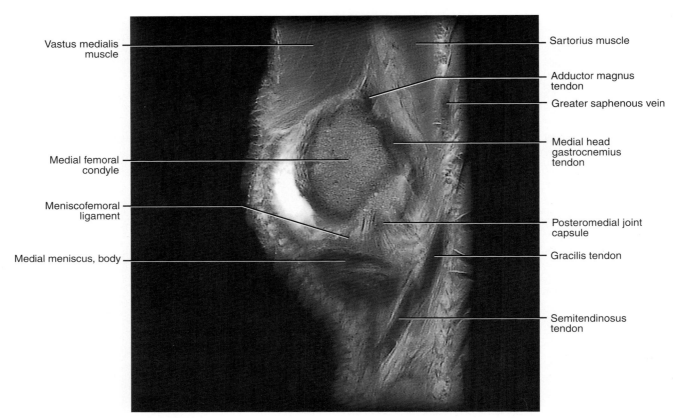

Vastus medialis muscle

Medial femoral condyle

Meniscofemoral ligament

Medial meniscus, body

Sartorius muscle

Adductor magnus tendon

Greater saphenous vein

Medial head gastrocnemius tendon

Posteromedial joint capsule

Gracilis tendon

Semitendinosus tendon

FIGURE 5-51

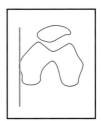

KNEE: SAGITTAL

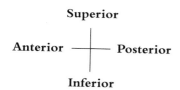

Superior

Anterior — Posterior

Inferior

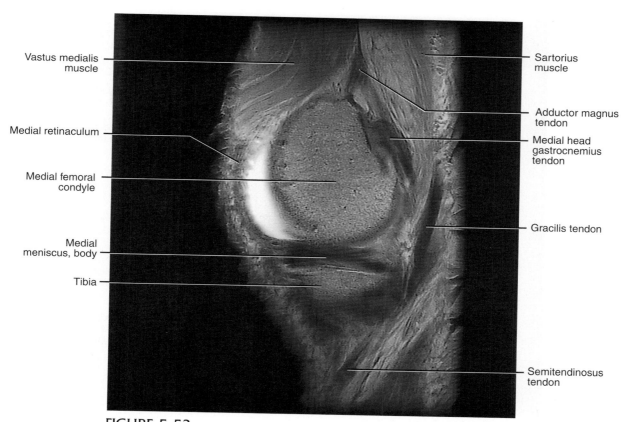

Vastus medialis muscle

Medial retinaculum

Medial femoral condyle

Medial meniscus, body

Tibia

Sartorius muscle

Adductor magnus tendon

Medial head gastrocnemius tendon

Gracilis tendon

Semitendinosus tendon

FIGURE 5-52

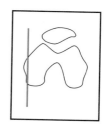

KNEE: SAGITTAL

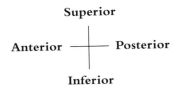

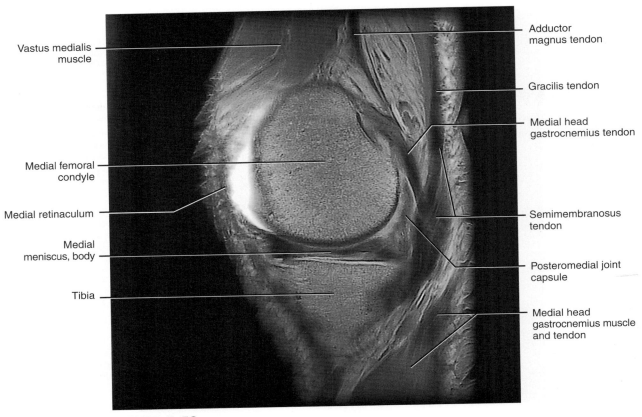

Vastus medialis muscle

Medial femoral condyle

Medial retinaculum

Medial meniscus, body

Tibia

Adductor magnus tendon

Gracilis tendon

Medial head gastrocnemius tendon

Semimembranosus tendon

Posteromedial joint capsule

Medial head gastrocnemius muscle and tendon

FIGURE 5-53

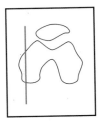

KNEE: SAGITTAL

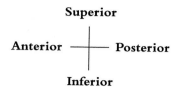

Superior

Anterior —— Posterior

Inferior

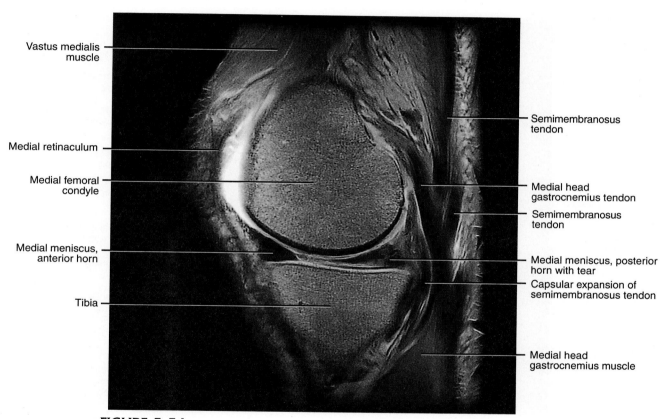

Vastus medialis muscle

Medial retinaculum

Medial femoral condyle

Medial meniscus, anterior horn

Tibia

Semimembranosus tendon

Medial head gastrocnemius tendon

Semimembranosus tendon

Medial meniscus, posterior horn with tear

Capsular expansion of semimembranosus tendon

Medial head gastrocnemius muscle

FIGURE 5-54

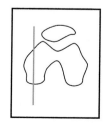

KNEE: SAGITTAL

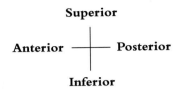

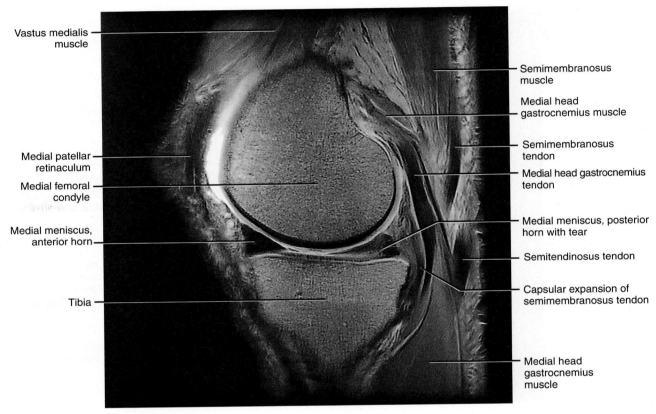

Vastus medialis
muscle

Semimembranosus
muscle

Medial head
gastrocnemius muscle

Semimembranosus
tendon

Medial patellar
retinaculum

Medial head gastrocnemius
tendon

Medial femoral
condyle

Medial meniscus, posterior
horn with tear

Medial meniscus,
anterior horn

Semitendinosus tendon

Capsular expansion of
semimembranosus tendon

Tibia

Medial head
gastrocnemius
muscle

FIGURE 5-55

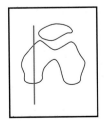

KNEE: SAGITTAL

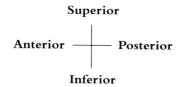

Superior

Anterior ——+—— Posterior

Inferior

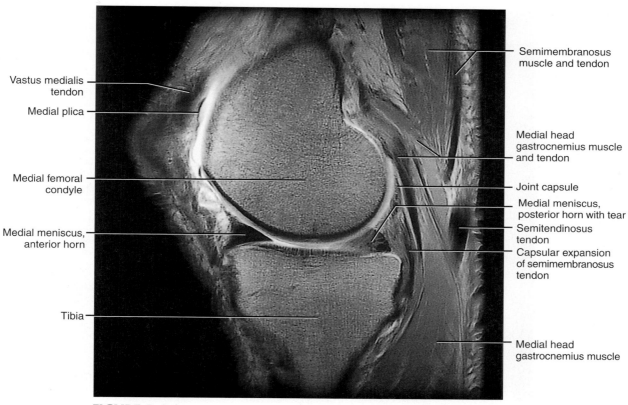

Vastus medialis tendon

Medial plica

Medial femoral condyle

Medial meniscus, anterior horn

Tibia

Semimembranosus muscle and tendon

Medial head gastrocnemius muscle and tendon

Joint capsule

Medial meniscus, posterior horn with tear

Semitendinosus tendon

Capsular expansion of semimembranosus tendon

Medial head gastrocnemius muscle

FIGURE 5-56

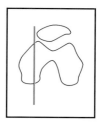

KNEE: SAGITTAL

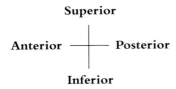

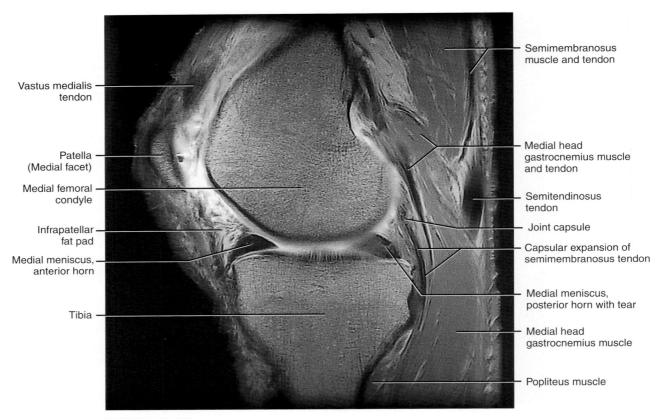

Vastus medialis tendon

Patella (Medial facet)

Medial femoral condyle

Infrapatellar fat pad

Medial meniscus, anterior horn

Tibia

Semimembranosus muscle and tendon

Medial head gastrocnemius muscle and tendon

Semitendinosus tendon

Joint capsule

Capsular expansion of semimembranosus tendon

Medial meniscus, posterior horn with tear

Medial head gastrocnemius muscle

Popliteus muscle

FIGURE 5-57

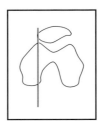

KNEE: SAGITTAL

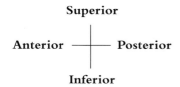

Superior

Anterior ┼ Posterior

Inferior

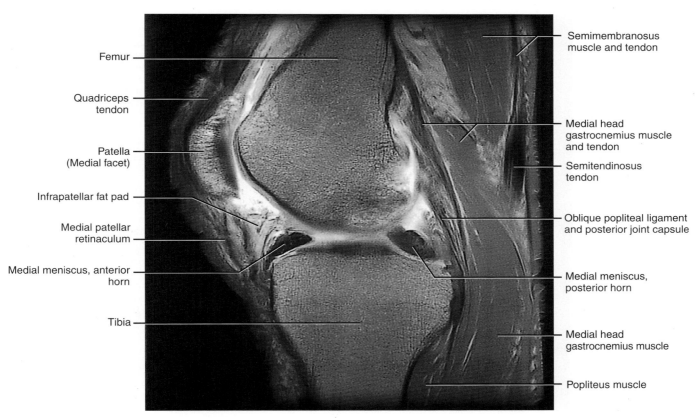

Femur

Quadriceps
tendon

Patella
(Medial facet)

Infrapatellar fat pad

Medial patellar
retinaculum

Medial meniscus, anterior
horn

Tibia

Semimembranosus
muscle and tendon

Medial head
gastrocnemius muscle
and tendon

Semitendinosus
tendon

Oblique popliteal ligament
and posterior joint capsule

Medial meniscus,
posterior horn

Medial head
gastrocnemius muscle

Popliteus muscle

FIGURE 5-58

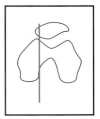

KNEE: SAGITTAL

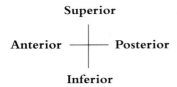

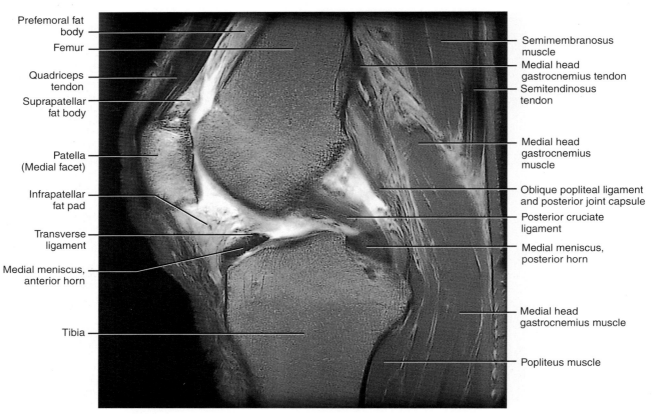

Prefemoral fat body

Femur

Quadriceps tendon

Suprapatellar fat body

Patella (Medial facet)

Infrapatellar fat pad

Transverse ligament

Medial meniscus, anterior horn

Tibia

Semimembranosus muscle

Medial head gastrocnemius tendon

Semitendinosus tendon

Medial head gastrocnemius muscle

Oblique popliteal ligament and posterior joint capsule

Posterior cruciate ligament

Medial meniscus, posterior horn

Medial head gastrocnemius muscle

Popliteus muscle

FIGURE 5-59

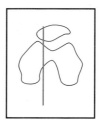

KNEE: SAGITTAL

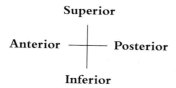

Superior

Anterior — Posterior

Inferior

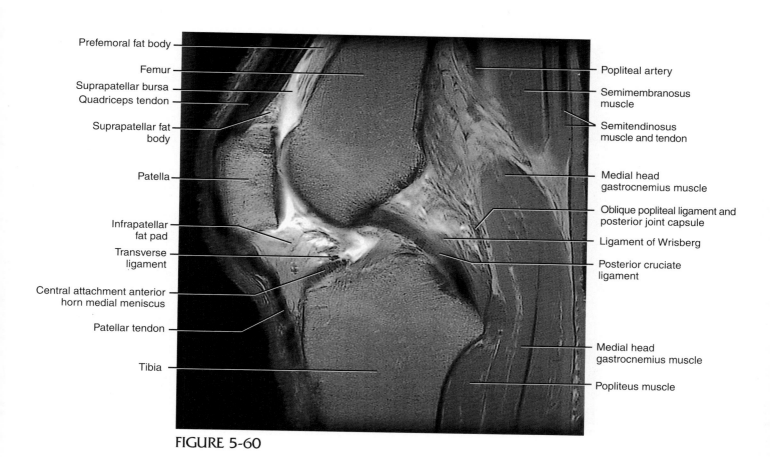

Prefemoral fat body

Femur

Suprapatellar bursa

Quadriceps tendon

Suprapatellar fat body

Patella

Infrapatellar fat pad

Transverse ligament

Central attachment anterior horn medial meniscus

Patellar tendon

Tibia

Popliteal artery

Semimembranosus muscle

Semitendinosus muscle and tendon

Medial head gastrocnemius muscle

Oblique popliteal ligament and posterior joint capsule

Ligament of Wrisberg

Posterior cruciate ligament

Medial head gastrocnemius muscle

Popliteus muscle

FIGURE 5-60

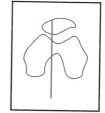

KNEE: SAGITTAL

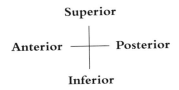

Superior

Anterior ─┼─ Posterior

Inferior

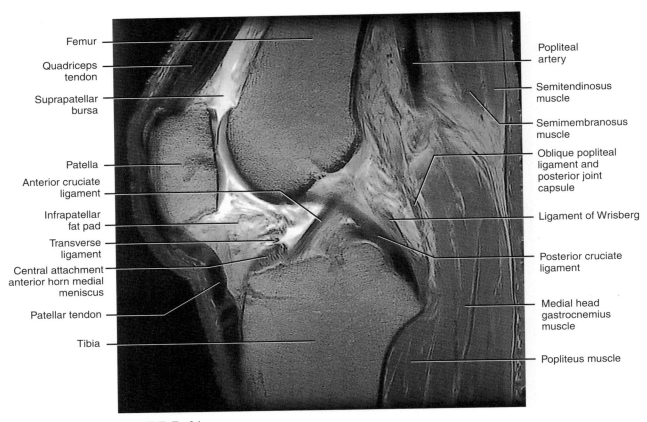

Femur

Quadriceps tendon

Suprapatellar bursa

Patella

Anterior cruciate ligament

Infrapatellar fat pad

Transverse ligament

Central attachment anterior horn medial meniscus

Patellar tendon

Tibia

Popliteal artery

Semitendinosus muscle

Semimembranosus muscle

Oblique popliteal ligament and posterior joint capsule

Ligament of Wrisberg

Posterior cruciate ligament

Medial head gastrocnemius muscle

Popliteus muscle

FIGURE 5-61

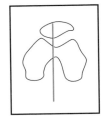

KNEE: SAGITTAL

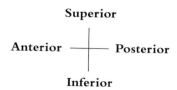

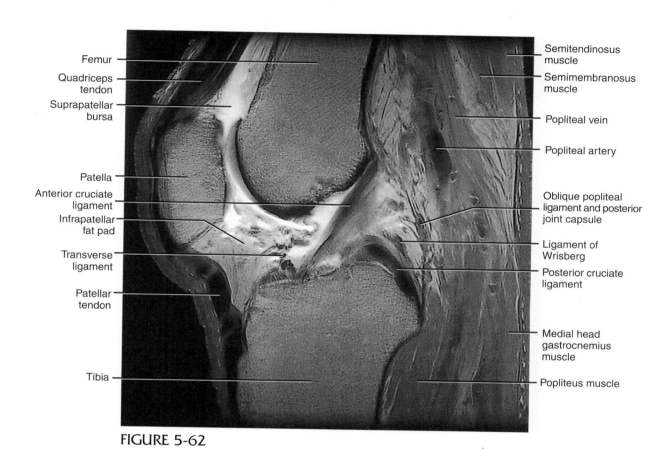

Femur

Quadriceps tendon

Suprapatellar bursa

Patella

Anterior cruciate ligament

Infrapatellar fat pad

Transverse ligament

Patellar tendon

Tibia

Semitendinosus muscle

Semimembranosus muscle

Popliteal vein

Popliteal artery

Oblique popliteal ligament and posterior joint capsule

Ligament of Wrisberg

Posterior cruciate ligament

Medial head gastrocnemius muscle

Popliteus muscle

FIGURE 5-62

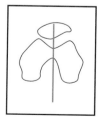

KNEE: SAGITTAL

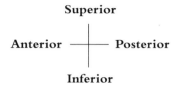

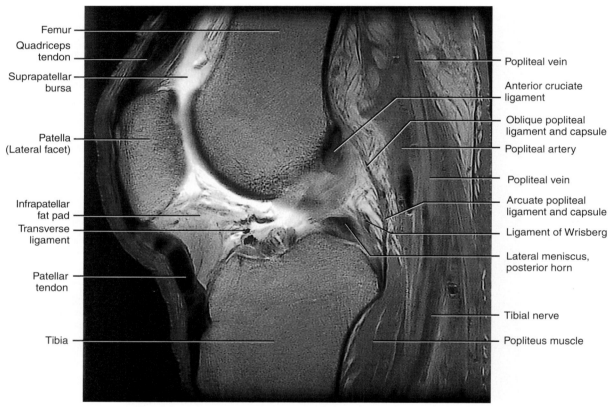

Femur

Quadriceps tendon

Suprapatellar bursa

Patella (Lateral facet)

Infrapatellar fat pad

Transverse ligament

Patellar tendon

Tibia

Popliteal vein

Anterior cruciate ligament

Oblique popliteal ligament and capsule

Popliteal artery

Popliteal vein

Arcuate popliteal ligament and capsule

Ligament of Wrisberg

Lateral meniscus, posterior horn

Tibial nerve

Popliteus muscle

FIGURE 5-63

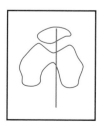

KNEE: SAGITTAL

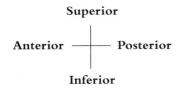

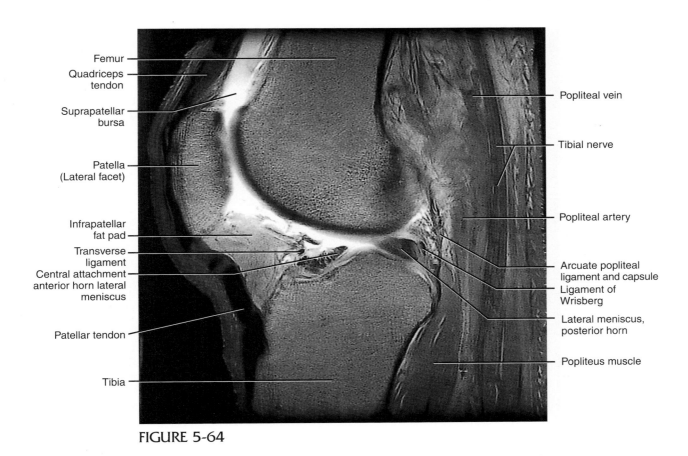

Femur

Quadriceps
tendon

Suprapatellar
bursa

Patella
(Lateral facet)

Infrapatellar
fat pad

Transverse
ligament

Central attachment
anterior horn lateral
meniscus

Patellar tendon

Tibia

Popliteal vein

Tibial nerve

Popliteal artery

Arcuate popliteal
ligament and capsule

Ligament of
Wrisberg

Lateral meniscus,
posterior horn

Popliteus muscle

FIGURE 5-64

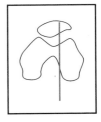

KNEE: SAGITTAL

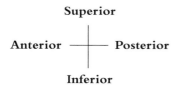

Superior

Anterior ——+—— Posterior

Inferior

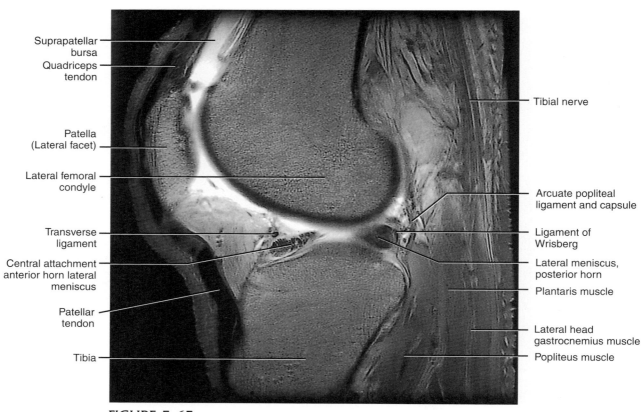

Suprapatellar bursa

Quadriceps tendon

Tibial nerve

Patella (Lateral facet)

Lateral femoral condyle

Arcuate popliteal ligament and capsule

Transverse ligament

Ligament of Wrisberg

Central attachment anterior horn lateral meniscus

Lateral meniscus, posterior horn

Patellar tendon

Plantaris muscle

Lateral head gastrocnemius muscle

Tibia

Popliteus muscle

FIGURE 5-65

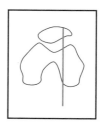

KNEE: SAGITTAL

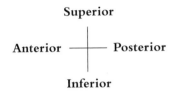

Superior

Anterior —— Posterior

Inferior

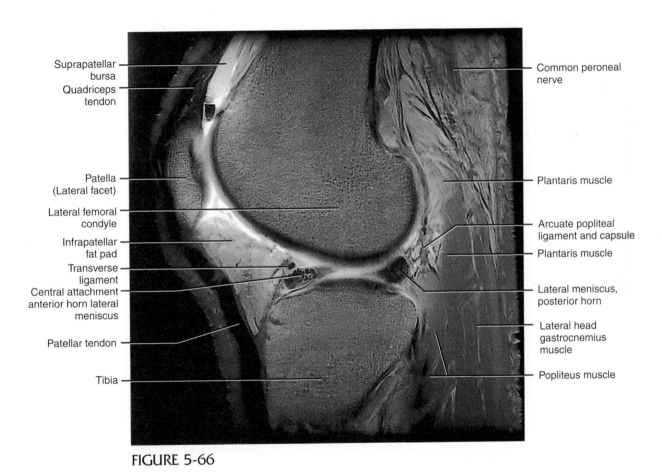

Suprapatellar bursa

Quadriceps tendon

Patella (Lateral facet)

Lateral femoral condyle

Infrapatellar fat pad

Transverse ligament

Central attachment anterior horn lateral meniscus

Patellar tendon

Tibia

Common peroneal nerve

Plantaris muscle

Arcuate popliteal ligament and capsule

Plantaris muscle

Lateral meniscus, posterior horn

Lateral head gastrocnemius muscle

Popliteus muscle

FIGURE 5-66

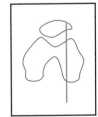

KNEE: SAGITTAL

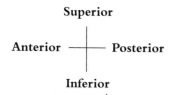

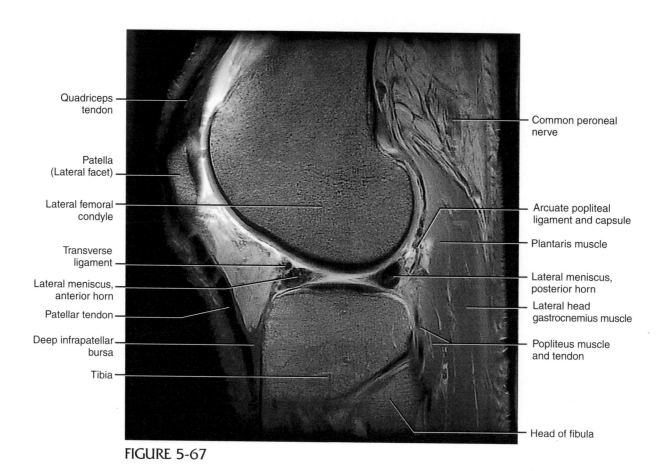

Quadriceps tendon

Patella (Lateral facet)

Lateral femoral condyle

Transverse ligament

Lateral meniscus, anterior horn

Patellar tendon

Deep infrapatellar bursa

Tibia

Common peroneal nerve

Arcuate popliteal ligament and capsule

Plantaris muscle

Lateral meniscus, posterior horn

Lateral head gastrocnemius muscle

Popliteus muscle and tendon

Head of fibula

FIGURE 5-67

KNEE: SAGITTAL

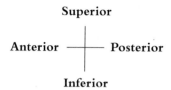

Superior

Anterior ——|—— **Posterior**

Inferior

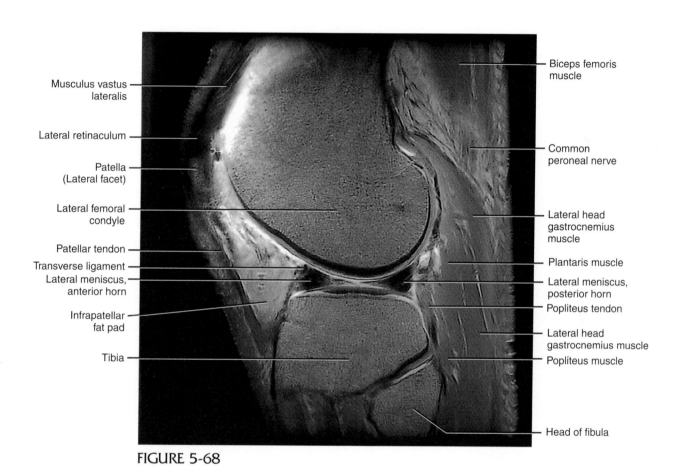

Musculus vastus lateralis

Lateral retinaculum

Patella (Lateral facet)

Lateral femoral condyle

Patellar tendon

Transverse ligament

Lateral meniscus, anterior horn

Infrapatellar fat pad

Tibia

Biceps femoris muscle

Common peroneal nerve

Lateral head gastrocnemius muscle

Plantaris muscle

Lateral meniscus, posterior horn

Popliteus tendon

Lateral head gastrocnemius muscle

Popliteus muscle

Head of fibula

FIGURE 5-68

KNEE: SAGITTAL

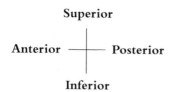

Superior

Anterior ——— Posterior

Inferior

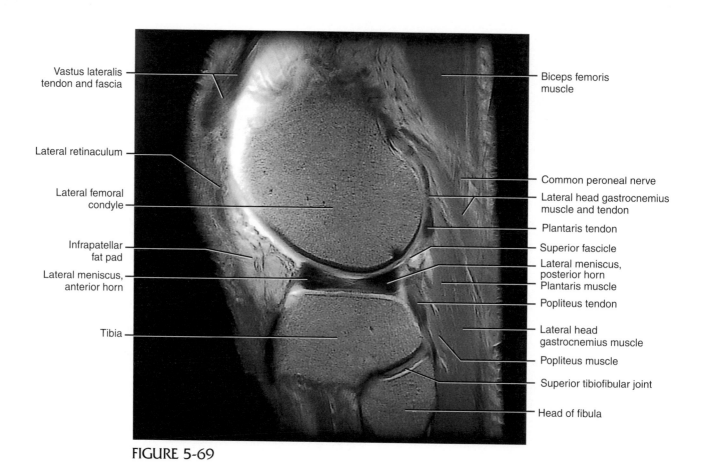

Vastus lateralis tendon and fascia

Lateral retinaculum

Lateral femoral condyle

Infrapatellar fat pad

Lateral meniscus, anterior horn

Tibia

Biceps femoris muscle

Common peroneal nerve

Lateral head gastrocnemius muscle and tendon

Plantaris tendon

Superior fascicle

Lateral meniscus, posterior horn

Plantaris muscle

Popliteus tendon

Lateral head gastrocnemius muscle

Popliteus muscle

Superior tibiofibular joint

Head of fibula

FIGURE 5-69

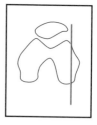

KNEE: SAGITTAL

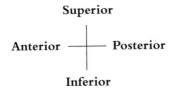

Superior

Anterior ─────┼───── Posterior

Inferior

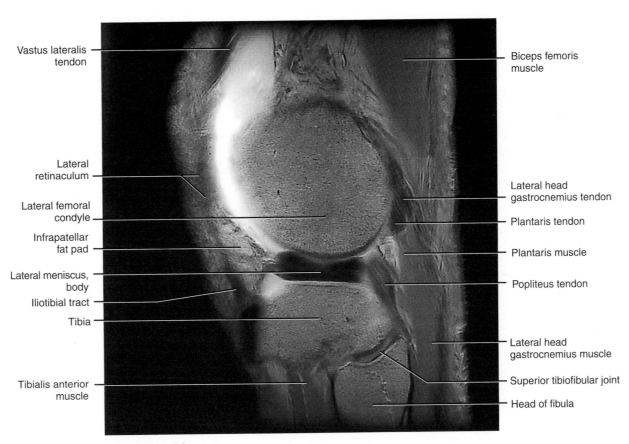

Vastus lateralis
tendon

Lateral
retinaculum

Lateral femoral
condyle

Infrapatellar
fat pad

Lateral meniscus,
body

Iliotibial tract

Tibia

Tibialis anterior
muscle

Biceps femoris
muscle

Lateral head
gastrocnemius tendon

Plantaris tendon

Plantaris muscle

Popliteus tendon

Lateral head
gastrocnemius muscle

Superior tibiofibular joint

Head of fibula

FIGURE 5-70

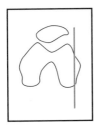

KNEE: SAGITTAL

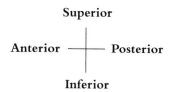

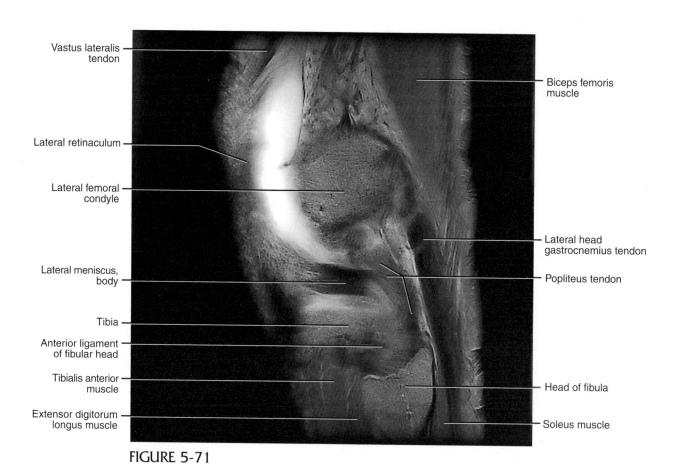

Vastus lateralis tendon

Lateral retinaculum

Lateral femoral condyle

Lateral meniscus, body

Tibia

Anterior ligament of fibular head

Tibialis anterior muscle

Extensor digitorum longus muscle

Biceps femoris muscle

Lateral head gastrocnemius tendon

Popliteus tendon

Head of fibula

Soleus muscle

FIGURE 5-71

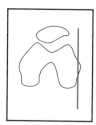

KNEE: SAGITTAL

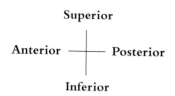

Superior

Anterior — Posterior

Inferior

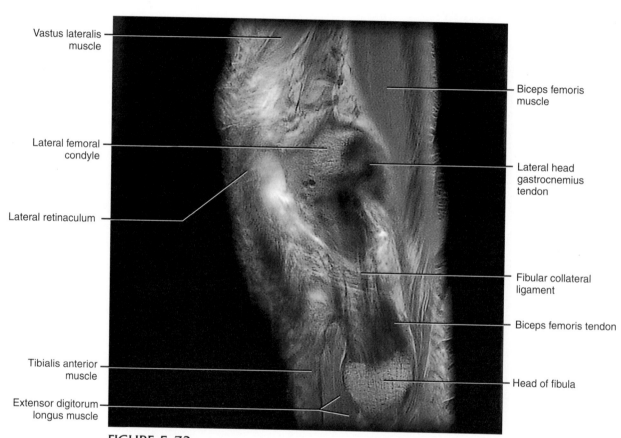

Vastus lateralis
muscle

Lateral femoral
condyle

Lateral retinaculum

Tibialis anterior
muscle

Extensor digitorum
longus muscle

Biceps femoris
muscle

Lateral head
gastrocnemius
tendon

Fibular collateral
ligament

Biceps femoris tendon

Head of fibula

FIGURE 5-72

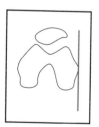

KNEE: SAGITTAL

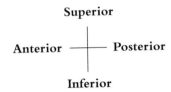

Vastus lateralis muscle

Iliotibial tract

Lateral retinaculum

Biceps femoris muscle and tendon

Fibular collateral ligament

Peroneus longus and extensor digitorum longus muscles

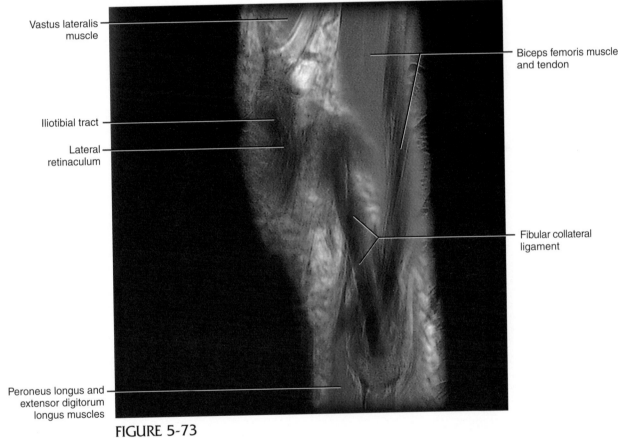

FIGURE 5-73

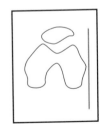

KNEE: SAGITTAL

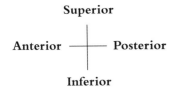

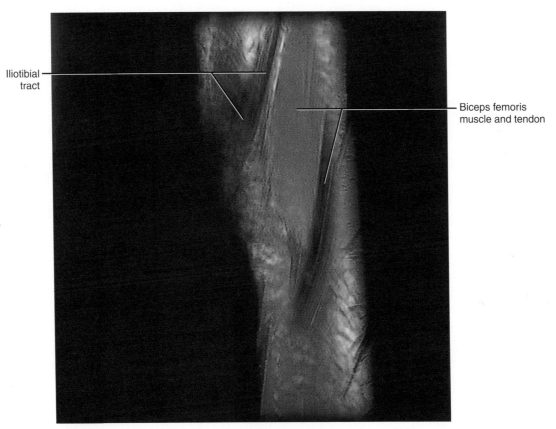

Iliotibial tract

Biceps femoris muscle and tendon

FIGURE 5-74

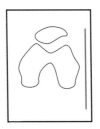

KNEE: MEDIAL COMPLEX, MEDIAL VIEW

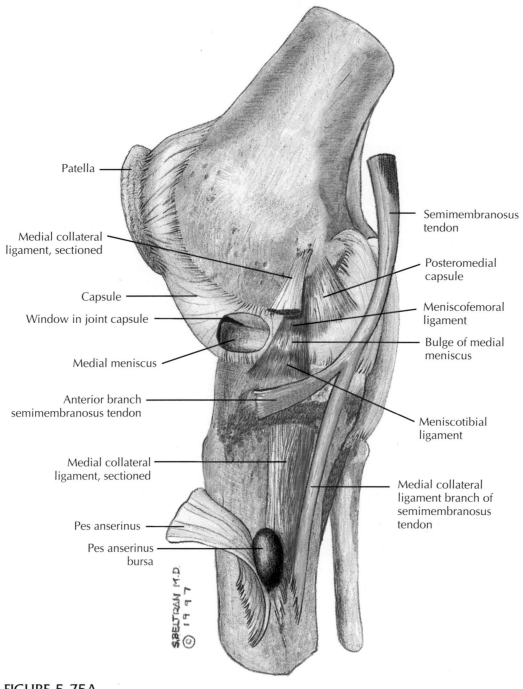

Patella

Medial collateral
ligament, sectioned

Capsule

Window in joint capsule

Medial meniscus

Anterior branch
semimembranosus tendon

Medial collateral
ligament, sectioned

Pes anserinus

Pes anserinus
bursa

Semimembranosus
tendon

Posteromedial
capsule

Meniscofemoral
ligament

Bulge of medial
meniscus

Meniscotibial
ligament

Medial collateral
ligament branch of
semimembranosus
tendon

A

FIGURE 5-75A

(A) Medial view of the knee with the pes anserinus cut and reflected. The tibial collateral ligament is
also sectioned to show the deep medial capsular ligament with meniscofemoral and meniscotibial
components and posteromedial capsule. For related MR, arthroscopy, and surgical anatomy images
see Figures 5-85 through 5-88.

KNEE: MEDIAL COMPLEX, MEDIAL VIEW

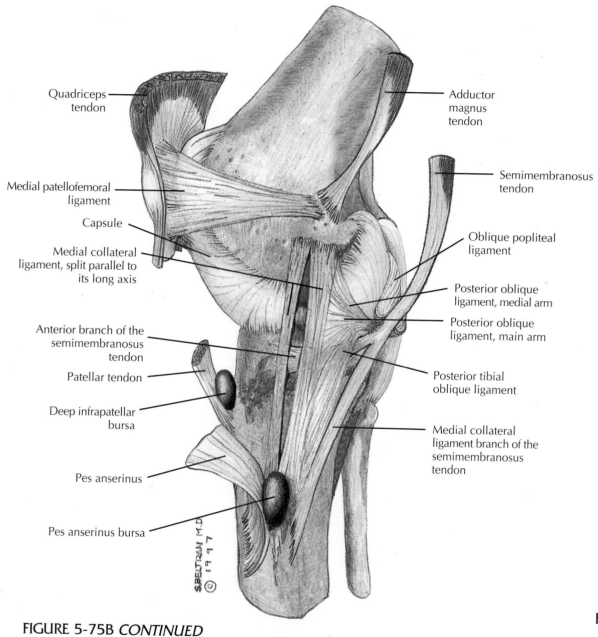

Quadriceps tendon

Adductor magnus tendon

Medial patellofemoral ligament

Semimembranosus tendon

Capsule

Oblique popliteal ligament

Medial collateral ligament, split parallel to its long axis

Posterior oblique ligament, medial arm

Posterior oblique ligament, main arm

Anterior branch of the semimembranosus tendon

Patellar tendon

Posterior tibial oblique ligament

Deep infrapatellar bursa

Medial collateral ligament branch of the semimembranosus tendon

Pes anserinus

Pes anserinus bursa

S.BELTRAN M.D. 1997 ©

FIGURE 5-75B *CONTINUED*

B

(B) The five arms of insertion of the semimembranosus tendon: (1) the attachment to the posteromedial aspect of the tibia just distal to the joint line; (2) the anterior attachment (anterior branch) to the tibia, deep to the tibial (medial) collateral and posterior oblique ligaments; (3) attachment of the tendon sheath to the posteromedial capsule, including an expansion to the posterior oblique ligament and posterior horn of the medial meniscus; (4) an oblique popliteal ligament attachment; and (5) a distal attachment to the fascia of the popliteus muscle and expansions to the posterior and posteromedial tibia (medial collateral ligament branch). Expansions to the oblique popliteal ligament, posteromedial capsule, anterior branch, and medial collateral ligament branch are shown, as is the joint capsule. The posterior oblique ligament represents the connection between the capsular attachment of the semimembranosus tendon and tibial collateral ligament. The fibers that extend over the semitendinosus tendon are also referred to as the posterior tibial oblique ligament. The tibial collateral ligament is split longitudinally to show the medial capsular layer. For related MR, arthroscopy, and surgical anatomy images see Figures 5-85 through 5-88.

KNEE: CAPSULE, MEDIAL VIEW

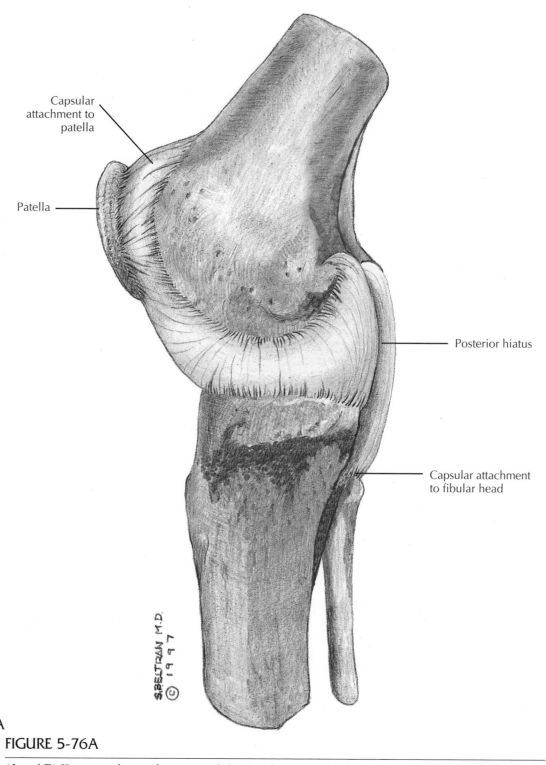

Capsular
attachment to
patella

Patella

Posterior hiatus

Capsular attachment
to fibular head

A

FIGURE 5-76A

(**A** and **B**) Knee capsular attachments, medial (**A**) and posteromedial (**B**) views.

KNEE: CAPSULE, POSTEROMEDIAL VIEW

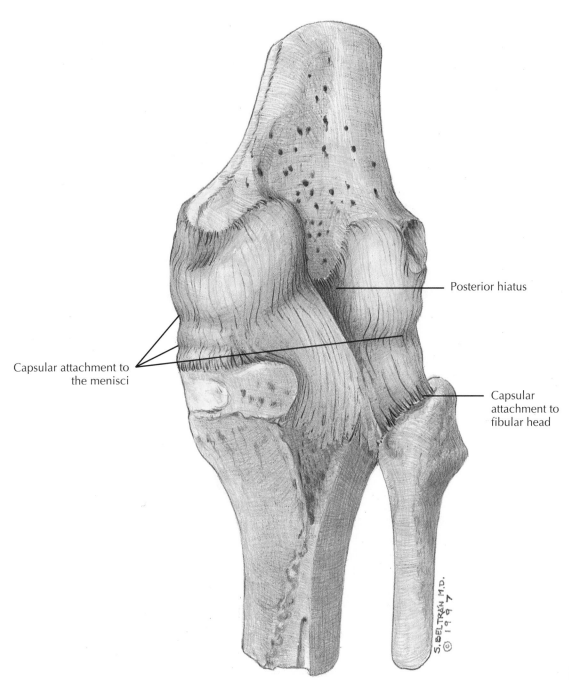

Posterior hiatus

Capsular attachment to
the menisci

Capsular
attachment to
fibular head

FIGURE 5-76B *CONTINUED*

B

KNEE: LATERAL COMPLEX, LATERAL VIEW

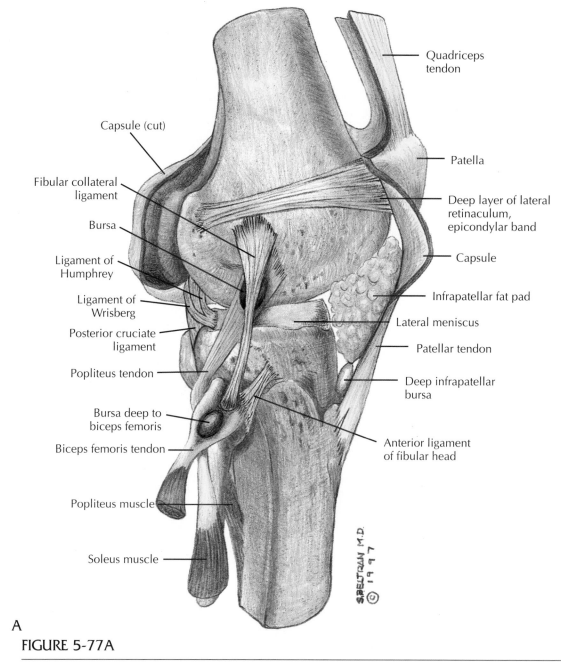

Quadriceps
tendon

Capsule (cut)

Fibular collateral
ligament

Bursa

Ligament of
Humphrey

Ligament of
Wrisberg

Posterior cruciate
ligament

Popliteus tendon

Bursa deep to
biceps femoris

Biceps femoris tendon

Popliteus muscle

Soleus muscle

Patella

Deep layer of lateral
retinaculum,
epicondylar band

Capsule

Infrapatellar fat pad

Lateral meniscus

Patellar tendon

Deep infrapatellar
bursa

Anterior ligament
of fibular head

A

FIGURE 5-77A

(A) Lateral view of the knee demonstrating the extracapsular course of the fibular collateral ligament from the lateral femoral epicondyle to its conjoined insertion with the biceps femoris tendon on the fibular head. The intracapsular popliteus tendon passes medial to the fibular collateral ligament. For related MR, arthroscopy, and surgical anatomy images see Figures 5-90 through 5-92.

KNEE: POPLITEOFIBULAR LIGAMENT, LATERAL VIEW

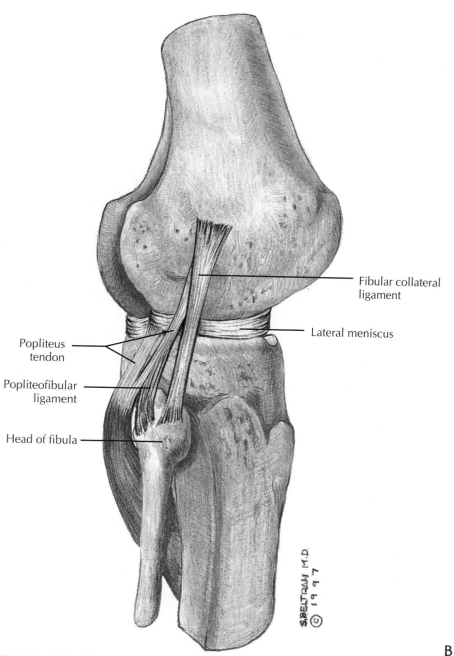

Fibular collateral
ligament

Lateral meniscus

Popliteus
tendon

Popliteofibular
ligament

Head of fibula

B

FIGURE 5-77B *CONTINUED*

(B) The recently rediscovered popliteofibular ligament originates from the posterior aspect of the fibula (posterior to the biceps insertion) and extends toward the junction of the popliteus muscle and tendon. Proximal to the musculotendinous junction of the popliteus, the popliteofibular ligament joins the popliteus tendon and is located deep to the lateral limb of the arcuate ligament. The popliteofibular ligament connects the fibula to the femur through the popliteus tendon and is biomechanically stronger than the fibular collateral ligament. The popliteal tendon attachments to the tibia and the popliteofibular ligament help resist posterior translation and varus and external rotation. For related MR, arthroscopy, and surgical anatomy images see Figures 5-90 through 5-92.

KNEE: ANTERIOR COMPLEX, ANTERIOR VIEW

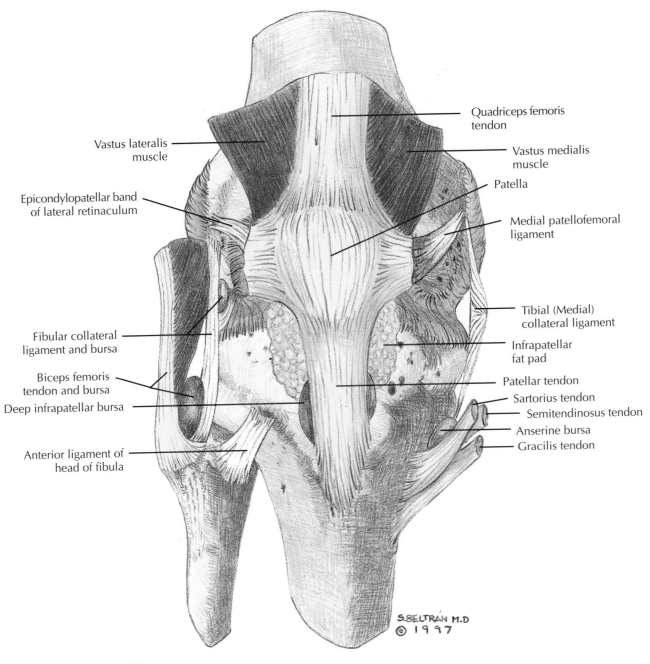

Vastus lateralis muscle

Epicondylopatellar band of lateral retinaculum

Fibular collateral ligament and bursa

Biceps femoris tendon and bursa

Deep infrapatellar bursa

Anterior ligament of head of fibula

Quadriceps femoris tendon

Vastus medialis muscle

Patella

Medial patellofemoral ligament

Tibial (Medial) collateral ligament

Infrapatellar fat pad

Patellar tendon

Sartorius tendon

Semitendinosus tendon

Anserine bursa

Gracilis tendon

S.BELTRÁN M.D
© 1997

A

FIGURE 5-78A

Anterior view of the knee. **(A)** The pes anserinus includes the semitendinosus, gracilis, and sartorius tendons. The anserine bursa is deep to the pes anserinus. The insertion of the pes anserinus is on the medial aspect of the tibia, distal to the tibial tuberosity. The lateral and medial retinaculum have superficial and deep layers. The deep layer of the lateral retinaculum consists of the epicondylopatellar band, the lateral patellotibial band, and the transverse ligament. The deep layer of the medial retinaculum consists of the medial patellofemoral ligament, the medial patellotibial ligament, and the patellomeniscal ligament. For related MR, arthroscopy, and surgical anatomy images see Figures 5-84 and 5-98.

KNEE: CAPSULE, ANTERIOR VIEW

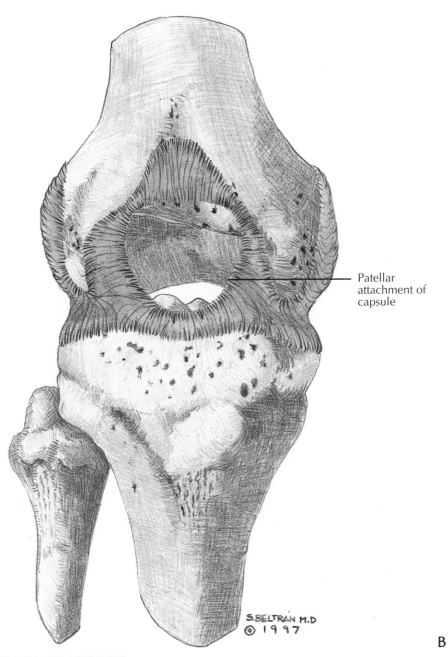

Patellar
attachment of
capsule

S.BELTRAN M.D
© 1997

B

FIGURE 5-78B *CONTINUED*

(B) The patellar attachment of the joint capsule is illustrated with anterior structures removed. For related MR, arthroscopy, and surgical anatomy images see Figures 5-84 and 5-98.

KNEE: JOINT INTERIOR, ANTERIOR VIEW

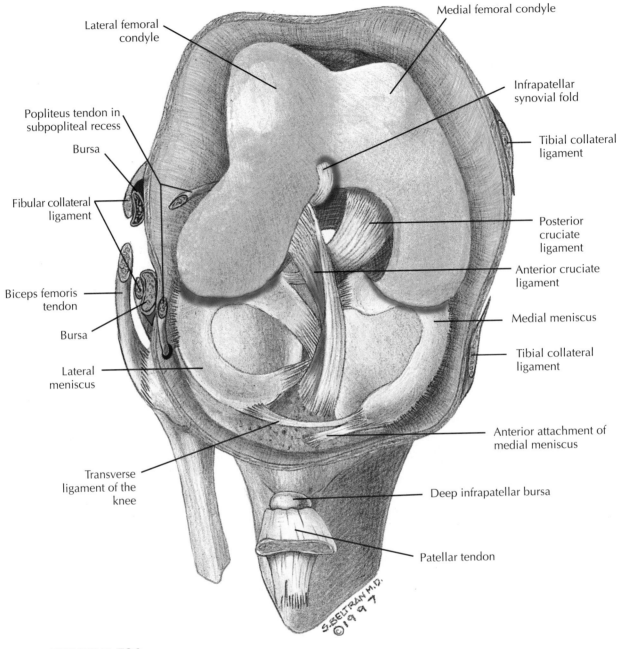

A

FIGURE 5-79A

(A) Anterior view of the joint interior with the knee in flexion. For related MR, arthroscopy, and surgical anatomy images see Figures 5-92 through 5-94, 5-96, and 5-99.

KNEE: JOINT INTERIOR, ANTEROSUPERIOR VIEW

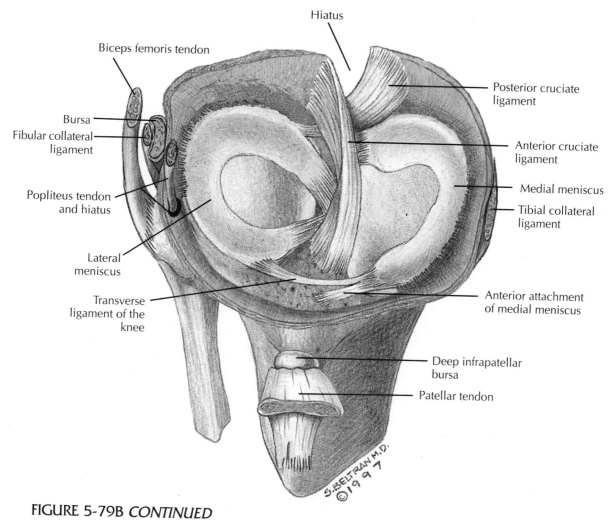

FIGURE 5-79B CONTINUED

B

(B) Anterosuperior view of the tibia with meniscal and cruciate attachments. The anterior cruciate ligament (ACL) and posterior cruciate ligament (PCL) are intracapsular and extrasynovial. Proximally, the ACL is attached to a fossa on the posteromedial aspect of the lateral femoral condyle. Distally, the ACL extends inferior and medial to the anterior tibial intercondylar area and attaches to a fossa anterior and lateral to the anterior tibial spine, between the anterior attachments of the menisci. The PCL originates in the lateral aspect of the medial femoral condyle, crosses the ACL, and attaches to the posterior intercondylar fossa of the tibia. For related MR, arthroscopy, and surgical anatomy images see Figures 5-92 through 5-94, 5-96, and 5-99.

KNEE: SUPERFICIAL DISSECTION, POSTERIOR VIEW

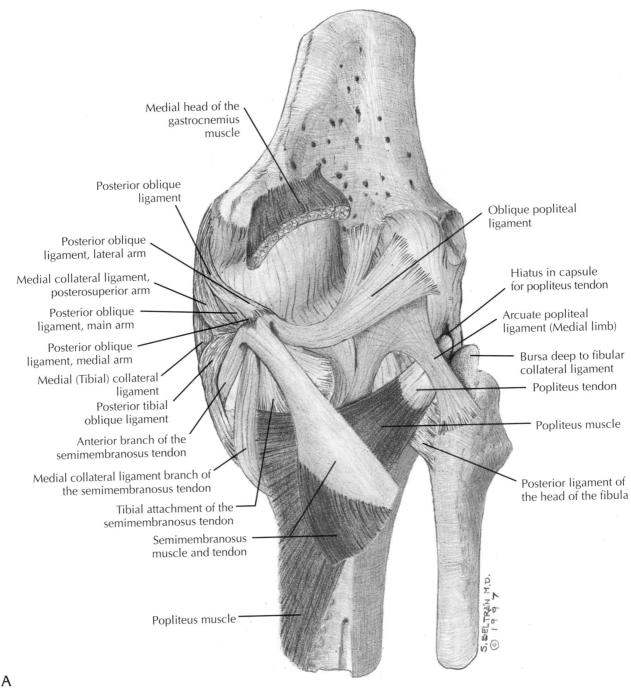

Medial head of the gastrocnemius muscle

Posterior oblique ligament

Posterior oblique ligament, lateral arm

Medial collateral ligament, posterosuperior arm

Posterior oblique ligament, main arm

Posterior oblique ligament, medial arm

Medial (Tibial) collateral ligament

Posterior tibial oblique ligament

Anterior branch of the semimembranosus tendon

Medial collateral ligament branch of the semimembranosus tendon

Tibial attachment of the semimembranosus tendon

Semimembranosus muscle and tendon

Popliteus muscle

Oblique popliteal ligament

Hiatus in capsule for popliteus tendon

Arcuate popliteal ligament (Medial limb)

Bursa deep to fibular collateral ligament

Popliteus tendon

Popliteus muscle

Posterior ligament of the head of the fibula

S. BELTRÁN M.D. © 1997

A

FIGURE 5-80A

(A and B) Posterior view of superficial (A) and deep (B) dissections. The semimembranosus tendon expansions, including the oblique popliteal ligament, are illustrated posteromedially. The posterior oblique ligament is shown with its main, lateral, and medial arms. The posterior tibial oblique ligament extends over the anterior branch of the semimembranosus tendon. The posterior tibial oblique ligament is formed by the posteroinferior fibers of the tibial collateral ligament. The posterior oblique ligament and posterior tibial oblique ligament fibers insert on the posterior tibial border. The arcuate popliteal ligament, the popliteus tendon, and the lateral collateral ligament components of the posterolateral corner are illustrated. The posterolateral complex also includes the popliteofibular ligament, the fabellofibular ligament, and the lateral head of the gastrocnemius muscle.

KNEE: DEEP DISSECTION, POSTERIOR VIEW

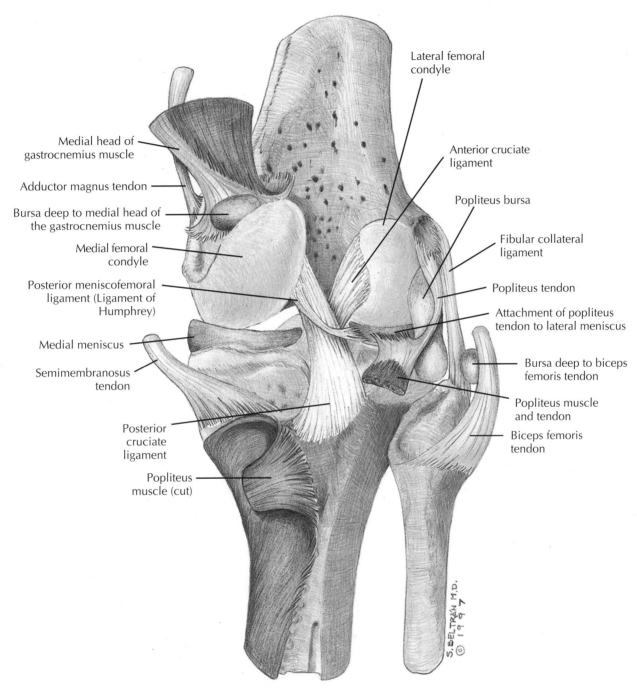

Lateral femoral condyle

Anterior cruciate ligament

Popliteus bursa

Fibular collateral ligament

Popliteus tendon

Attachment of popliteus tendon to lateral meniscus

Bursa deep to biceps femoris tendon

Popliteus muscle and tendon

Biceps femoris tendon

Medial head of gastrocnemius muscle

Adductor magnus tendon

Bursa deep to medial head of the gastrocnemius muscle

Medial femoral condyle

Posterior meniscofemoral ligament (Ligament of Humphrey)

Medial meniscus

Semimembranosus tendon

Posterior cruciate ligament

Popliteus muscle (cut)

S. BELTRAN M.D. © 1997

B

FIGURE 5-80B *CONTINUED*

The proximal attachment of the anterior cruciate ligament and the distal attachment of the posterior cruciate ligament are illustrated in the deep dissection (part **B**). The posterior meniscofemoral ligament (the ligament of Wrisberg) connects the posterior horn of the lateral meniscus to the lateral aspect of the medial
femoral condyle near the origin of the posterior cruciate ligament. For related MR, arthroscopy, and surgical anatomy images see Figures 5-88, 5-90 through 5-92, and 5-96.

KNEE: TIBIA, ANTEROSUPERIOR VIEW

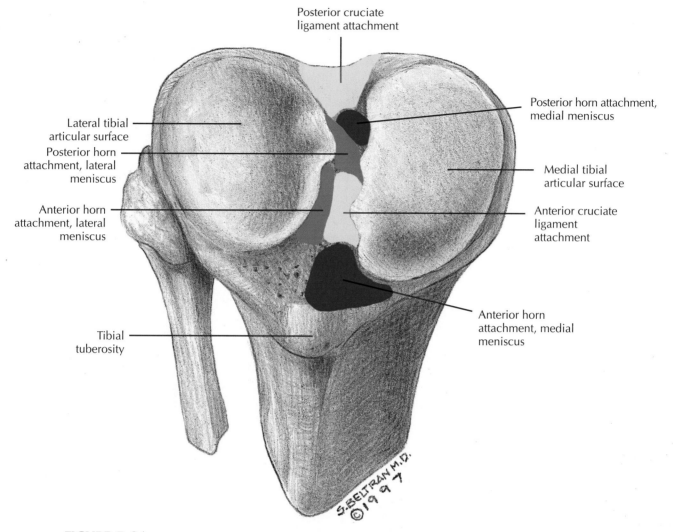

FIGURE 5-81

Anterosuperior view of the tibia with the menisci, cruciate, and collateral ligaments removed. The tibial attachments of the lateral and medial menisci and anterior and posterior cruciate ligaments are mapped on the tibial surface. Anterior to the tibial attachment of the anterior cruciate ligament, the anterior horn of the medial meniscus is attached to the area of the intercondylar fossa of the tibia. The attachment of the posterior horn of the medial meniscus is located at the posterior intercondylar fossa of the tibia between the attachments of the posterior horn of the lateral meniscus and the posterior cruciate ligament. The anterior horn of the lateral meniscus is attached between the tibial intercondylar eminence and the anterior attachment of the anterior cruciate ligament. The posterior horn of the lateral meniscus is attached between the tibial intercondylar eminence and the posterior horn of the medial meniscus. For related MR, arthroscopy, and surgical anatomy images see Figure 5-92 through 5-94 and 5-96.

KNEE: MENISCI, ANTEROLATERAL VIEW

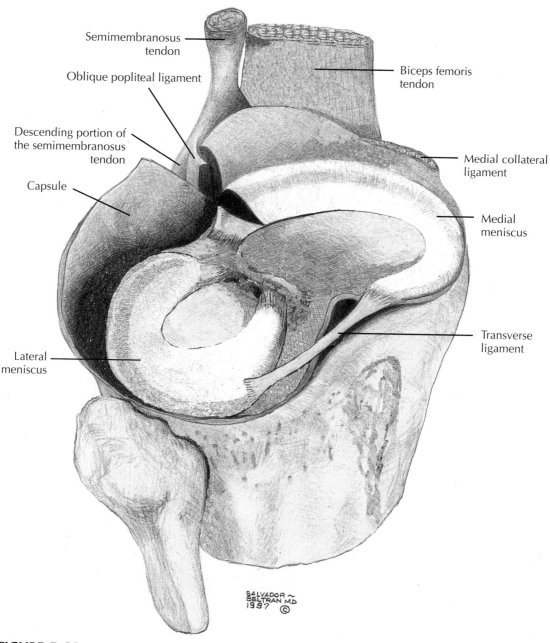

Semimembranosus tendon

Oblique popliteal ligament

Descending portion of the semimembranosus tendon

Capsule

Lateral meniscus

Biceps femoris tendon

Medial collateral ligament

Medial meniscus

Transverse ligament

FIGURE 5-82

Anterolateral and superior view of the medial and lateral menisci. The semicircular medial meniscus has a wide posterior horn, narrows anteriorly, and has a more open C-shaped configuration than the more circular lateral meniscus. The lateral meniscus is relatively symmetric in width from anterior to posterior. The posterior fibers of the anterior horn attachment of the medial meniscus attach to the transverse ligament. The transverse ligament of the knee connects the anterior horns of the medial and lateral menisci. The oblique popliteal ligament, which reinforces the posterior capsule, is seen through the cut capsule. For related MR, arthroscopy, and surgical anatomy images see Figures 5-93 through 5-95.

KNEE: POSTEROMEDIAL CORNER, SUPERIOR VIEW

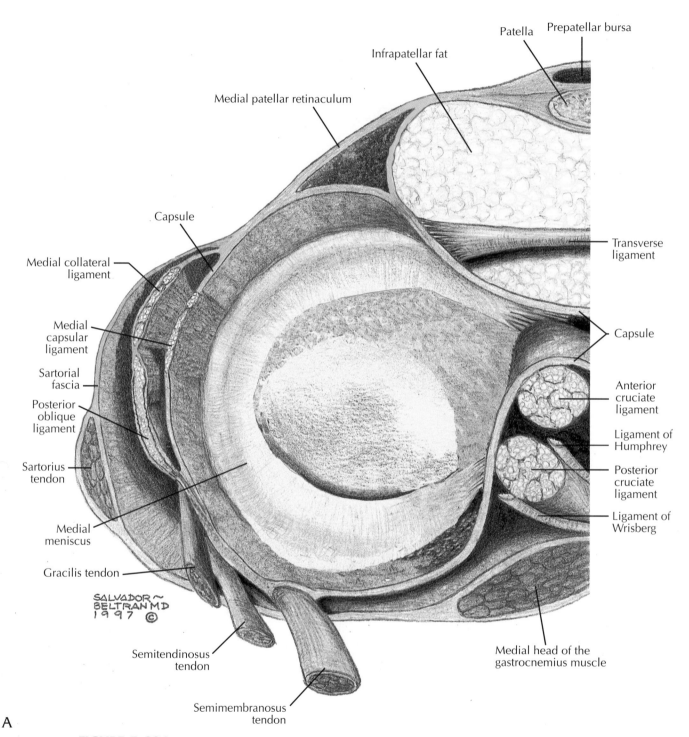

A

FIGURE 5-83A

(A and B) Axial (superior) views of posteromedial (A) and posterolateral (B) knee anatomy. The postero-medial corner receives an important contribution from the semimembranosus tendon. The sartorial fascia (layer I), superficial tibial collateral ligament (layer II), and medial capsular ligament (layer III) merge ante-riorly. The medial patellar retinaculum is formed from the fusion of layers I and II. Posteriorly, layers II and III merge to form the posterior oblique ligament. The posteromedial corner resists valgus laxity in knee extension. For related MR, arthroscopy, and surgical anatomy images see Figures 5-85 through 5-95.

KNEE: POSTEROLATERAL CORNER, SUPERIOR VIEW

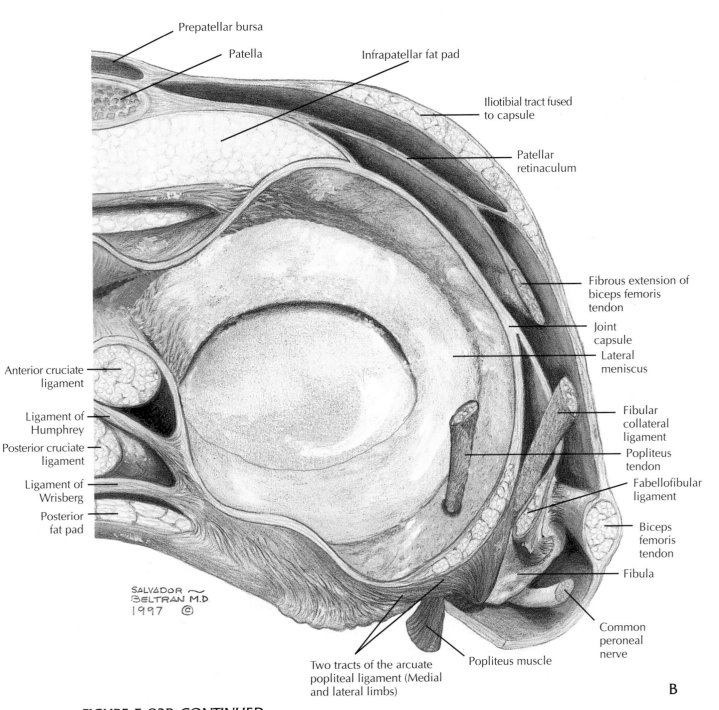

Prepatellar bursa

Patella

Infrapatellar fat pad

Iliotibial tract fused to capsule

Patellar retinaculum

Fibrous extension of biceps femoris tendon

Joint capsule

Lateral meniscus

Fibular collateral ligament

Popliteus tendon

Fabellofibular ligament

Biceps femoris tendon

Fibula

Common peroneal nerve

Popliteus muscle

Two tracts of the arcuate popliteal ligament (Medial and lateral limbs)

Posterior fat pad

Ligament of Wrisberg

Posterior cruciate ligament

Ligament of Humphrey

Anterior cruciate ligament

SALVADOR ~ BELTRAN M.D 1997 ©

B

FIGURE 5-83B *CONTINUED*

The arcuate ligament, fibular collateral ligament, fabellofibular ligament, and popliteus tendon components of the posterolateral complex are shown in the axial (superior) view of the anatomy of the posterolateral knee (part **B**). The arcuate ligament spans the posterolateral joint and extends distally, parallel with the fibular collateral ligament. The Y-shaped arcuate ligament has medial and lateral limbs. The arcuate ligament and posterolateral complex stabilize the posterolateral aspect of the knee against varus and external rotation. The popliteofibular ligament portion of the posterolateral complex is also seen in part **B** of Figure 5-77. For related MR, arthroscopy, and surgical anatomy images see Figures 5-85 through 5-95.

KNEE: ARCIFORM INTERMEDIATE OBLIQUE LAYERS

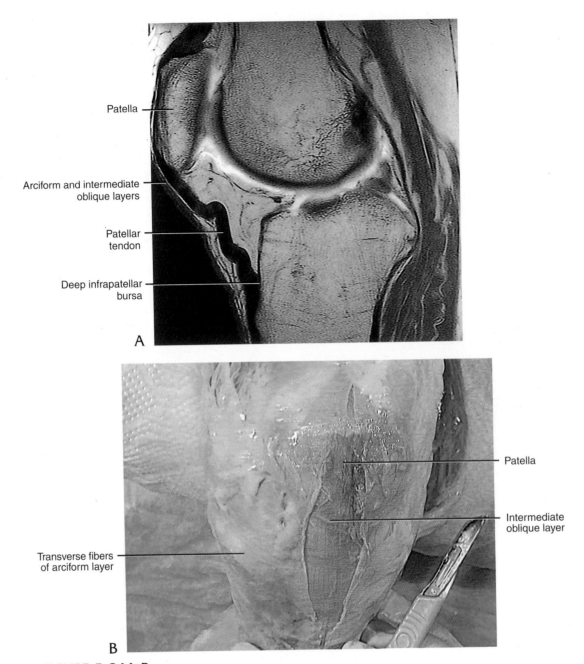

FIGURE 5-84A,B

(A) T1-weighted sagittal image with hypointensity of the arciform and intermediate oblique layers of the knee. The bursa between the arciform and intermediate oblique layers is collapsed. **(B)** Corresponding dissection with the transverse fibers of the arciform layer divided to expose the intermediate oblique layer. **(C)** T1-weighted coronal image with attachment of the proximal patellar tendon and quadriceps tendon. **(D and E)** Corresponding dissection showing the intermediate oblique fibers **(D)** and the long tract of the rectus femoris fibers **(E)**. The intermediate oblique layer attenuates distal to the patella. Note that the long fibers of the rectus are seen after sectioning the more superficial intermediate oblique layer.

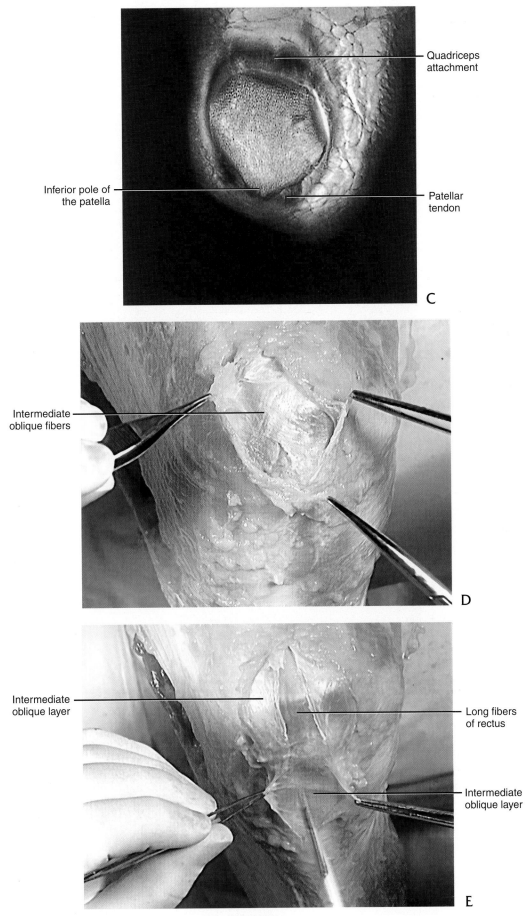

Quadriceps
attachment

Inferior pole of
the patella

Patellar
tendon

C

Intermediate
oblique fibers

D

Intermediate
oblique layer

Long fibers
of rectus

Intermediate
oblique layer

E

FIGURE 5-84C–E *CONTINUED*

KNEE: PES ANSERINUS

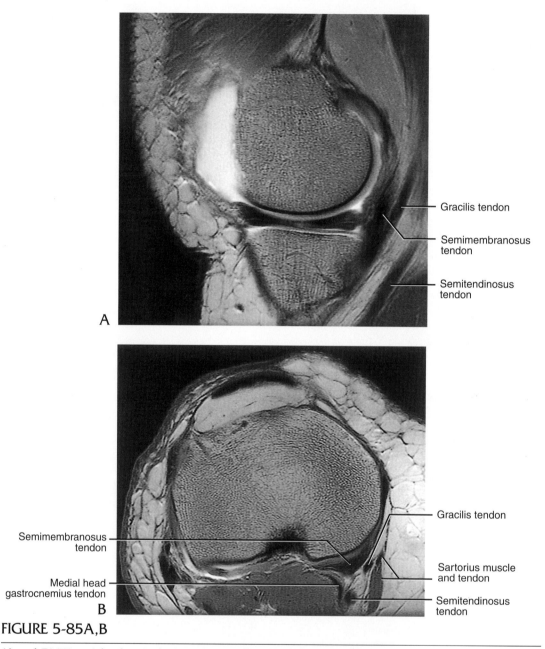

A

B

Gracilis tendon

Semimembranosus tendon

Semitendinosus tendon

Semimembranosus tendon

Medial head gastrocnemius tendon

Gracilis tendon

Sartorius muscle and tendon

Semitendinosus tendon

FIGURE 5-85A,B

(**A** and **B**) T1-weighted sagittal (**A**) and axial (**B**) MR arthrograms of the pes anserinus tendons. The pes anserinus tendons (the semitendinosus, gracilis, and sartorius tendons) as well as the tendons of the semimembranosus and medial head of the gastrocnemius are best seen on part **B**, the axial image.

KNEE: PES ANSERINUS

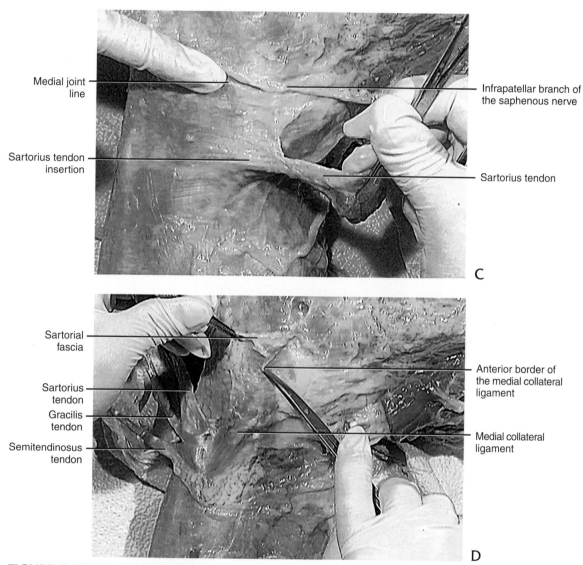

Medial joint line

Sartorius tendon insertion

Infrapatellar branch of the saphenous nerve

Sartorius tendon

C

Sartorial fascia

Sartorius tendon

Gracilis tendon

Semitendinosus tendon

Anterior border of the medial collateral ligament

Medial collateral ligament

D

FIGURE 5-85C,D *CONTINUED*

(C) The more superficial sartorius tendon of the pes anserinus group is exposed. The infrapatellar branch of the saphenous nerve is shown at the level of the medial joint line. **(D)** The medial collateral ligament is exposed deep to the reflected pes anserinus tendons.

KNEE: PES ANSERINUS

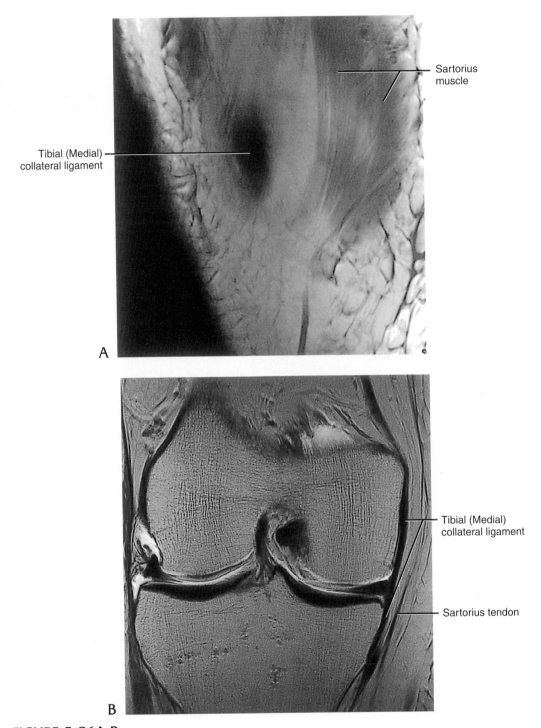

FIGURE 5-86A,B

(**A** and **B**) T1-weighted sagittal (**A**) and coronal (**B**) MR arthrograms showing the anterior fibers of the medial collateral ligament and the sartorius muscle in the sagittal plane (part **A**) and the posterior fibers of the medial collateral ligament and sartorius tendon in the coronal plane (part **B**). (**C**) Superficial exposure of the medial side of the knee showing corresponding longitudinal fibers of the sartorial fascia, which run in two directions in a basket-weave mesh. The more superficial fibers are perpendicular to the longitudinal fibers of the sartorial fascia, which are shown parallel to the sartorius muscle. The pes anserinus is demonstrated at the distal end of the sartorius.

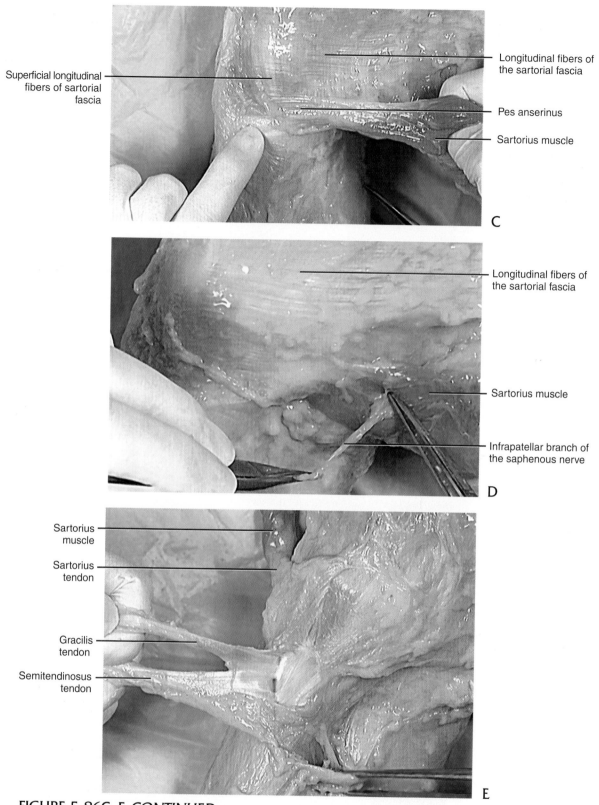

Superficial longitudinal fibers of sartorial fascia

Longitudinal fibers of the sartorial fascia

Pes anserinus

Sartorius muscle

C

Longitudinal fibers of the sartorial fascia

Sartorius muscle

Infrapatellar branch of the saphenous nerve

D

Sartorius muscle

Sartorius tendon

Gracilis tendon

Semitendinosus tendon

E

FIGURE 5-86C–E *CONTINUED*

(D) The infrapatellar branch of the saphenous nerve exits through the sartorius muscle. The sensory branch (not shown) exits below the sartorius muscle. The saphenous nerve leaves Hunter's canal by passing between the sartorius and gracilis. The infrapatellar branch is given off by piercing the sartorius muscle before the saphenous nerve exits the canal. **(E)** With the more superficial sartorius retracted, the gracilis and semitendinosus tendons can be identified. Retracting the pes tendons allows visualization of the medial collateral ligament. The anserine bursa lies between the pes anserinus tendons and the medial collateral ligament.

KNEE: MEDIAL COLLATERAL LIGAMENT
AND POSTERIOR OBLIQUE LIGAMENT

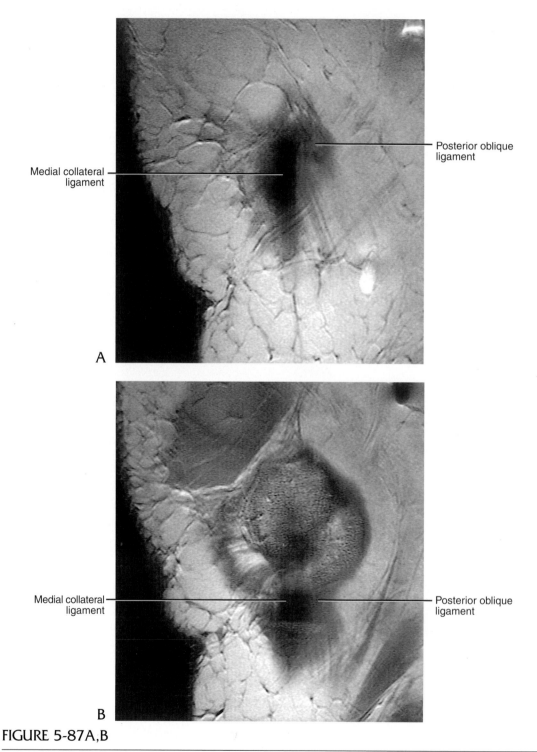

FIGURE 5-87A,B

(A and B) T1-weighted sagittal images showing the medial collateral ligament and posterior oblique ligament. Part **A** is medial to part **B**.

KNEE: MEDIAL COLLATERAL LIGAMENT AND POSTERIOR OBLIQUE LIGAMENT

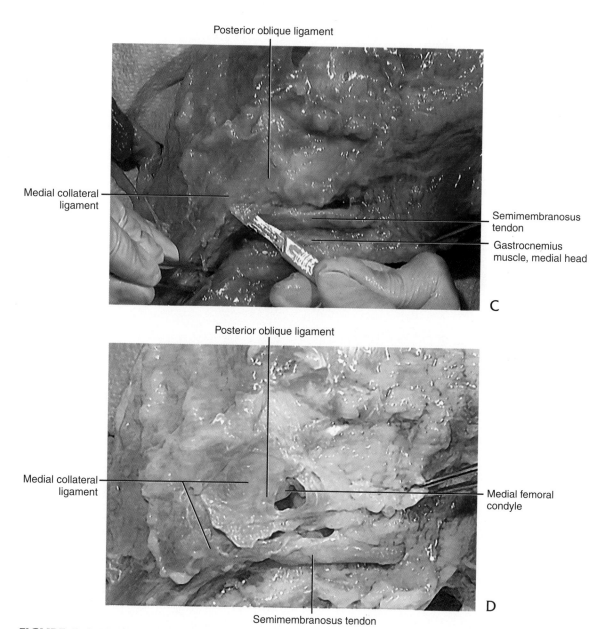

Posterior oblique ligament

Medial collateral ligament

Semimembranosus tendon

Gastrocnemius muscle, medial head

C

Posterior oblique ligament

Medial collateral ligament

Medial femoral condyle

Semimembranosus tendon

D

FIGURE 5-87C,D *CONTINUED*

(**C** and **D**) Corresponding dissections showing the connection between the oblique fibers of the superficial medial collateral ligament and the semimembranosus.

KNEE: SEMIMEMBRANOSUS ATTACHMENTS

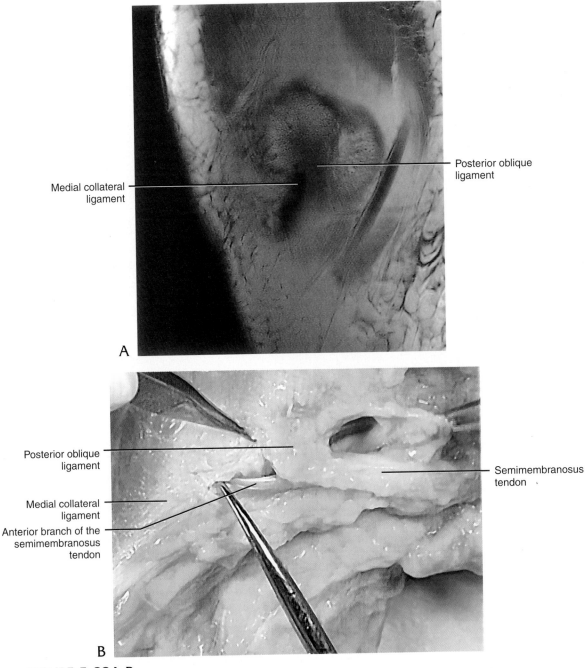

FIGURE 5-88A,B

(A) Medial collateral and posterior oblique ligaments on a T1-weighted sagittal MR image. **(B)** The anterior branch of the semimembranosus and posterior oblique ligament are demonstrated on a corresponding medial dissection. The anterior branch passes deep to the posterior oblique ligament.

KNEE: SEMIMEMBRANOSUS ATTACHMENTS

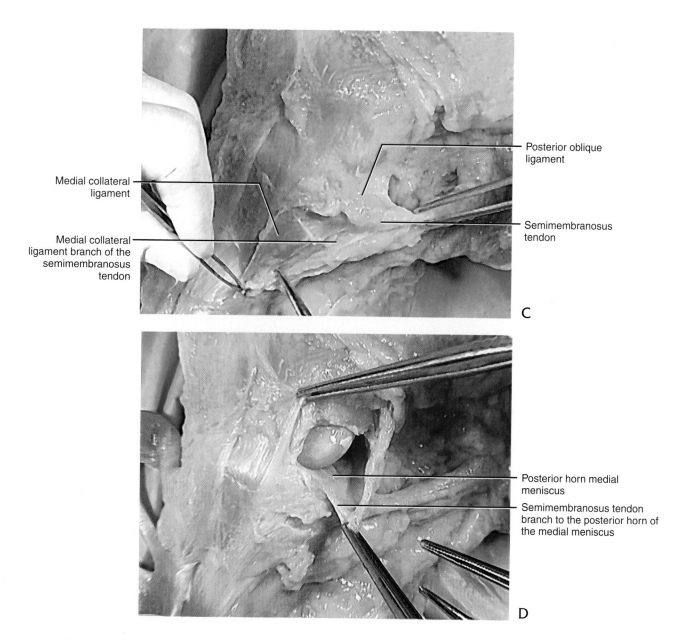

Medial collateral ligament

Medial collateral ligament branch of the semimembranosus tendon

Posterior oblique ligament

Semimembranosus tendon

C

Posterior horn medial meniscus

Semimembranosus tendon branch to the posterior horn of the medial meniscus

D

FIGURE 5-88C,D *CONTINUED*

(C) The medial collateral branch of the semimembranosus tendon is posterior and parallel to the medial collateral ligament. (D) The attachment of the semimembranosus to the posterior horn of the medial meniscus is shown through the posteromedial capsular arthrotomy.

KNEE: ILIOTIBIAL TRACT AND BICEPS FEMORIS

A

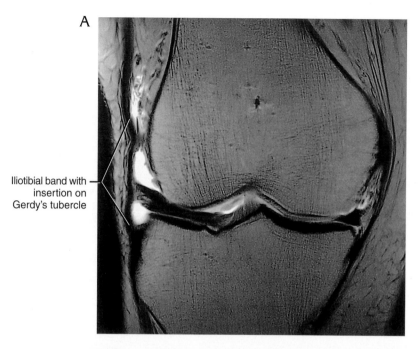

Iliotibial band with insertion on Gerdy's tubercle

B

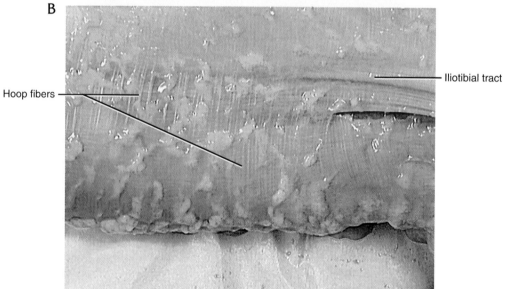

Hoop fibers

Iliotibial tract

FIGURE 5-89A,B

(A and B) The iliotibial band is shown on a T1-weighted coronal MR image (A) and a corresponding lateral superficial dissection (B). The iliotibial band or tract is a thickening of the fascia lata and inserts into a facet on the anterolateral condylar surface of the tibia. The superficial hoop fibers create a circumferential supporting envelope.

KNEE: ILIOTIBIAL TRACT AND BICEPS FEMORIS

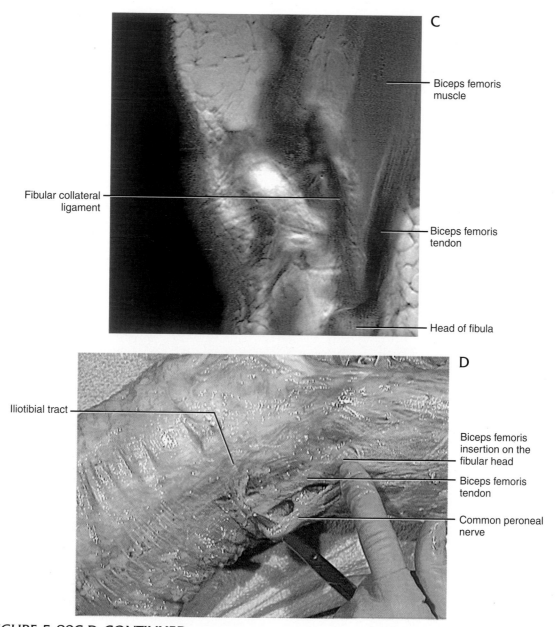

C

Biceps femoris
muscle

Fibular collateral
ligament

Biceps femoris
tendon

Head of fibula

D

Iliotibial tract

Biceps femoris
insertion on the
fibular head

Biceps femoris
tendon

Common peroneal
nerve

FIGURE 5-89C,D *CONTINUED*

(C) Lateral T1-weighted sagittal MR arthrogram showing the lateral collateral ligament and the biceps femoris tendon converging on the fibular head to create a "V-shaped" configuration. **(D)** The corresponding dissection demonstrates the biceps femoris insertion and exposure of the peroneal nerve. The long head and short head components of the biceps femoris form a single tendon, which inserts anterior to the styloid process of the fibula and across the tibiofibular joint. The insertion of the biceps femoris is folded around the anterior aspect of the distal fibular collateral ligament. The common peroneal nerve is medial to the biceps tendon.

KNEE: BICEPS FEMORIS
AND LATERAL COLLATERAL LIGAMENT

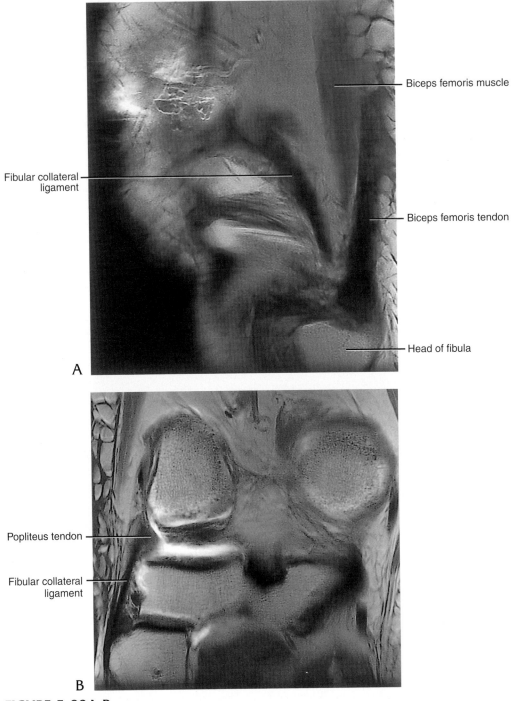

FIGURE 5-90A,B

(A) T1-weighted coronal MR arthrogram showing the lateral collateral ligament. **(B)** T1-weighted sagittal MR arthrogram showing the lateral (fibular) collateral ligament and popliteus tendon.

KNEE: BICEPS FEMORIS AND LATERAL COLLATERAL LIGAMENT

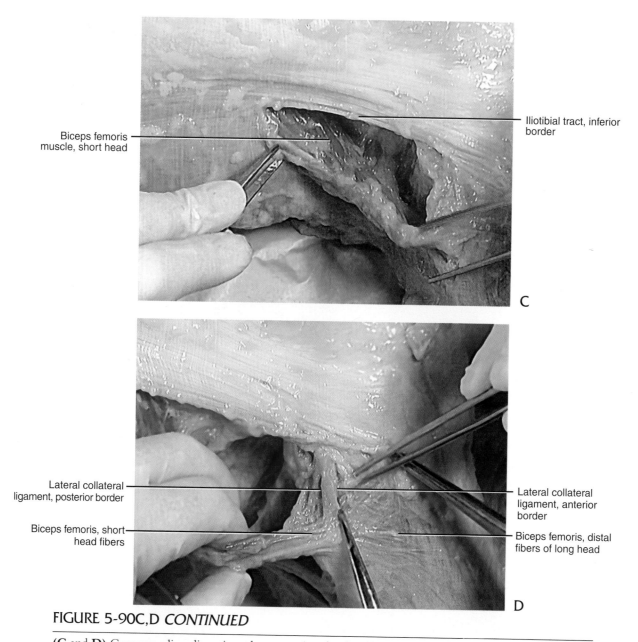

Biceps femoris muscle, short head

Iliotibial tract, inferior border

C

Lateral collateral ligament, posterior border

Biceps femoris, short head fibers

Lateral collateral ligament, anterior border

Biceps femoris, distal fibers of long head

D

FIGURE 5-90C,D *CONTINUED*

(**C** and **D**) Corresponding dissections demonstrating the short head fibers of the biceps femoris muscle (**C**) and the exposure of the lateral collateral ligament (**D**). The short head fibers blend with the posterior inferior border of the lateral collateral ligament. The muscle fibers of the short head also fuse with the long head.

KNEE: POPLITEUS TENDON

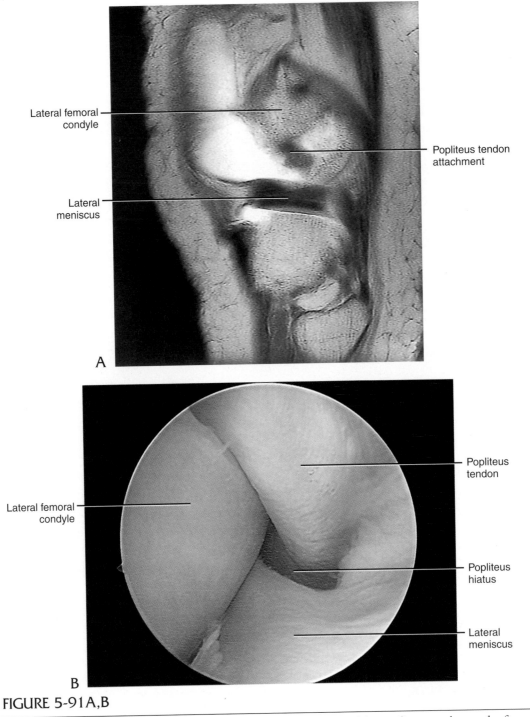

FIGURE 5-91A,B

(A) T1-weighted sagittal MR arthrogram illustrating the attachment of the popliteus tendon to the fossa on the lateral femoral condylar surface. (B) Corresponding arthroscopic view of the popliteus tendon entering the knee joint through the popliteus hiatus.

KNEE: POPLITEUS TENDON

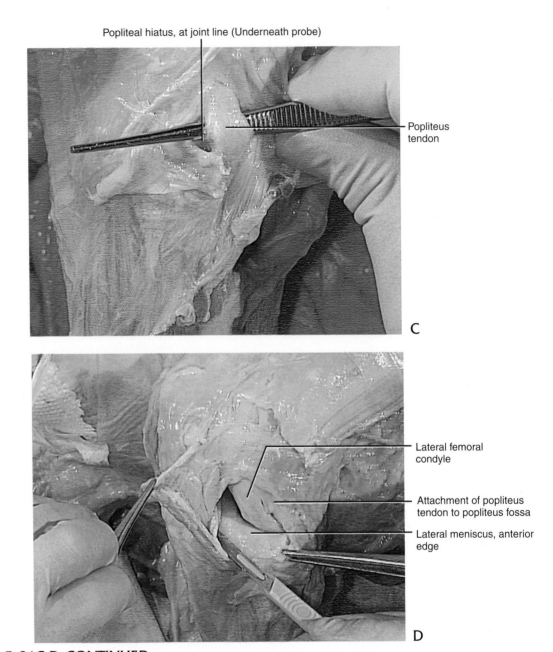

Popliteal hiatus, at joint line (Underneath probe)

Popliteus
tendon

C

Lateral femoral
condyle

Attachment of popliteus
tendon to popliteus fossa

Lateral meniscus, anterior
edge

D

FIGURE 5-91C,D *CONTINUED*

(**C** and **D**) Corresponding lateral dissections showing the location of the popliteal hiatus (**C**) and the insertion of the popliteus tendon onto the popliteal fossa of the femur, anterior and inferior to the lateral collateral ligament (**D**).

KNEE: POPLITEUS TENDON

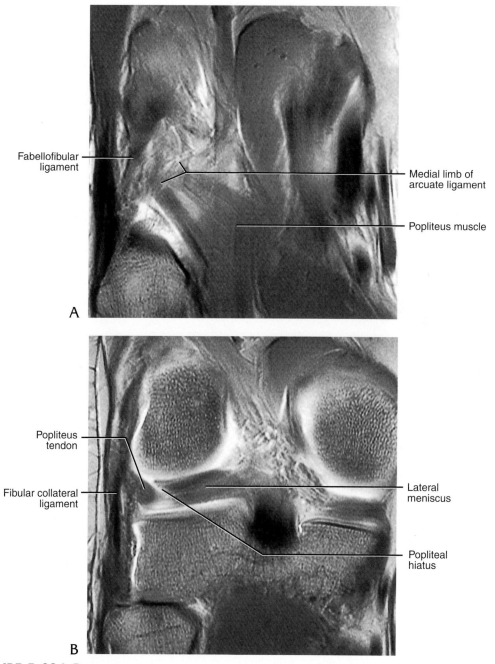

FIGURE 5-92A,B

T1-weighted coronal MR arthrographic images of the fabellofibular ligament and medial limb of the arcuate ligament (**A**) and the fibular collateral ligament and the popliteus tendon and hiatus (**B**) (the image in part **A** is more posterior than the image in part **B**). The fabellofibular ligament, when present, functions as the lateral limb of the arcuate ligament.

KNEE: POPLITEUS TENDON

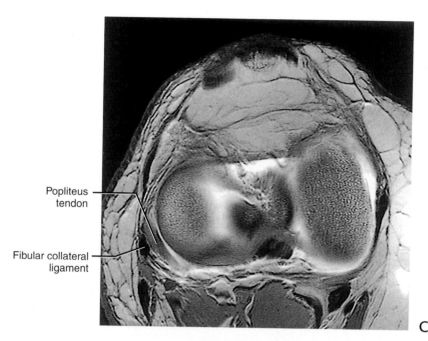

Popliteus tendon

Fibular collateral ligament

C

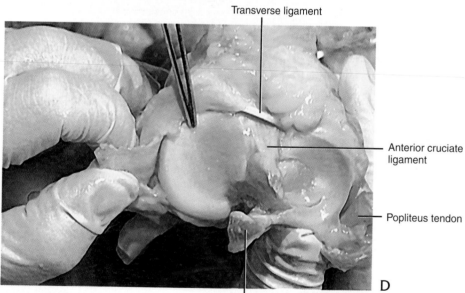

Transverse ligament

Anterior cruciate ligament

Popliteus tendon

Posterior cruciate ligament

D

FIGURE 5-92C,D *CONTINUED*

(C) The popliteus tendon is easily identified at the level of the lateral meniscus deep to the lateral collateral ligament in the axial plane on this T1-weighted arthrographic image. **(D)** Corresponding superior view of the tibial plateau shows the relationship of the lateral meniscus to the popliteal hiatus.

KNEE: MENISCUS

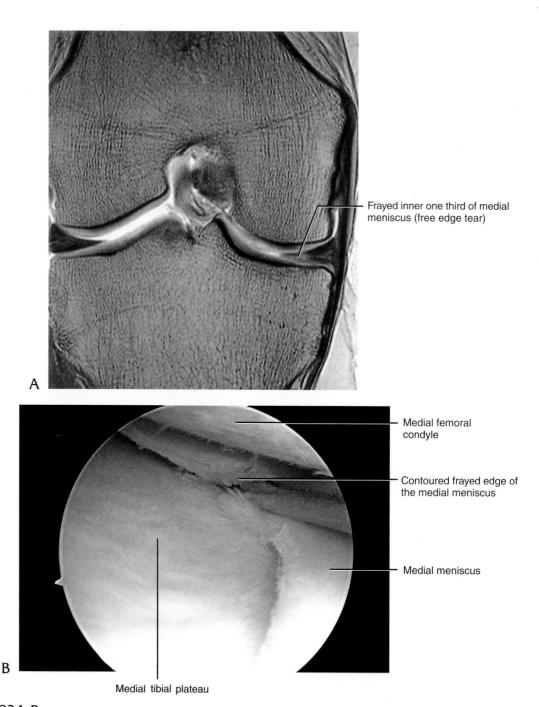

A — Frayed inner one third of medial meniscus (free edge tear)

B

Medial femoral condyle

Contoured frayed edge of the medial meniscus

Medial meniscus

Medial tibial plateau

FIGURE 5-93A,B

(A) Increased signal intensity in a frayed medial meniscal apex on a T1-weighted coronal image. The peripheral two-thirds of the meniscus is normal, except for intrasubstance signal intensity representing mucinous degeneration. **(B)** Arthroscopic contouring of the frayed posterior horn of the medial meniscus.

KNEE: MENISCUS

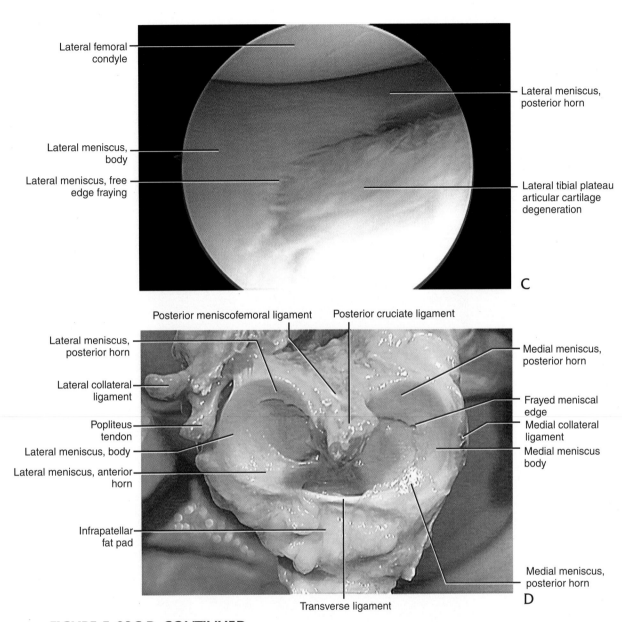

Lateral femoral condyle

Lateral meniscus, posterior horn

Lateral meniscus, body

Lateral meniscus, free edge fraying

Lateral tibial plateau articular cartilage degeneration

C

Posterior meniscofemoral ligament

Posterior cruciate ligament

Lateral meniscus, posterior horn

Medial meniscus, posterior horn

Lateral collateral ligament

Frayed meniscal edge

Medial collateral ligament

Popliteus tendon

Medial meniscus body

Lateral meniscus, body

Lateral meniscus, anterior horn

Infrapatellar fat pad

Medial meniscus, posterior horn

Transverse ligament

D

FIGURE 5-93C,D *CONTINUED*

(C) Less prominent degeneration is shown arthroscopically on the free edge of the central one-third of the lateral meniscus. **(D)** Medial meniscus contour irregularity is evident on superior surface viewing of the dissected menisci.

KNEE: MENISCUS

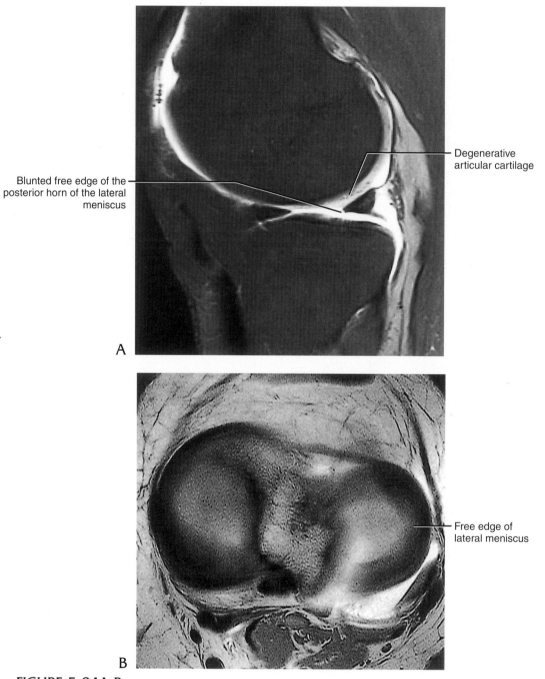

Degenerative
articular cartilage

Blunted free edge of the
posterior horn of the lateral
meniscus

A

Free edge of
lateral meniscus

B

FIGURE 5-94A,B

(**A** and **B**) The blunted apex of the posterior horn of the lateral meniscus is seen on a fat-suppressed T2-weighted MR arthrogram (**A**) and on a T1-weighted axial MR arthrogram (**B**). Degenerative articular cartilage can be visualized in the lateral compartment (part **A**).

KNEE: MENISCUS

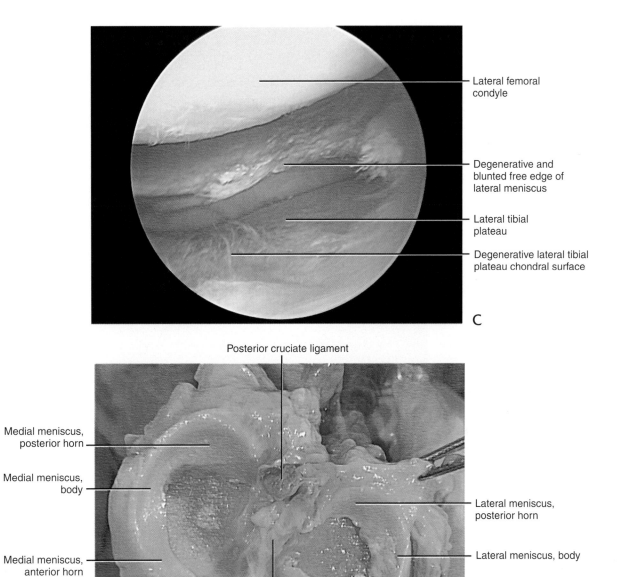

Lateral femoral condyle

Degenerative and blunted free edge of lateral meniscus

Lateral tibial plateau

Degenerative lateral tibial plateau chondral surface

C

Posterior cruciate ligament

Medial meniscus, posterior horn

Medial meniscus, body

Medial meniscus, anterior horn

Lateral meniscus, posterior horn

Lateral meniscus, body

Lateral meniscus, anterior horn

D

Anterior cruciate ligament

FIGURE 5-94C,D *CONTINUED*

(**C** and **D**) Arthroscopic view (**C**) and corresponding dissection (**D**) of the degenerative free edge of the lateral meniscus.

KNEE: MENISCUS

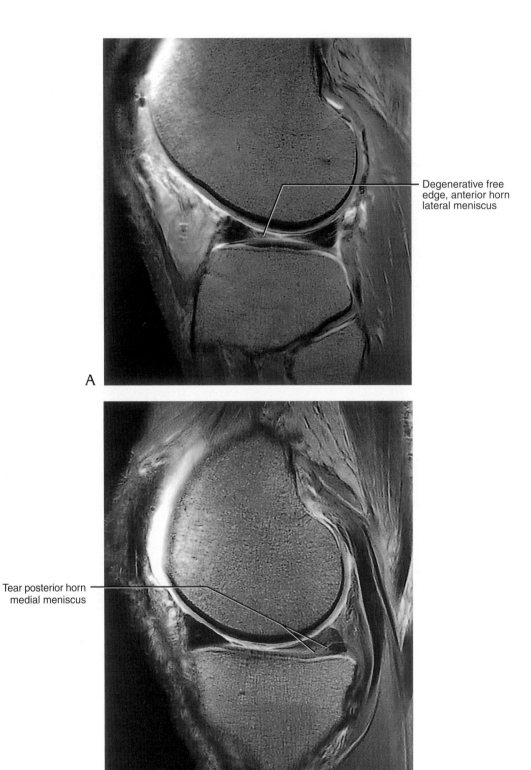

Degenerative free
edge, anterior horn
lateral meniscus

Tear posterior horn
medial meniscus

A

B

FIGURE 5-95A,B

(A) T1-weighted sagittal MR arthrographic image showing free-edge fraying at the junction of the anterior horn and the body of the lateral meniscus. **(B)** A tear of the posterior horn of the medial meniscus as seen on a T1-weighted sagittal MR arthrogram. There is irregularity of the inner two-thirds of the inferior leaf of the posterior horn or the medial meniscus.

KNEE: MENISCUS

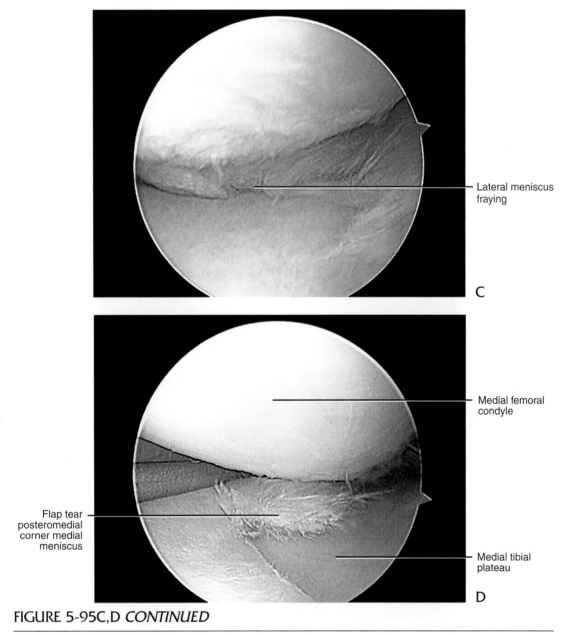

Lateral meniscus
fraying

C

Medial femoral
condyle

Flap tear
posteromedial
corner medial
meniscus

Medial tibial
plateau

D

FIGURE 5-95C,D *CONTINUED*

(**C** and **D**) Corresponding arthroscopic views of the frayed lateral meniscus (**C**) and a flap tear of the medial meniscus (**D**).

KNEE: CRUCIATE LIGAMENTS

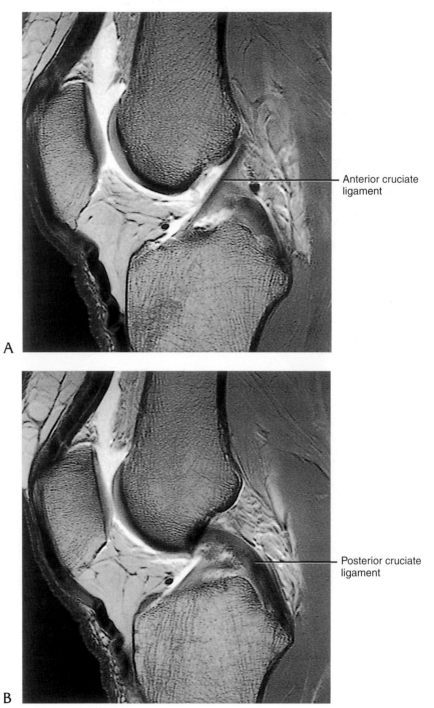

Anterior cruciate
ligament

A

Posterior cruciate
ligament

B

FIGURE 5-96A,B

(**A** and **B**) T1-weighted sagittal MR arthrograms depicting the anterior cruciate ligament (ACL) (**A**) and the posterior cruciate ligament (PCL) (**B**) (the image in part **A** is lateral to the image in part **B**). The posterior extent of the origin of the ACL from the posteromedial aspect of the lateral femoral condyle can be appreciated in the sagittal plane. The PCL attaches onto an inclined recessed shelf, posterior and inferior to the articular surface of the tibia.

KNEE: CRUCIATE LIGAMENTS

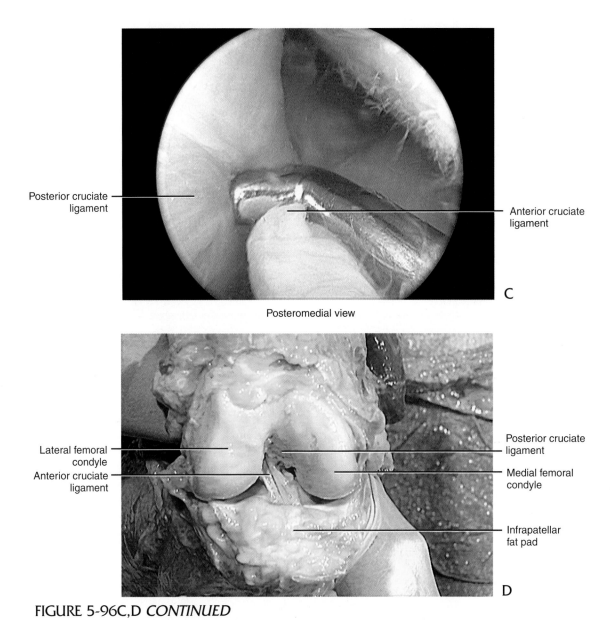

Posterior cruciate
ligament

Anterior cruciate
ligament

C

Posteromedial view

Lateral femoral
condyle

Posterior cruciate
ligament

Anterior cruciate
ligament

Medial femoral
condyle

Infrapatellar
fat pad

D

FIGURE 5-96C,D *CONTINUED*

(**C** and **D**) The ACL and PCL on corresponding arthroscopy (posteromedial view) (**C**) and anterior dissection with the knee in flexion (**D**).

KNEE: PATELLOFEMORAL JOINT

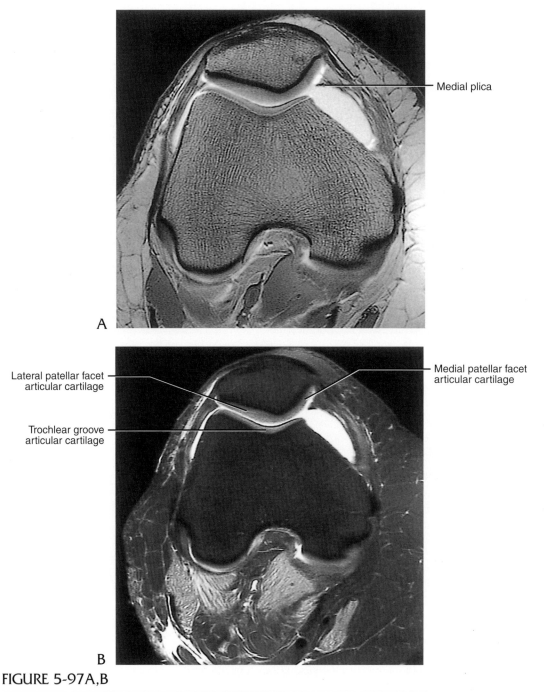

FIGURE 5-97A,B

(A and B) T1-weighted (A) and fat-suppressed T2-weighted (B) axial MR arthrographic images of the patellofemoral joint. The fat-suppressed T2-weighted contrast (part B) is superior for demonstrating articular cartilage detail of the patellar facets. A small medial plica is present.

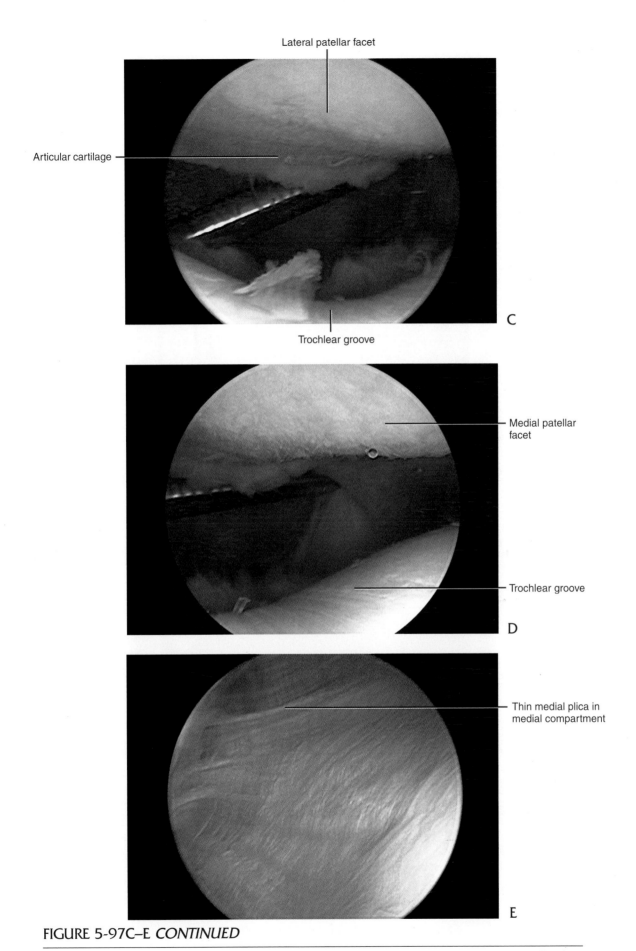

Lateral patellar facet

Articular cartilage

Trochlear groove

C

Medial patellar facet

Trochlear groove

D

Thin medial plica in medial compartment

E

FIGURE 5-97C–E *CONTINUED*

(**C, D,** and **E**) Corresponding arthrographic views of the lateral patellar facet **(C)**, the medial patellar facet and the trochlear groove **(D)**, and the medial plica **(E)**.

KNEE: MEDIAL AND LATERAL COMPARTMENT

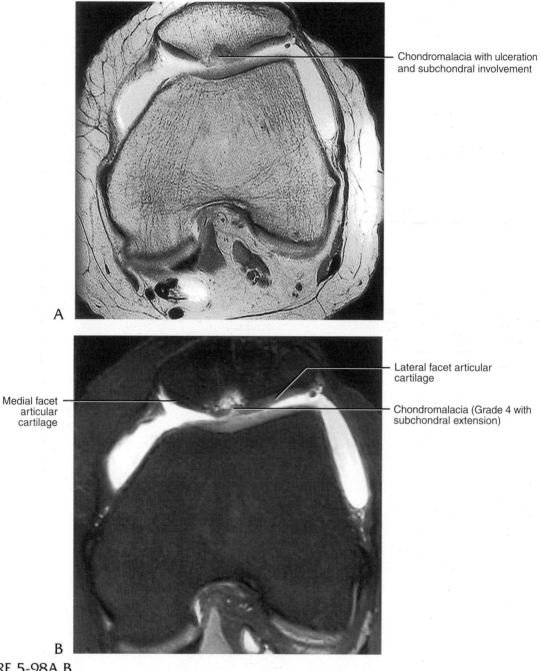

Chondromalacia with ulceration and subchondral involvement

A

Lateral facet articular cartilage

Medial facet articular cartilage

Chondromalacia (Grade 4 with subchondral extension)

B

FIGURE 5-98A,B

(A and B) T1-weighted (A) and fat-suppressed T2-weighted (B) axial MR images illustrating chondromalacia (with subchondral erosion) of the patellar ridge and medial aspect of the lateral patellar facet. (C and D) The full thickness chondral lesion is appreciated on a corresponding arthroscopic image (C) and on the surgical view of the patella (D). (E) The trochlear groove surface is shown with the knee flexed in an anterior exposure. The medial femoral condyle is longer than the lateral condyle and is oriented toward the lateral aspect of the knee, as it extends from posterior to anterior. Arthroscopy is more sensitive than the gross specimen for assessing superficial chondral fibrillation of the trochlear groove at an early stage.

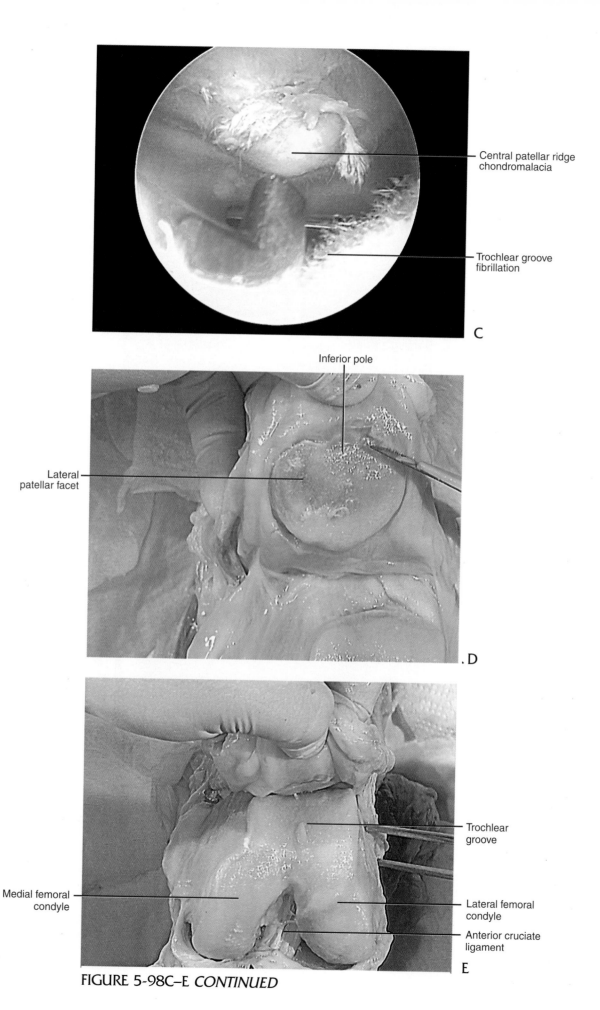

Central patellar ridge chondromalacia

Trochlear groove fibrillation

C

Inferior pole

Lateral patellar facet

.D

Trochlear groove

Medial femoral condyle

Lateral femoral condyle

Anterior cruciate ligament

E

FIGURE 5-98C–E CONTINUED

KNEE: MEDIAL AND LATERAL COMPARTMENT

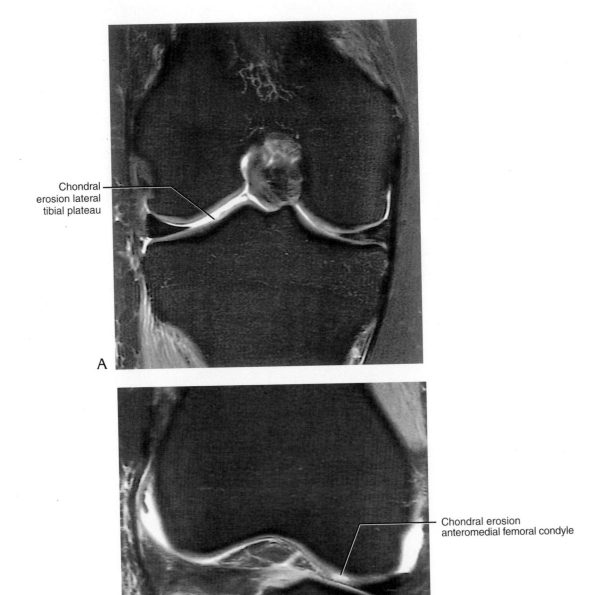

Chondral erosion lateral tibial plateau

A

Chondral erosion anteromedial femoral condyle

B

FIGURE 5-99A,B

(**A** and **B**) Fat-suppressed T2-weighted coronal MR arthrograms showing chondral erosions of the lateral tibial plateau (**A**) and the anteromedial femoral condyle (**B**) (the image in part **A** is more posterior than the image in part **B**). (**C** and **D**) Corresponding arthroscopic images of the lateral tibial plateau (**C**) and medial femoral condylar erosions (**D**). (**E**) The chondral defect is seen on the lateral aspect of the medial femoral condyle on a corresponding gross view of the distal femur. This specimen also shows that the trochlear groove is continuous with the intercondylar notch inferiorly and posteriorly.

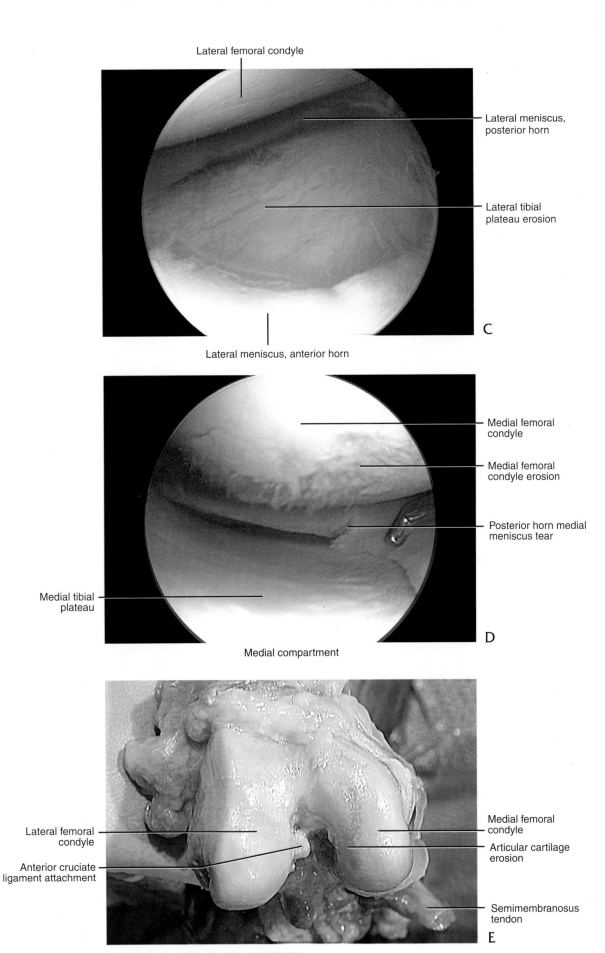

Lateral femoral condyle

Lateral meniscus, posterior horn

Lateral tibial plateau erosion

Lateral meniscus, anterior horn

C

Medial femoral condyle

Medial femoral condyle erosion

Posterior horn medial meniscus tear

Medial tibial plateau

Medial compartment

D

Lateral femoral condyle

Anterior cruciate ligament attachment

Medial femoral condyle

Articular cartilage erosion

Semimembranosus tendon

E

FIGURE 5-99C–E *CONTINUED*

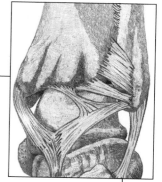

C H A P T E R 6

THE ANKLE AND FOOT

David W. Stoller

Richard D. Ferkel

Salvador Beltran

ANKLE ARTHROSCOPY AND DISSECTION
   Anterior Ankle Examination
   Central Ankle Examination
   Posterior Ankle Examination

MR NORMAL ANATOMY
COLOR ANATOMIC ILLUSTRATIONS
MR, ARTHROSCOPY, AND SURGICAL
   CORRELATION

———— ANKLE ARTHROSCOPY ————

PROPER PORTAL PLACEMENT is critical in the performance of good diagnostic and therapeutic arthroscopy. Ankle arthroscopy portals include anterior portals, posterior portals, and transmalleolar portals (Table 6-1).

Three primary anterior portals are used in arthroscopy of the ankle: anteromedial, anterolateral, and anterocentral. The anterocentral portal is not commonly used. Posterior portals are routinely used in ankle arthroscopy and may be established posteromedial, posterolateral, or directly through the Achilles tendon (transachilles portal). The transachilles portal, however, does not allow easy manipulation of arthroscopy instruments, and its use may lead to increased morbidity in the Achilles tendon region. Transmalleolar portals may be used for various operative techniques to gain better access to osteochondral lesions of the talar dome.

The anteromedial portal is always established first, because it is easier to access, has less risk of injury to neurovascular structures, and is most reproducible. The location of the anterolateral portal varies, depending on the location of the primary pathology in the ankle, and it should not be established first. The posterolateral portal is always established, not only to facilitate inflow, but also to permit visualization of the posterior structures. The arthroscope is maneuvered under the medial notch of Harty until the posterior capsule and posterior ligaments are visualized.

The ankle joint can be divided into anterior and posterior cavities, each of which can then be subdivided further into three compartments. A 21-point systematic examination (as developed by Ferkel) is performed of the anterior, central, and posterior ankle joint. The anteromedial portal is al-

TABLE 6–1. Portals and the nearest anatomy at risk

Portal	Tendons	Nerves	Vessels
Anterior approaches			
Anterolateral	Extensor digitorum, peroneus tertius	Superficial peroneal	
Anteromedial	Anterior tibialis	Saphenous	Greater saphenous vein
Anterocentral	Extensors	Deep peroneal	Dorsalis pedis artery
Posterior approaches			
Posterolateral	Peroneal	Sural	Small saphenous vein
Posteromedial	Posterior tibial, flexor digitorum, flexor hallucis	Tibial	Posterior tibial artery
Transachilles	Achilles		
Transmalleolar			
Medial	None	Saphenous	Saphenous
Lateral	Extensor	Superficial peroneal, deep peroneal	Anterior, tibial

ways used for the initial arthroscopic examination, and then the anterolateral and posterolateral portals are used.

Anterior Ankle Examination

The first structure visualized during the anterior examination (see the illustration of an eight-point anterior examination) is the deep portion of the deltoid ligament. It arises from the tip of the medial malleolus and its fibers run vertically down to the medial trochlear surface of the talus (area 1). This is an area where ossicles may be hidden. The articular surface of the tip of the medial malleolus (as it corresponds and articulates with the medial talar dome), the posterior recess, and the posterior ligament are also found in area 1. Area 2, the medial gutter, is defined as the area from the deltoid ligament to below the medial dome of the talus. Area 3, the medial talar dome, is where the tibial plafond and the medial malleolus meet. The tibia articulates with the medial dome of the talus and is termed the medial corner of the ankle. At the medial articular notch (the notch of Harty), the arthroscope may be maneuvered most easily into the central and posterior aspects of the joint without scuffing the articular surfaces. Area 4 is where the medial talus articulates with the tibial plafond. The anterior tibial lip has hyaline cartilage that extends from the undersurface of the tibial plafond around the anterior corner superiorly. Between the anterior tibial lip and the capsular reflection there is a periosteum-covered subchondral bone, the synovial recess. This is where tibial osteophytes develop and where synovium and capsule become adherent at the margins of the osteophyte. The fifth and sixth areas of the anterior ankle examination are the lateral talus and the talofibular articulation (area 5). This area is called the trifurcation, as it includes the distal lateral tibial plafond, the lateral talar dome, and the fibula. It is bounded by the anterior inferior tibiofibular ligament superiorly and is often the site of soft tissue and bony pathology. The syndesmotic, or anterior inferior tibiofibular, ligament courses at a 45° angle from the lateral portion of the distal tibia to the fibula, just below the level of the lateral talus (area 6). About 20% of the

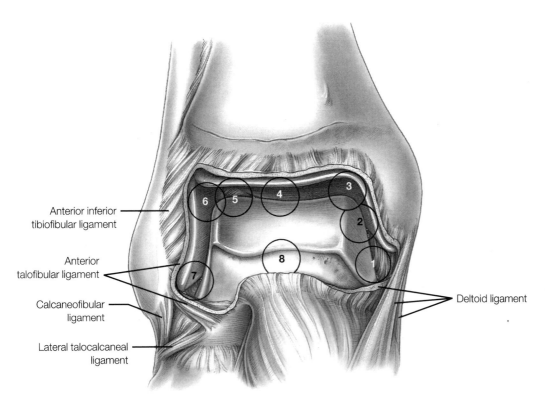

Eight-point anterior examination, viewed from the anteromedial portal.

anterior inferior tibiofibular ligament is intraarticular. Behind this thick, strong ligament is a synovial recess as well as the tibiofibular articulation. This is often the site of synovitis, particularly after inversion ankle sprains. Anteriorly the seventh area is the lateral gutter, a space between the medial border of the fibular articulation and the lateral border of the talar articulation. The lateral gutter extends below the anterior inferior tibiofibular ligament to the anterior talofibular ligament. This is often the site of chondromalacia, as well as ossicles at the tip of the fibula within the ligament substance. The anterior talofibular ligament represents a capsular reflection running from the tip of the fibula to the inferolateral portion of the talus. Soft tissue impingement often occurs within this space. The anterior gutter (area 8) represents the anterior capsular reflection of the ankle as it inserts along the talar neck. There is a normal bare area proximal to the capsular insertion. A synovial recess can also be found at the anterior inferior aspect of the talar dome. In this area anterior talar osteophytes may articulate or impinge against osteophytes of the anterior talar lip.

Central Ankle Examination

After the anterior ankle evaluation is complete the arthroscope is maneuvered through the medial tibial notch to evaluate the central portion of the tibiotalar articulation (see the illustration of a six-point central examination). Area 9 is the medial dome of the talus, with the tibial plafond as it bends into the medial malleolar region. This is an area where osteochondral lesions of the talus often begin. Area 10 is the central portion of the tibia and talus. The articulation of the lateral talar dome with the distal tibia and fibula and the syndesmotic articulation is in area 11. Synovitis or synovial nodules may compress against this articulation and produce pain.

Posterior Ankle Examination

Several posterior structures are visualized with the arthroscope initially in the central portion of the ankle. With the arthrosocpe laterally, the posterior inferior tibiofibular ligament is visualized as it runs obliquely at about a 45° angle from the posterior tibia to the fibula (area 12). Just medial and inferior to this ligament is the transverse tibiofibular ligament (area 13). There is usually a small gap between the transverse tibiofibular ligament and the posterior inferior tibiofibular ligament. A separate tibial slip may run from the posterior talofibular ligament to the transverse tibiofibular ligament. Medial to the transverse tibiofibular ligament is the capsular reflection of the flexor hallucis longus tendon (area 14). The posterior examination continues from the posterolateral portal (see the illustration of a seven-point posterior examination).

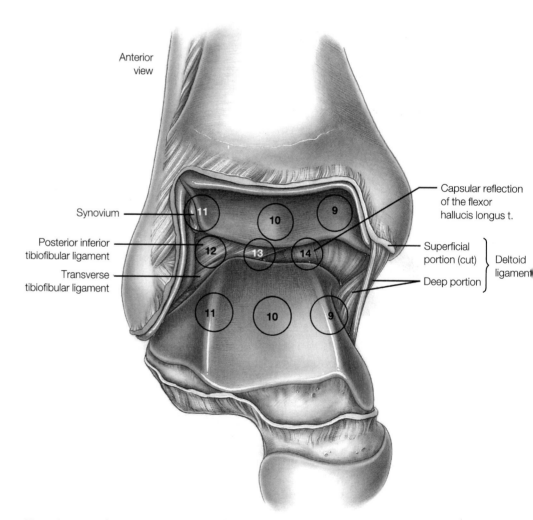

Six-point central examination, viewed from the anteromedial portal. The arthroscope is maneuvered from a central to a posterior position to examine the posterior capsular structures.

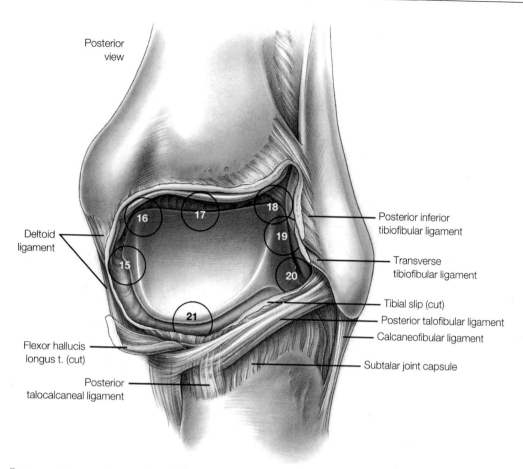

Posterior view

Deltoid ligament

Flexor hallucis longus t. (cut)

Posterior talocalcaneal ligament

Posterior inferior tibiofibular ligament

Transverse tibiofibular ligament

Tibial slip (cut)

Posterior talofibular ligament

Calcaneofibular ligament

Subtalar joint capsule

Seven-point posterior examination, viewed from the posterolateral portal.

The deltoid ligament and posteromedial gutter are visualized in area 15. The posteromedial talar dome and tibial plafond are evaluated and assessed for osteochondral lesions (area 16). The central talus and distal tibia are seen in area 17. The transverse tibiofibular ligament, together with the posterior inferior tibiofibular ligament, forms a posterior labrum over the posterior tibial lip. Areas 18 and 19 consist of the lateral talar dome, the posterior tibia, and the posterior talofibular articulation. Synovitis and other soft tissue pathology can be seen in the area of the posterior inferior tibiofibular ligament and transverse tibiofibular ligament (area 18). The posterior talofibular articulation is rarely the site of pathology (area 19). Area 20 is the lateral gutter, where the inferior portions of the fibula and talus articulate. Area 21 is the posterior gutter with synovial and capsular reflections.

SURGICAL DISSECTION OF THE ANKLE

The skin of the ankle and foot consists of a dense connective tissue and a dermis that is arranged in reticular and papillary layers. The arrangement of connective tissue bundles in the reticular layer gives rise to various patterns of tension lines (Langer's lines). The septa on the plantar surface of the foot divide the subcutaneous fat into small chambers that act as protective shock absorbers.

Several bony landmarks and soft tissue structures are easily palpated on the ankle, including:

- the lateral malleolus
- the medial malleolus
- the anterior joint line
- the posterior joint line
- the sinus tarsi

Foot landmarks include:

- the tarsal bones, including the base of the fifth metatarsal
- the navicular tuberosity
- the midfoot and forefoot joints

Tendon landmarks easy to identify and palpate include:

- the extensor tibialis (tibialis anterior)
- the extensor digitorum
- the Achilles tendon
- the tibialis posterior tendon
- the flexor tendons
- the peroneal tendons

The nerves that cross the ankle and foot are the superficial peroneal nerve, the sural nerve, and the saphenous nerve. The superficial peroneal nerve arises from the common peroneal nerve and divides into the intermediate and medial dorsal cutaneous nerves. The sural nerve, which passes 1.5 cm below the tip of the lateral malleolus, divides into lateral and medial terminal branches at the base of the fifth metatarsal. The saphenous nerve passes over the anterior aspect of the medial malleolus (medial to the great saphenous vein) and crosses over the anteromedial joint capsule.

The deep fascial layer contains the flexor and extensor tendons of the foot and ankle as well as the two deep neurovascular structures. The anterior compartment of the leg contains the tibialis anterior muscle, the extensor hallucis and extensor digitorum longus muscles, and their blood supply (the anterior tibial vessels) and innervation (the deep peroneal nerve). The deep peroneal nerve arises from the common peroneal nerve, reaches the anterior intermuscular septum, and joins the anterior tibial artery in the proximal third of the leg. It lies lateral to the artery and terminates into lateral and medial branches in the dorsum of the foot. On the medial aspect of the ankle, the tarsal tunnel contains—from anterior to posterior—the posterior tibial tendon, the flexor digitorum longus tendon, the posterior tibial artery and venae comitantes, the tibial nerve, and the flexor hallucis longus tendon. The posterior tibial nerve divides into medial and lateral plantar nerves as it exits the tarsal tunnel. On the lateral aspect of the ankle, the peroneus brevis grooves the lateral malleolus, curving distally to its insertion on the tuberosity of the fifth metatarsal. The peroneus longus lies posterior to the brevis and runs in a groove on the plantar surface of the foot to insert onto the first metatarsal and medial cuneiform.

The ligaments that make up the tibiofibular syndesmosis are the anterior and posterior inferior tibiofibular ligaments, the transverse tibiofibular ligament, and the interosseous membrane. The anterior inferior tibiofibular ligament may be two or three bands or multifascicular. Approximately 20% of the ligament is seen intraarticularly via the arthroscope. The posterior inferior tibiofibular ligament is quadrilateral in shape and smaller than its anterior counterpart. The transverse tibiofibular ligament runs medial to the posterior inferior tibiofibular ligament and forms a true posterior labrum, deepening the tibial articulating surface of the talus. During plantar flexion, this ligament can be injured or torn as it is tightly squeezed between the posterior tibial margin and the posterior talofibular ligament. The transverse tibiofibular ligament also forms the attachment for the tibial slip. The interosseous membrane consists of numerous short fibrous bands running from the tibia to the fibula.

The deltoid ligament consists of superficial and deep fibers. The tibiocalcaneal ligament is the strongest component of the superficial deltoid ligament. The posterior talotibial (deep layer) is the strongest component in the entire medial complex. The deep portion or layer is intraarticular and covered only by synovium.

The lateral collateral ligamentous complex consists of three distinct structures: the anterior talofibular ligament, the calcaneofibular ligament, and the posterior talofibular ligament. The anterior talofibular ligament runs from the lateral malleolus to insert onto the talus. The anterior talofibular ligament is closely related to the capsule of the talofibular joint and is the most frequently injured of the lateral ligaments. The calcaneofibular ligament is the largest of the three collateral ligaments and can be seen through visualization of the subtalar joint. The posterior talofibular ligament is intracapsular, but extrasynovial. The tibial slip (posterior intermalleolar ligament) runs from the posterior talofibular ligament and inserts on the transverse tibiofibular ligament.

Synovial folds, or plicae, are membranes that invest the deep surfaces of the ligaments. Plicae occur at the anterior and posterior tibiofibular junctions, the inferior tibiofibular syndesmosis, and the medial and lateral talomalleolar spaces.

At the level of the distal tibia, the flat tendon of the tibialis anterior lies on the anterior tibial crest. Adjacent and just lateral to the tibialis anterior tendon is the tendon of the extensor hallucis longus muscle. The anterior tibial vessels and the deep peroneal nerve are between, and deep to, the two tendons, directly on the tibial surface. Posteromedially, the posterior tibial vessels and the tibial nerve lie deep to the soleus muscle, between the flexor hallucis longus and the flexor digitorum muscles.

At the level of the ankle joint, the anterior tibial vessels and the deep peroneal nerve lie between the extensor hallucis longus tendon and the first tendon of the extensor digitorum longus. The structures that pass anterior to the ankle joint—from the medial to the lateral side—include the tibialis anterior tendon, the extensor hallucis longus tendon, the anterior tibial artery and the venae comitantes, the deep peroneal nerve, the extensor digitorum longus tendon, and the peroneus tertius tendon. The posterior tibial neurovascular bundle is located behind the posteromedial aspect of the tibia, between the flexor digitorum longus and flexor hallucis longus tendons.

ANKLE: CORONAL

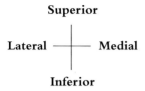

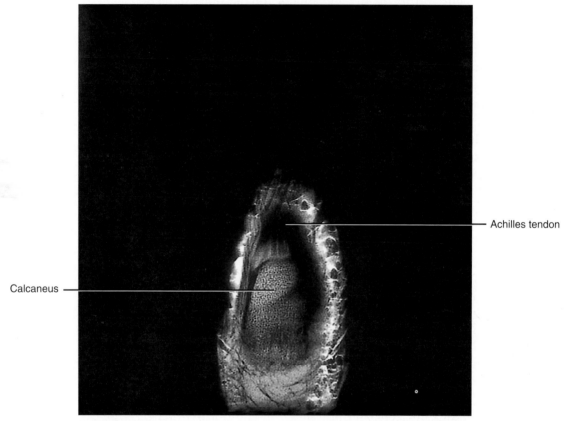

Achilles tendon

Calcaneus

FIGURE 6-1

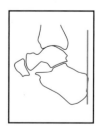

ANKLE: CORONAL

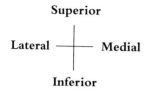

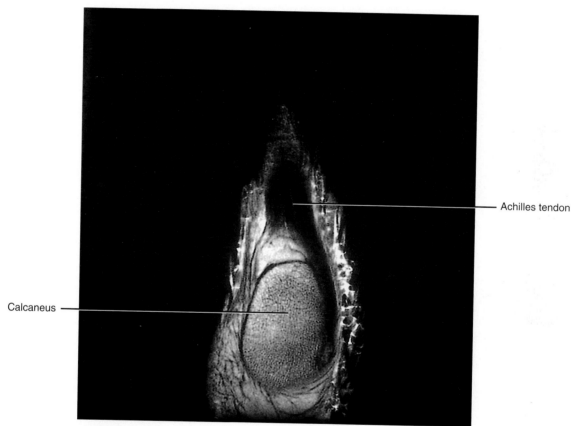

Achilles tendon

Calcaneus

FIGURE 6-2

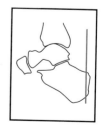

ANKLE: CORONAL

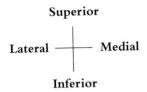

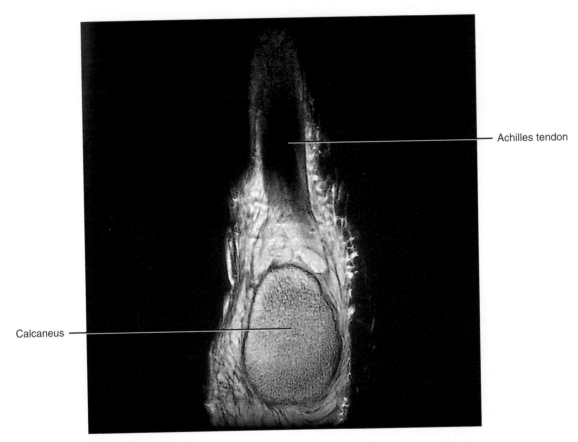

Achilles tendon

Calcaneus

FIGURE 6-3

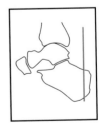

ANKLE: CORONAL

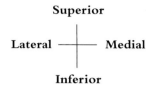

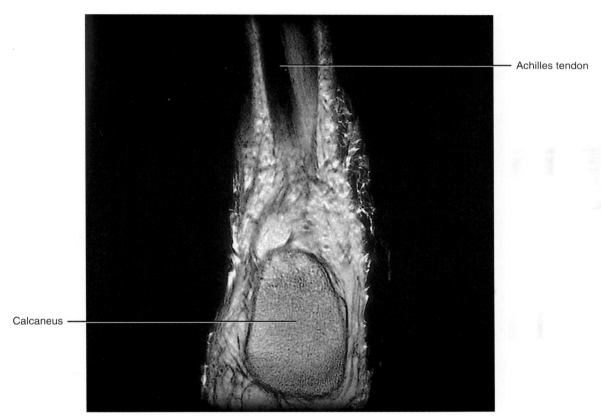

FIGURE 6-4

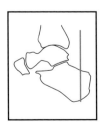

ANKLE: CORONAL

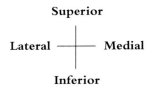

Superior

Lateral ─────┼───── Medial

Inferior

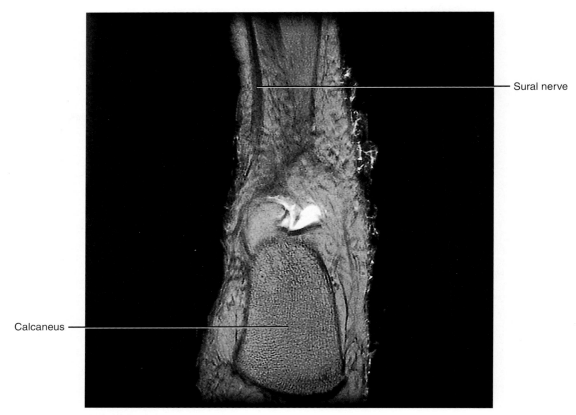

Sural nerve

Calcaneus

FIGURE 6-5

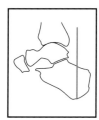

ANKLE: CORONAL

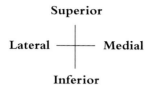

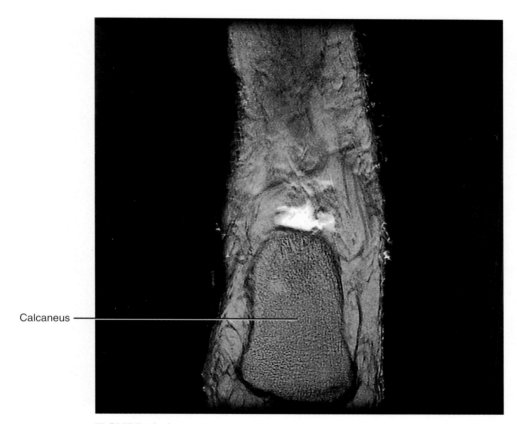

Calcaneus

FIGURE 6-6

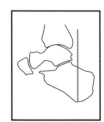

ANKLE: CORONAL

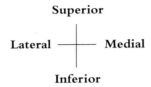

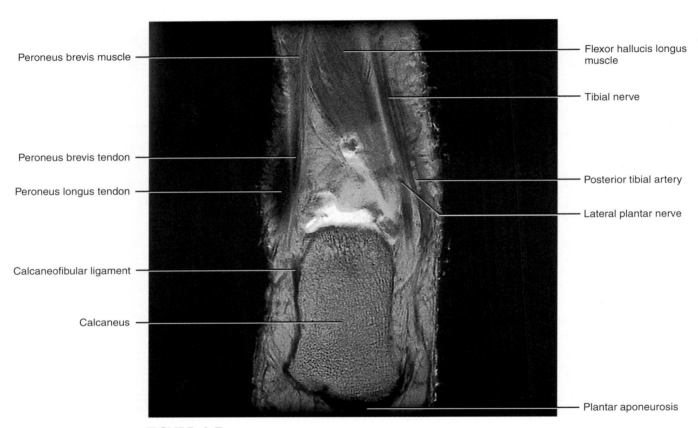

Peroneus brevis muscle

Peroneus brevis tendon

Peroneus longus tendon

Calcaneofibular ligament

Calcaneus

Flexor hallucis longus muscle

Tibial nerve

Posterior tibial artery

Lateral plantar nerve

Plantar aponeurosis

FIGURE 6-7

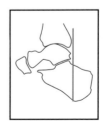

ANKLE: CORONAL

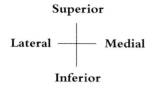

Superior

Lateral —|— Medial

Inferior

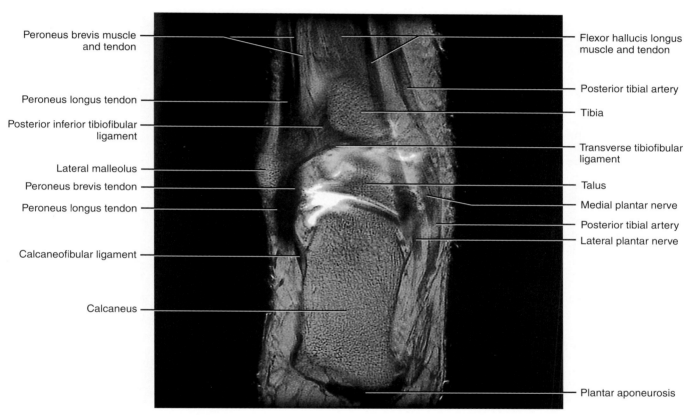

Peroneus brevis muscle
and tendon

Flexor hallucis longus
muscle and tendon

Posterior tibial artery

Peroneus longus tendon

Tibia

Posterior inferior tibiofibular
ligament

Transverse tibiofibular
ligament

Lateral malleolus

Peroneus brevis tendon

Talus

Medial plantar nerve

Peroneus longus tendon

Posterior tibial artery

Lateral plantar nerve

Calcaneofibular ligament

Calcaneus

Plantar aponeurosis

FIGURE 6-8

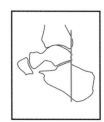

ANKLE: CORONAL

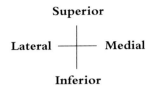

Superior
|
Lateral ——+—— Medial
|
Inferior

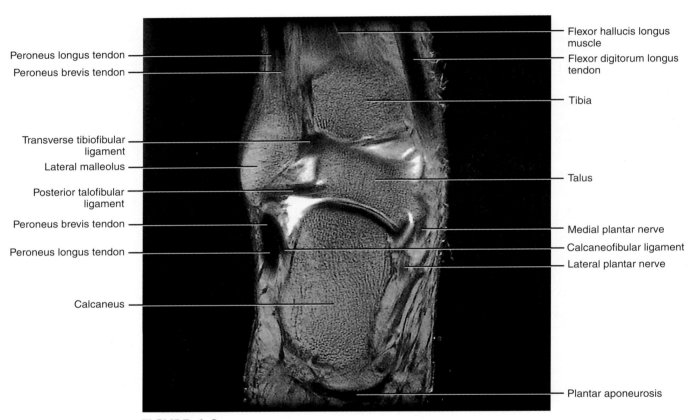

Peroneus longus tendon

Peroneus brevis tendon

Transverse tibiofibular ligament

Lateral malleolus

Posterior talofibular ligament

Peroneus brevis tendon

Peroneus longus tendon

Calcaneus

Flexor hallucis longus muscle

Flexor digitorum longus tendon

Tibia

Talus

Medial plantar nerve

Calcaneofibular ligament

Lateral plantar nerve

Plantar aponeurosis

FIGURE 6-9

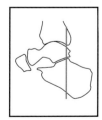

ANKLE: CORONAL

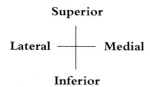

Superior

Lateral —+— Medial

Inferior

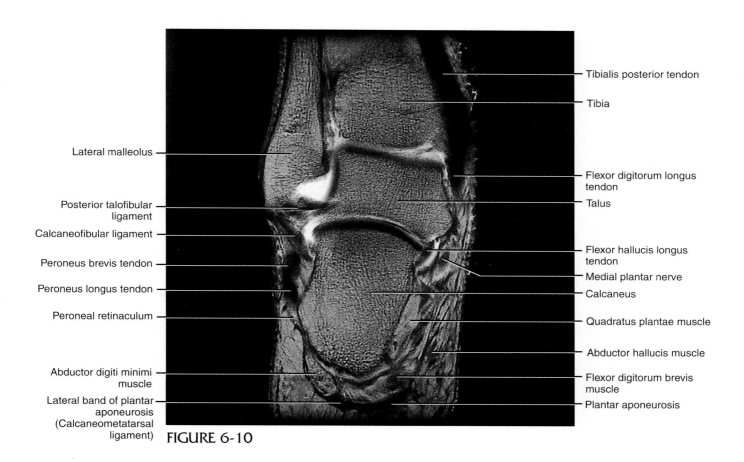

Tibialis posterior tendon

Tibia

Lateral malleolus

Flexor digitorum longus tendon

Posterior talofibular ligament

Talus

Calcaneofibular ligament

Peroneus brevis tendon

Flexor hallucis longus tendon

Peroneus longus tendon

Medial plantar nerve

Calcaneus

Peroneal retinaculum

Quadratus plantae muscle

Abductor hallucis muscle

Abductor digiti minimi muscle

Flexor digitorum brevis muscle

Lateral band of plantar aponeurosis (Calcaneometatarsal ligament)

Plantar aponeurosis

FIGURE 6-10

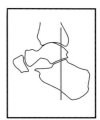

ANKLE: CORONAL

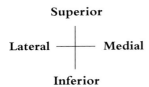

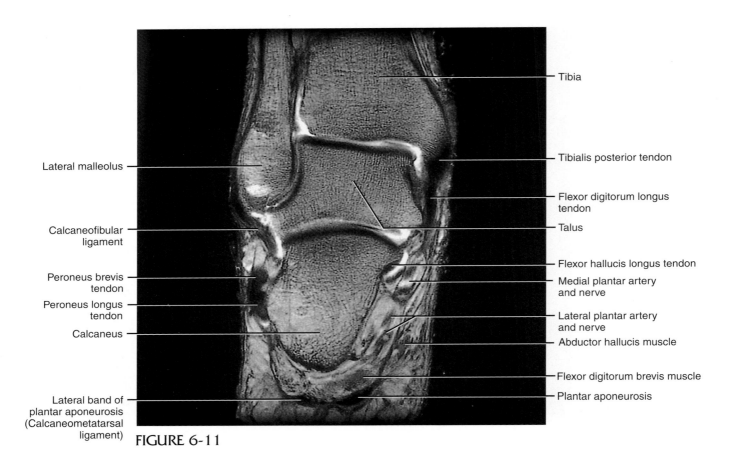

Tibia

Tibialis posterior tendon

Flexor digitorum longus tendon

Talus

Flexor hallucis longus tendon

Medial plantar artery and nerve

Lateral plantar artery and nerve

Abductor hallucis muscle

Flexor digitorum brevis muscle

Plantar aponeurosis

Lateral malleolus

Calcaneofibular ligament

Peroneus brevis tendon

Peroneus longus tendon

Calcaneus

Lateral band of plantar aponeurosis (Calcaneometatarsal ligament)

FIGURE 6-11

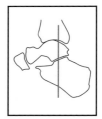

ANKLE: CORONAL

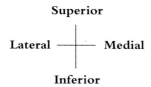

Superior

Lateral ——┼—— Medial

Inferior

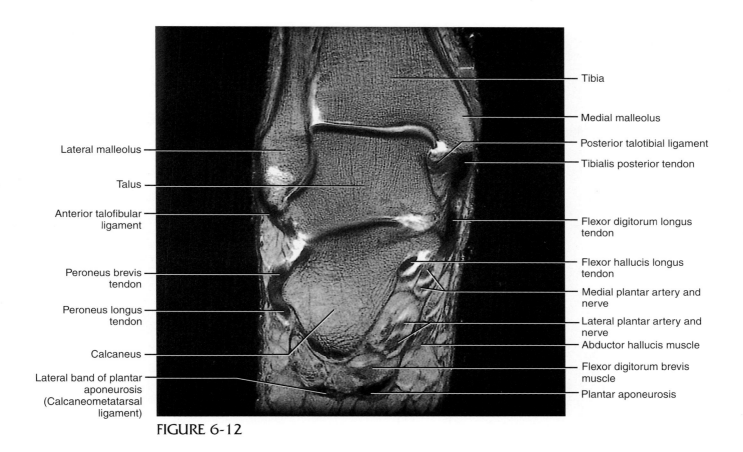

Lateral malleolus ———

Talus ———

Anterior talofibular ligament ———

Peroneus brevis tendon ———

Peroneus longus tendon ———

Calcaneus ———

Lateral band of plantar aponeurosis (Calcaneometatarsal ligament) ———

——— Tibia

——— Medial malleolus

——— Posterior talotibial ligament

——— Tibialis posterior tendon

——— Flexor digitorum longus tendon

——— Flexor hallucis longus tendon

——— Medial plantar artery and nerve

——— Lateral plantar artery and nerve

——— Abductor hallucis muscle

——— Flexor digitorum brevis muscle

——— Plantar aponeurosis

FIGURE 6-12

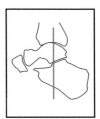

ANKLE: CORONAL

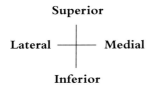

Superior

Lateral —|— Medial

Inferior

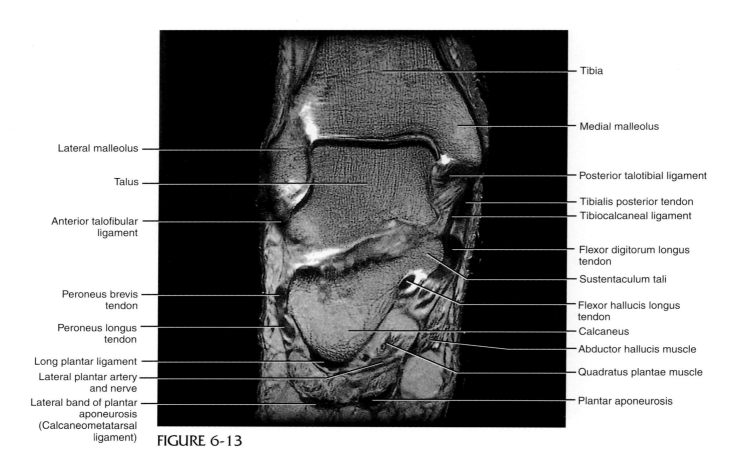

Lateral malleolus

Talus

Anterior talofibular ligament

Peroneus brevis tendon

Peroneus longus tendon

Long plantar ligament

Lateral plantar artery and nerve

Lateral band of plantar aponeurosis (Calcaneometatarsal ligament)

Tibia

Medial malleolus

Posterior talotibial ligament

Tibialis posterior tendon

Tibiocalcaneal ligament

Flexor digitorum longus tendon

Sustentaculum tali

Flexor hallucis longus tendon

Calcaneus

Abductor hallucis muscle

Quadratus plantae muscle

Plantar aponeurosis

FIGURE 6-13

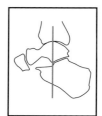

ANKLE: CORONAL

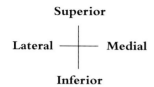

Superior

Lateral —|— Medial

Inferior

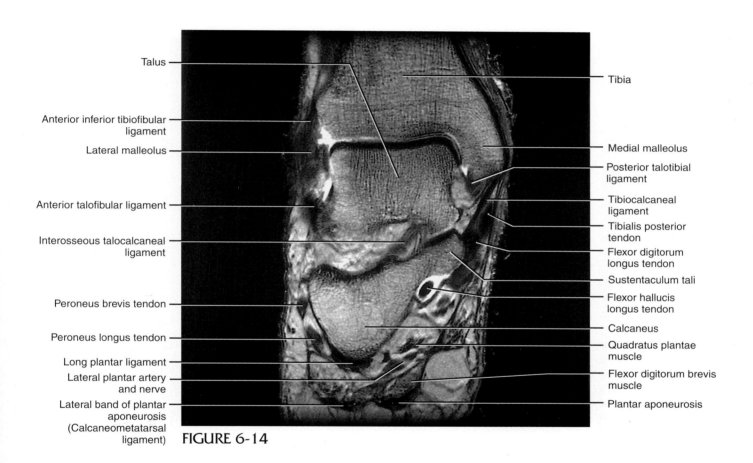

Talus

Anterior inferior tibiofibular ligament

Lateral malleolus

Anterior talofibular ligament

Interosseous talocalcaneal ligament

Peroneus brevis tendon

Peroneus longus tendon

Long plantar ligament

Lateral plantar artery and nerve

Lateral band of plantar aponeurosis (Calcaneometatarsal ligament)

Tibia

Medial malleolus

Posterior talotibial ligament

Tibiocalcaneal ligament

Tibialis posterior tendon

Flexor digitorum longus tendon

Sustentaculum tali

Flexor hallucis longus tendon

Calcaneus

Quadratus plantae muscle

Flexor digitorum brevis muscle

Plantar aponeurosis

FIGURE 6-14

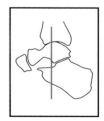

ANKLE: CORONAL

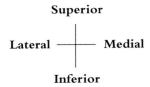

Superior

Lateral ———|——— Medial

Inferior

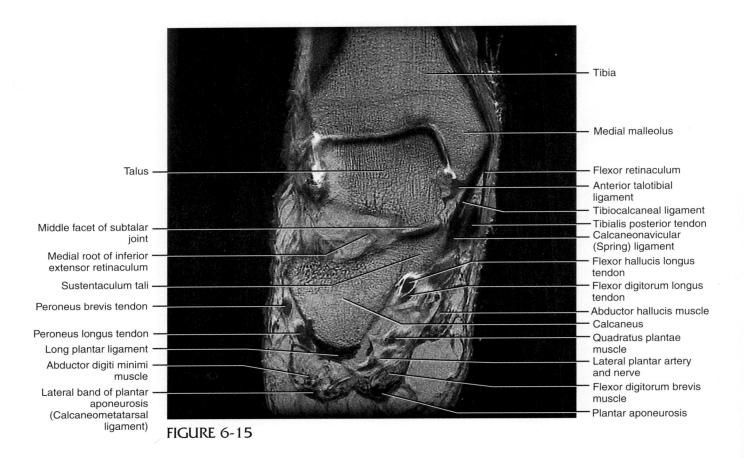

Talus

Middle facet of subtalar joint

Medial root of inferior extensor retinaculum

Sustentaculum tali

Peroneus brevis tendon

Peroneus longus tendon

Long plantar ligament

Abductor digiti minimi muscle

Lateral band of plantar aponeurosis (Calcaneometatarsal ligament)

Tibia

Medial malleolus

Flexor retinaculum

Anterior talotibial ligament

Tibiocalcaneal ligament

Tibialis posterior tendon

Calcaneonavicular (Spring) ligament

Flexor hallucis longus tendon

Flexor digitorum longus tendon

Abductor hallucis muscle

Calcaneus

Quadratus plantae muscle

Lateral plantar artery and nerve

Flexor digitorum brevis muscle

Plantar aponeurosis

FIGURE 6-15

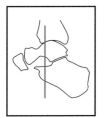

ANKLE: CORONAL

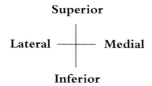

Superior

Lateral —|— Medial

Inferior

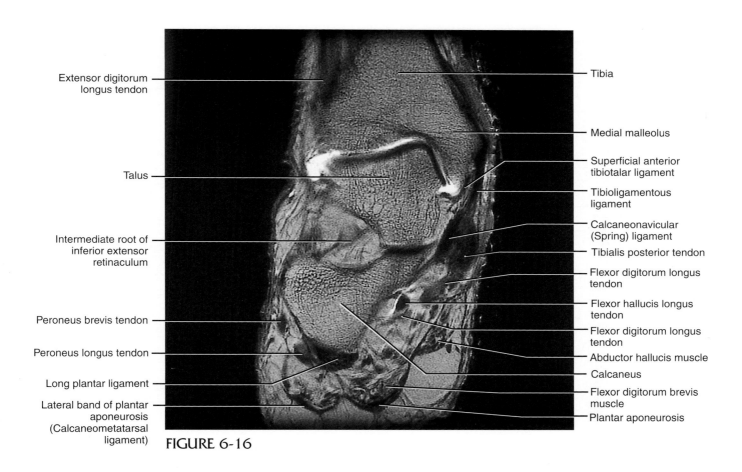

Extensor digitorum longus tendon

Talus

Intermediate root of inferior extensor retinaculum

Peroneus brevis tendon

Peroneus longus tendon

Long plantar ligament

Lateral band of plantar aponeurosis (Calcaneometatarsal ligament)

Tibia

Medial malleolus

Superficial anterior tibiotalar ligament

Tibioligamentous ligament

Calcaneonavicular (Spring) ligament

Tibialis posterior tendon

Flexor digitorum longus tendon

Flexor hallucis longus tendon

Flexor digitorum longus tendon

Abductor hallucis muscle

Calcaneus

Flexor digitorum brevis muscle

Plantar aponeurosis

FIGURE 6-16

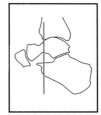

ANKLE: CORONAL

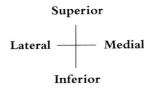

Superior

Lateral ——— Medial

Inferior

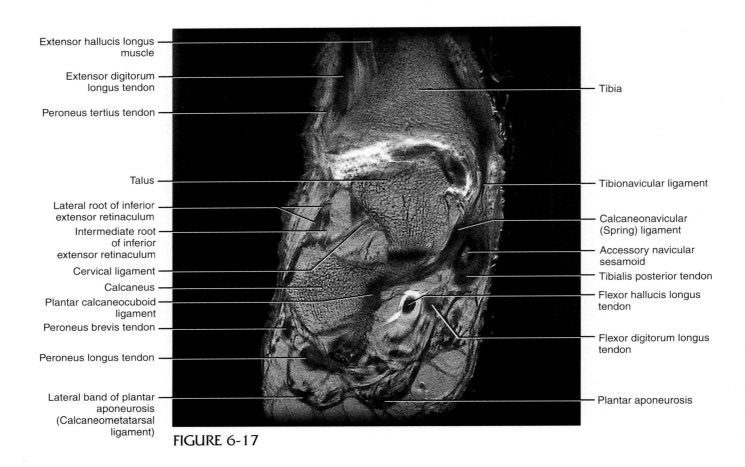

Extensor hallucis longus muscle

Extensor digitorum longus tendon

Peroneus tertius tendon

Talus

Lateral root of inferior extensor retinaculum

Intermediate root of inferior extensor retinaculum

Cervical ligament

Calcaneus

Plantar calcaneocuboid ligament

Peroneus brevis tendon

Peroneus longus tendon

Lateral band of plantar aponeurosis (Calcaneometatarsal ligament)

Tibia

Tibionavicular ligament

Calcaneonavicular (Spring) ligament

Accessory navicular sesamoid

Tibialis posterior tendon

Flexor hallucis longus tendon

Flexor digitorum longus tendon

Plantar aponeurosis

FIGURE 6-17

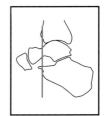

ANKLE: CORONAL

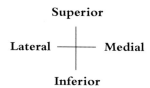

Superior

Lateral —— Medial

Inferior

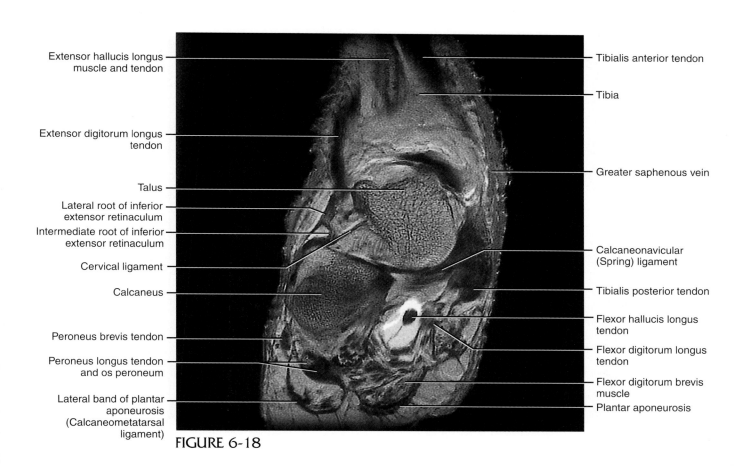

Extensor hallucis longus muscle and tendon

Extensor digitorum longus tendon

Talus

Lateral root of inferior extensor retinaculum

Intermediate root of inferior extensor retinaculum

Cervical ligament

Calcaneus

Peroneus brevis tendon

Peroneus longus tendon and os peroneum

Lateral band of plantar aponeurosis (Calcaneometatarsal ligament)

Tibialis anterior tendon

Tibia

Greater saphenous vein

Calcaneonavicular (Spring) ligament

Tibialis posterior tendon

Flexor hallucis longus tendon

Flexor digitorum longus tendon

Flexor digitorum brevis muscle

Plantar aponeurosis

FIGURE 6-18

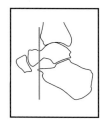

ANKLE: CORONAL

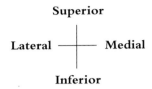

Superior

Lateral ——|—— **Medial**

Inferior

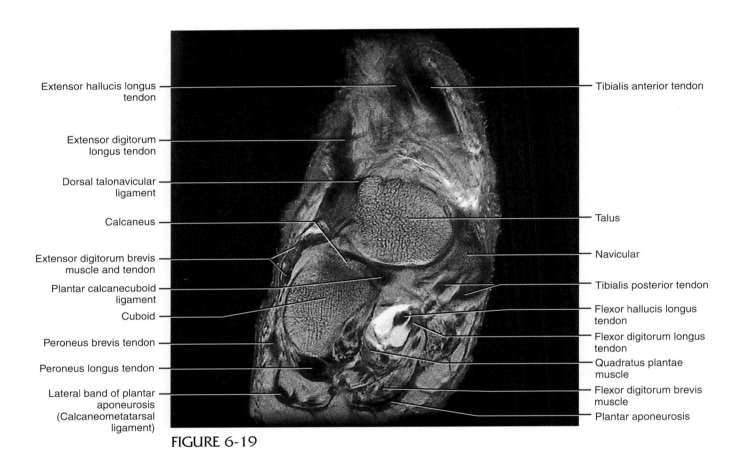

Extensor hallucis longus tendon

Extensor digitorum longus tendon

Dorsal talonavicular ligament

Calcaneus

Extensor digitorum brevis muscle and tendon

Plantar calcanecuboid ligament

Cuboid

Peroneus brevis tendon

Peroneus longus tendon

Lateral band of plantar aponeurosis (Calcaneometatarsal ligament)

Tibialis anterior tendon

Talus

Navicular

Tibialis posterior tendon

Flexor hallucis longus tendon

Flexor digitorum longus tendon

Quadratus plantae muscle

Flexor digitorum brevis muscle

Plantar aponeurosis

FIGURE 6-19

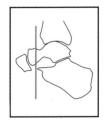

ANKLE: CORONAL

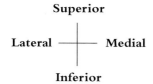

Superior

Lateral —— Medial

Inferior

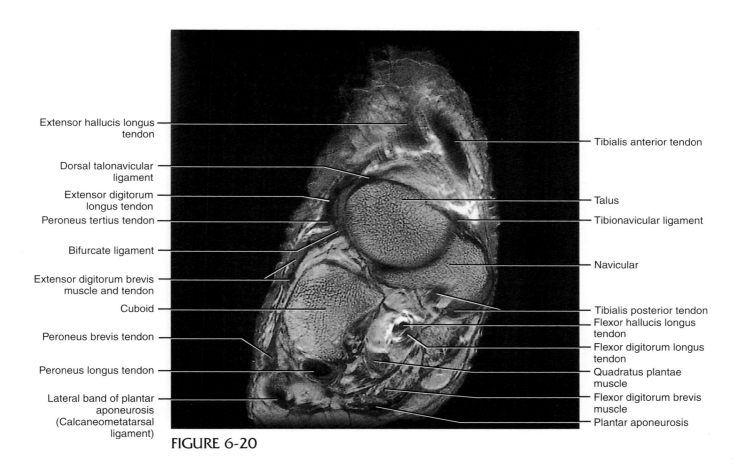

Extensor hallucis longus tendon

Dorsal talonavicular ligament

Extensor digitorum longus tendon

Peroneus tertius tendon

Bifurcate ligament

Extensor digitorum brevis muscle and tendon

Cuboid

Peroneus brevis tendon

Peroneus longus tendon

Lateral band of plantar aponeurosis (Calcaneometatarsal ligament)

Tibialis anterior tendon

Talus

Tibionavicular ligament

Navicular

Tibialis posterior tendon

Flexor hallucis longus tendon

Flexor digitorum longus tendon

Quadratus plantae muscle

Flexor digitorum brevis muscle

Plantar aponeurosis

FIGURE 6-20

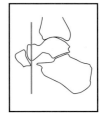

ANKLE: CORONAL

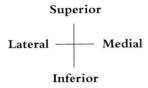

Superior

Lateral ——+—— Medial

Inferior

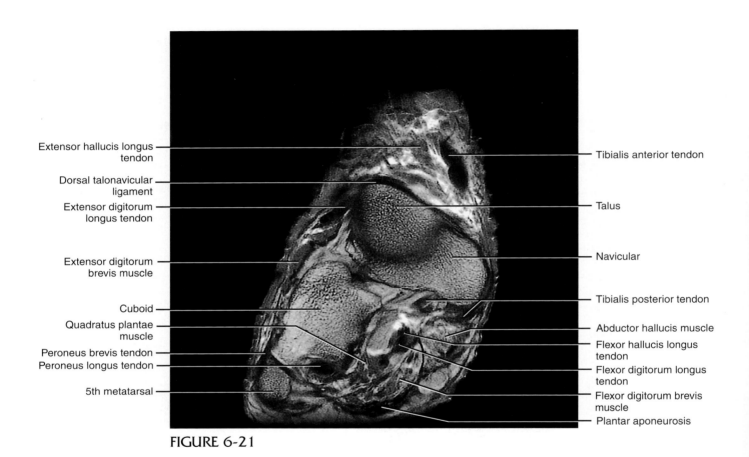

Extensor hallucis longus
tendon

Dorsal talonavicular
ligament

Extensor digitorum
longus tendon

Extensor digitorum
brevis muscle

Cuboid

Quadratus plantae
muscle

Peroneus brevis tendon

Peroneus longus tendon

5th metatarsal

Tibialis anterior tendon

Talus

Navicular

Tibialis posterior tendon

Abductor hallucis muscle

Flexor hallucis longus
tendon

Flexor digitorum longus
tendon

Flexor digitorum brevis
muscle

Plantar aponeurosis

FIGURE 6-21

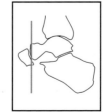

ANKLE: CORONAL

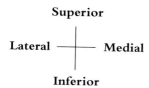

Superior

Lateral — Medial

Inferior

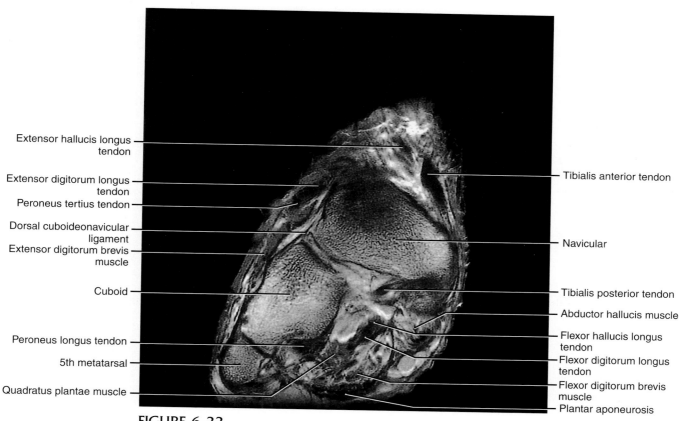

Extensor hallucis longus tendon

Extensor digitorum longus tendon

Peroneus tertius tendon

Dorsal cuboideonavicular ligament

Extensor digitorum brevis muscle

Cuboid

Peroneus longus tendon

5th metatarsal

Quadratus plantae muscle

Tibialis anterior tendon

Navicular

Tibialis posterior tendon

Abductor hallucis muscle

Flexor hallucis longus tendon

Flexor digitorum longus tendon

Flexor digitorum brevis muscle

Plantar aponeurosis

FIGURE 6-22

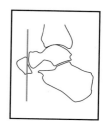

ANKLE: CORONAL

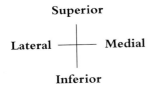

Superior

Lateral —┼— Medial

Inferior

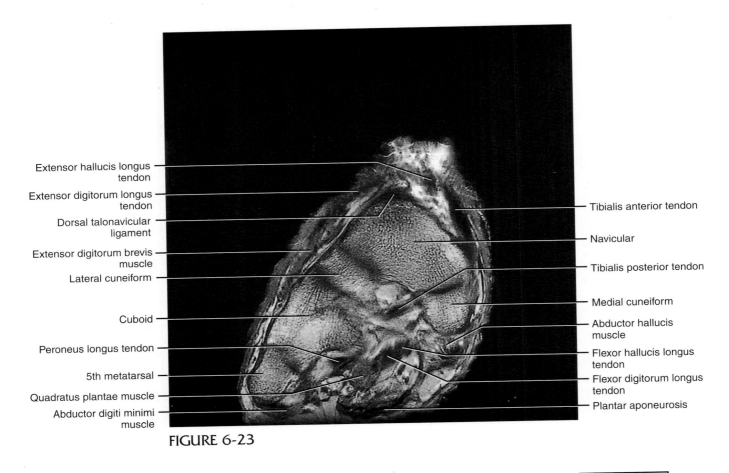

Extensor hallucis longus tendon

Extensor digitorum longus tendon

Dorsal talonavicular ligament

Extensor digitorum brevis muscle

Lateral cuneiform

Cuboid

Peroneus longus tendon

5th metatarsal

Quadratus plantae muscle

Abductor digiti minimi muscle

Tibialis anterior tendon

Navicular

Tibialis posterior tendon

Medial cuneiform

Abductor hallucis muscle

Flexor hallucis longus tendon

Flexor digitorum longus tendon

Plantar aponeurosis

FIGURE 6-23

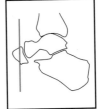

ANKLE: CORONAL

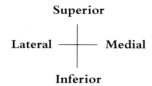

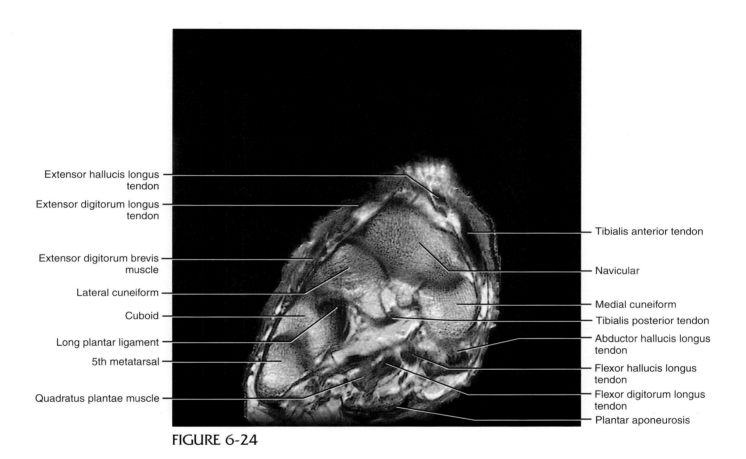

Extensor hallucis longus tendon

Extensor digitorum longus tendon

Extensor digitorum brevis muscle

Lateral cuneiform

Cuboid

Long plantar ligament

5th metatarsal

Quadratus plantae muscle

Tibialis anterior tendon

Navicular

Medial cuneiform

Tibialis posterior tendon

Abductor hallucis longus tendon

Flexor hallucis longus tendon

Flexor digitorum longus tendon

Plantar aponeurosis

FIGURE 6-24

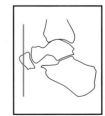

ANKLE: AXIAL

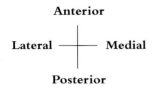

Anterior

Lateral ——— Medial

Posterior

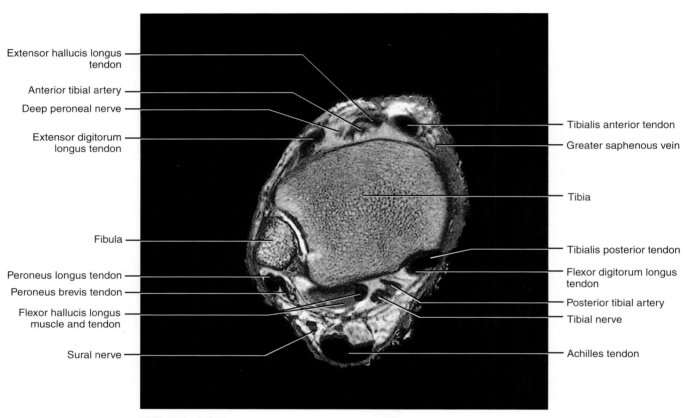

Extensor hallucis longus tendon

Anterior tibial artery

Deep peroneal nerve

Extensor digitorum longus tendon

Tibialis anterior tendon

Greater saphenous vein

Tibia

Fibula

Tibialis posterior tendon

Peroneus longus tendon

Flexor digitorum longus tendon

Peroneus brevis tendon

Posterior tibial artery

Flexor hallucis longus muscle and tendon

Tibial nerve

Sural nerve

Achilles tendon

FIGURE 6-25

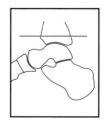

ANKLE: AXIAL

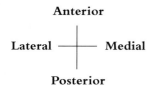

Anterior

Lateral ──┼── Medial

Posterior

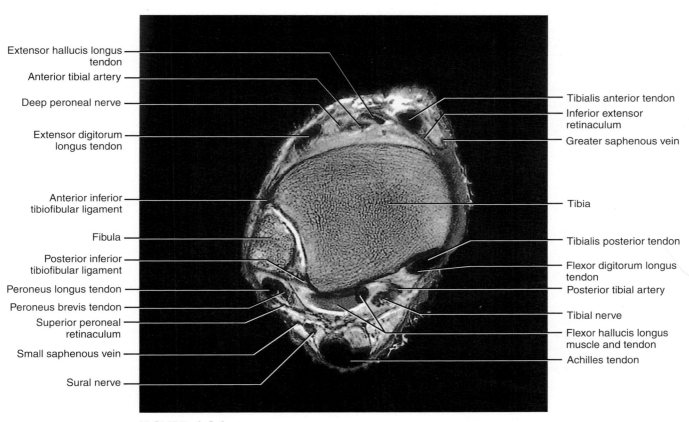

Extensor hallucis longus tendon

Anterior tibial artery

Deep peroneal nerve

Extensor digitorum longus tendon

Anterior inferior tibiofibular ligament

Fibula

Posterior inferior tibiofibular ligament

Peroneus longus tendon

Peroneus brevis tendon

Superior peroneal retinaculum

Small saphenous vein

Sural nerve

Tibialis anterior tendon

Inferior extensor retinaculum

Greater saphenous vein

Tibia

Tibialis posterior tendon

Flexor digitorum longus tendon

Posterior tibial artery

Tibial nerve

Flexor hallucis longus muscle and tendon

Achilles tendon

FIGURE 6-26

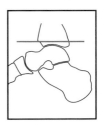

ANKLE: AXIAL

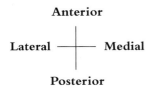

Anterior

Lateral ——┼—— Medial

Posterior

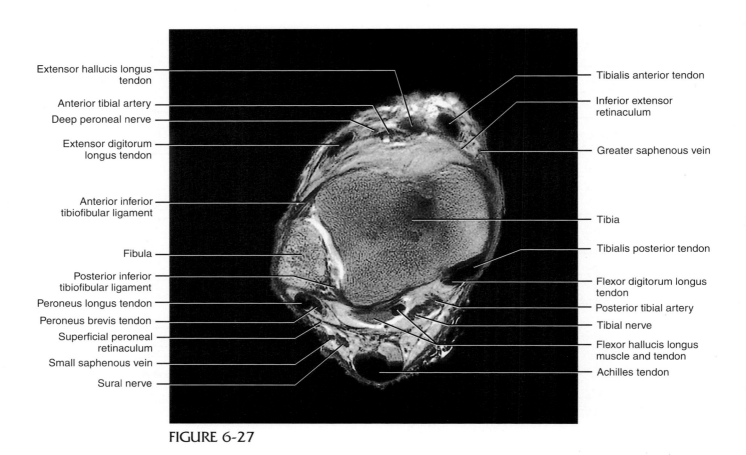

Extensor hallucis longus tendon

Anterior tibial artery

Deep peroneal nerve

Extensor digitorum longus tendon

Anterior inferior tibiofibular ligament

Fibula

Posterior inferior tibiofibular ligament

Peroneus longus tendon

Peroneus brevis tendon

Superficial peroneal retinaculum

Small saphenous vein

Sural nerve

Tibialis anterior tendon

Inferior extensor retinaculum

Greater saphenous vein

Tibia

Tibialis posterior tendon

Flexor digitorum longus tendon

Posterior tibial artery

Tibial nerve

Flexor hallucis longus muscle and tendon

Achilles tendon

FIGURE 6-27

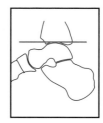

ANKLE: AXIAL

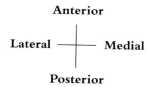

Anterior

Lateral — Medial

Posterior

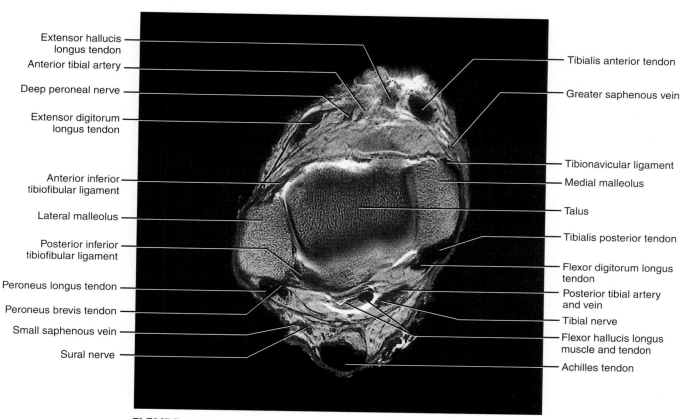

Extensor hallucis longus tendon

Anterior tibial artery

Deep peroneal nerve

Extensor digitorum longus tendon

Anterior inferior tibiofibular ligament

Lateral malleolus

Posterior inferior tibiofibular ligament

Peroneus longus tendon

Peroneus brevis tendon

Small saphenous vein

Sural nerve

Tibialis anterior tendon

Greater saphenous vein

Tibionavicular ligament

Medial malleolus

Talus

Tibialis posterior tendon

Flexor digitorum longus tendon

Posterior tibial artery and vein

Tibial nerve

Flexor hallucis longus muscle and tendon

Achilles tendon

FIGURE 6-28

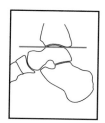

ANKLE: AXIAL

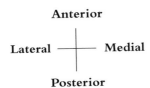

Anterior

Lateral —— Medial

Posterior

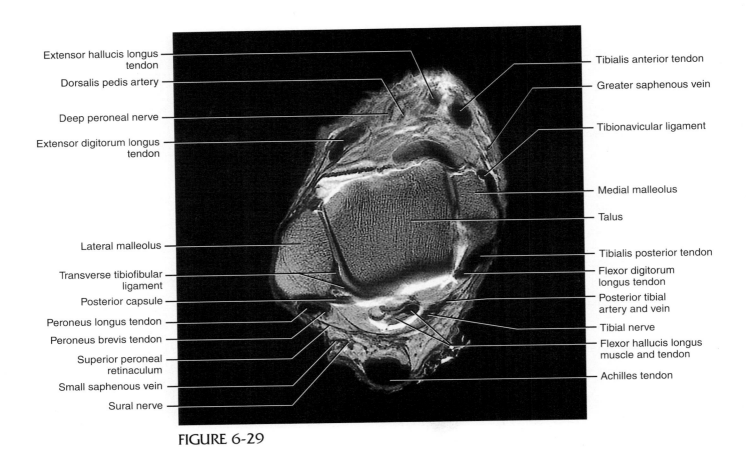

Extensor hallucis longus tendon

Dorsalis pedis artery

Deep peroneal nerve

Extensor digitorum longus tendon

Lateral malleolus

Transverse tibiofibular ligament

Posterior capsule

Peroneus longus tendon

Peroneus brevis tendon

Superior peroneal retinaculum

Small saphenous vein

Sural nerve

Tibialis anterior tendon

Greater saphenous vein

Tibionavicular ligament

Medial malleolus

Talus

Tibialis posterior tendon

Flexor digitorum longus tendon

Posterior tibial artery and vein

Tibial nerve

Flexor hallucis longus muscle and tendon

Achilles tendon

FIGURE 6-29

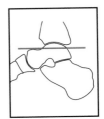

ANKLE: AXIAL

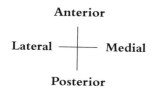

Anterior

Lateral ─┼─ Medial

Posterior

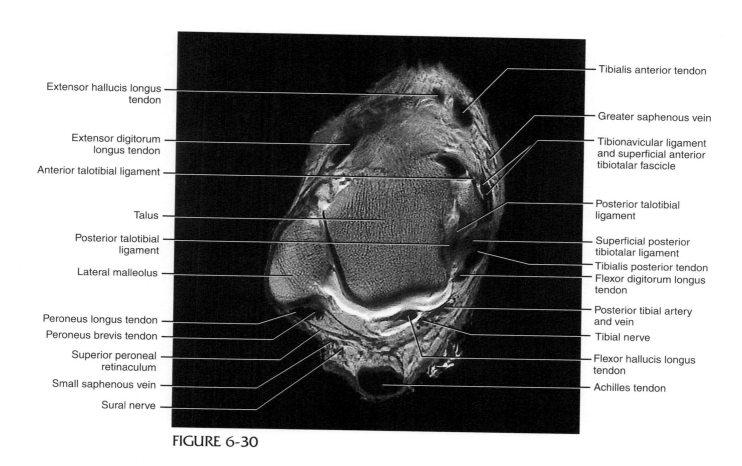

Extensor hallucis longus tendon

Extensor digitorum longus tendon

Anterior talotibial ligament

Talus

Posterior talotibial ligament

Lateral malleolus

Peroneus longus tendon

Peroneus brevis tendon

Superior peroneal retinaculum

Small saphenous vein

Sural nerve

Tibialis anterior tendon

Greater saphenous vein

Tibionavicular ligament and superficial anterior tibiotalar fascicle

Posterior talotibial ligament

Superficial posterior tibiotalar ligament

Tibialis posterior tendon

Flexor digitorum longus tendon

Posterior tibial artery and vein

Tibial nerve

Flexor hallucis longus tendon

Achilles tendon

FIGURE 6-30

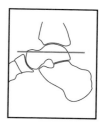

ANKLE: AXIAL

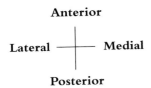

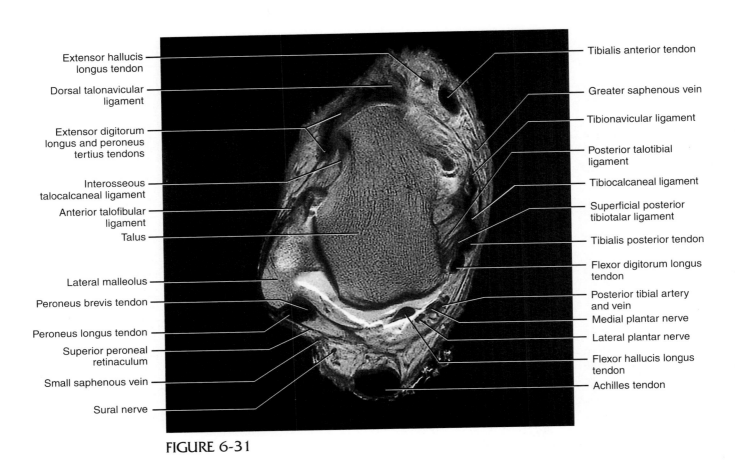

Extensor hallucis longus tendon

Dorsal talonavicular ligament

Extensor digitorum longus and peroneus tertius tendons

Interosseous talocalcaneal ligament

Anterior talofibular ligament

Talus

Lateral malleolus

Peroneus brevis tendon

Peroneus longus tendon

Superior peroneal retinaculum

Small saphenous vein

Sural nerve

Tibialis anterior tendon

Greater saphenous vein

Tibionavicular ligament

Posterior talotibial ligament

Tibiocalcaneal ligament

Superficial posterior tibiotalar ligament

Tibialis posterior tendon

Flexor digitorum longus tendon

Posterior tibial artery and vein

Medial plantar nerve

Lateral plantar nerve

Flexor hallucis longus tendon

Achilles tendon

FIGURE 6-31

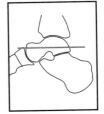

ANKLE: AXIAL

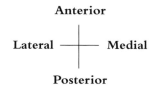

Anterior

Lateral ——|—— Medial

Posterior

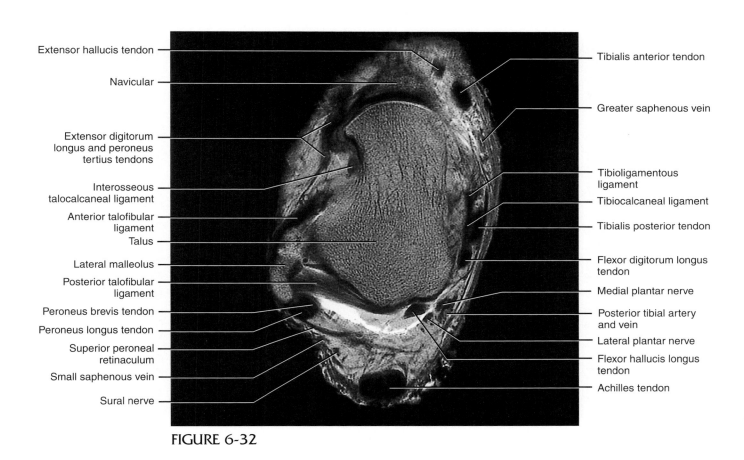

Extensor hallucis tendon

Navicular

Extensor digitorum longus and peroneus tertius tendons

Interosseous talocalcaneal ligament

Anterior talofibular ligament

Talus

Lateral malleolus

Posterior talofibular ligament

Peroneus brevis tendon

Peroneus longus tendon

Superior peroneal retinaculum

Small saphenous vein

Sural nerve

Tibialis anterior tendon

Greater saphenous vein

Tibioligamentous ligament

Tibiocalcaneal ligament

Tibialis posterior tendon

Flexor digitorum longus tendon

Medial plantar nerve

Posterior tibial artery and vein

Lateral plantar nerve

Flexor hallucis longus tendon

Achilles tendon

FIGURE 6-32

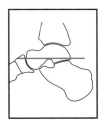

ANKLE: AXIAL

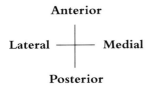

Anterior

Lateral —— Medial

Posterior

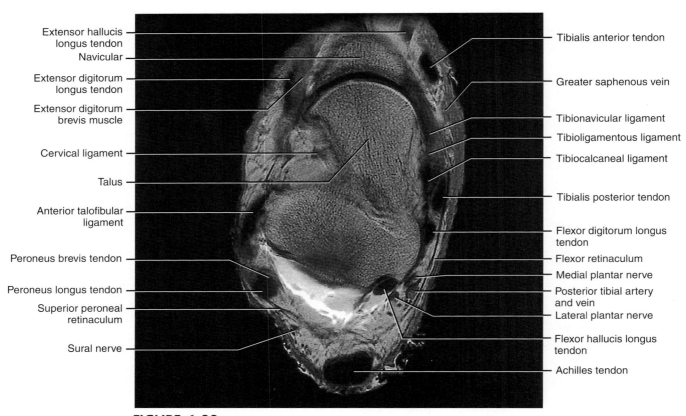

Extensor hallucis longus tendon
Navicular
Extensor digitorum longus tendon
Extensor digitorum brevis muscle
Cervical ligament
Talus
Anterior talofibular ligament
Peroneus brevis tendon
Peroneus longus tendon
Superior peroneal retinaculum
Sural nerve

Tibialis anterior tendon
Greater saphenous vein
Tibionavicular ligament
Tibioligamentous ligament
Tibiocalcaneal ligament
Tibialis posterior tendon
Flexor digitorum longus tendon
Flexor retinaculum
Medial plantar nerve
Posterior tibial artery and vein
Lateral plantar nerve
Flexor hallucis longus tendon
Achilles tendon

FIGURE 6-33

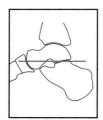

ANKLE: AXIAL

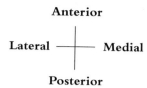

Intermediate cuneiform

Dorsal cuneonavicular ligament

Extensor digitorum longus tendon

Extensor digitorum brevis muscle

Talus

Intermediate root of extensor retinaculum

Cervical ligament

Interosseous talocalcaneal ligament

Talus

Calcaneofibular ligament

Peroneus brevis tendon

Peroneus longus tendon

Peroneal retinaculum

Sural nerve

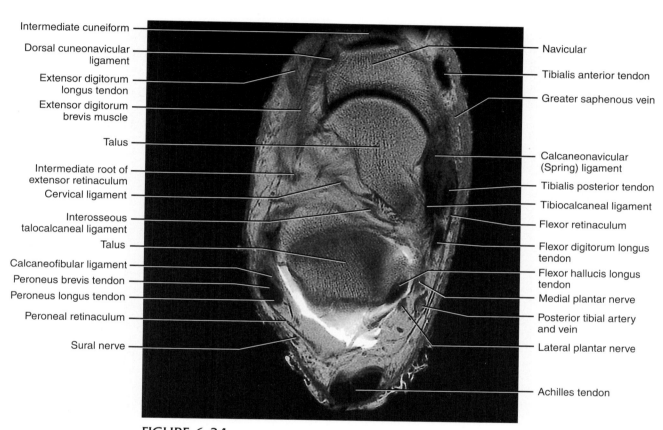

Navicular

Tibialis anterior tendon

Greater saphenous vein

Calcaneonavicular (Spring) ligament

Tibialis posterior tendon

Tibiocalcaneal ligament

Flexor retinaculum

Flexor digitorum longus tendon

Flexor hallucis longus tendon

Medial plantar nerve

Posterior tibial artery and vein

Lateral plantar nerve

Achilles tendon

FIGURE 6-34

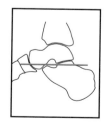

ANKLE: AXIAL

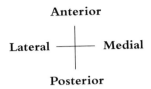

Anterior

Lateral — Medial

Posterior

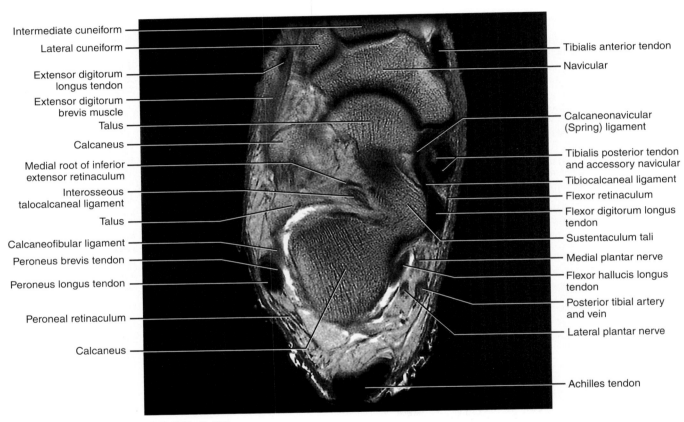

Intermediate cuneiform

Lateral cuneiform

Extensor digitorum longus tendon

Extensor digitorum brevis muscle

Talus

Calcaneus

Medial root of inferior extensor retinaculum

Interosseous talocalcaneal ligament

Talus

Calcaneofibular ligament

Peroneus brevis tendon

Peroneus longus tendon

Peroneal retinaculum

Calcaneus

Tibialis anterior tendon

Navicular

Calcaneonavicular (Spring) ligament

Tibialis posterior tendon and accessory navicular

Tibiocalcaneal ligament

Flexor retinaculum

Flexor digitorum longus tendon

Sustentaculum tali

Medial plantar nerve

Flexor hallucis longus tendon

Posterior tibial artery and vein

Lateral plantar nerve

Achilles tendon

FIGURE 6-35

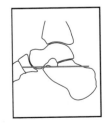

ANKLE: AXIAL

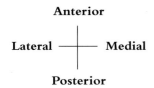

Anterior

Lateral ——— Medial

Posterior

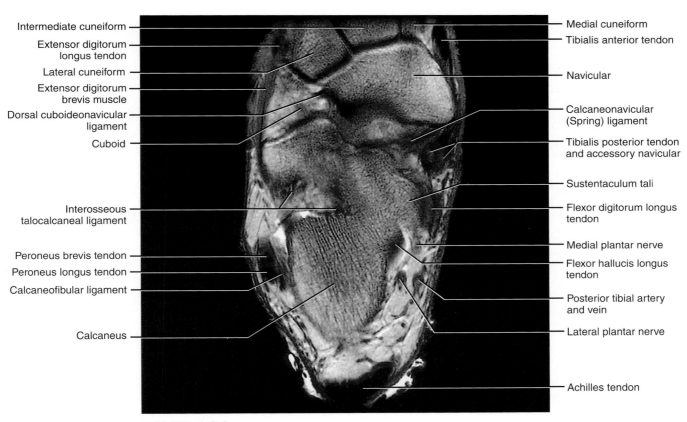

Intermediate cuneiform

Extensor digitorum
longus tendon

Lateral cuneiform

Extensor digitorum
brevis muscle

Dorsal cuboideonavicular
ligament

Cuboid

Interosseous
talocalcaneal ligament

Peroneus brevis tendon

Peroneus longus tendon

Calcaneofibular ligament

Calcaneus

Medial cuneiform

Tibialis anterior tendon

Navicular

Calcaneonavicular
(Spring) ligament

Tibialis posterior tendon
and accessory navicular

Sustentaculum tali

Flexor digitorum longus
tendon

Medial plantar nerve

Flexor hallucis longus
tendon

Posterior tibial artery
and vein

Lateral plantar nerve

Achilles tendon

FIGURE 6-36

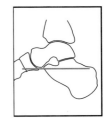

ANKLE: AXIAL

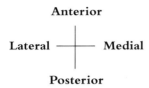

Anterior

Lateral —+— Medial

Posterior

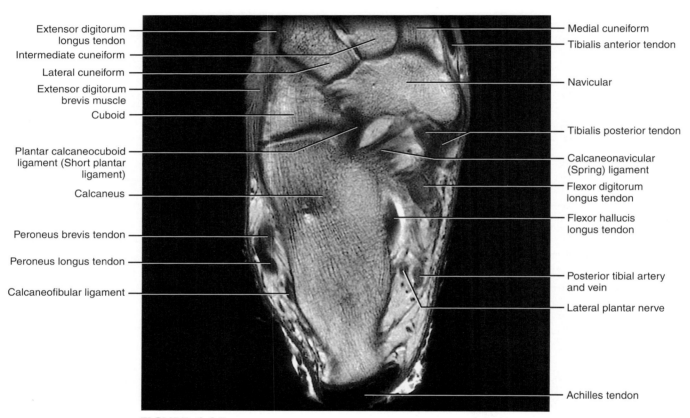

Extensor digitorum longus tendon

Intermediate cuneiform

Lateral cuneiform

Extensor digitorum brevis muscle

Cuboid

Plantar calcaneocuboid ligament (Short plantar ligament)

Calcaneus

Peroneus brevis tendon

Peroneus longus tendon

Calcaneofibular ligament

Medial cuneiform

Tibialis anterior tendon

Navicular

Tibialis posterior tendon

Calcaneonavicular (Spring) ligament

Flexor digitorum longus tendon

Flexor hallucis longus tendon

Posterior tibial artery and vein

Lateral plantar nerve

Achilles tendon

FIGURE 6-37

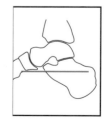

ANKLE: AXIAL

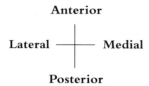

Anterior

Lateral —— Medial

Posterior

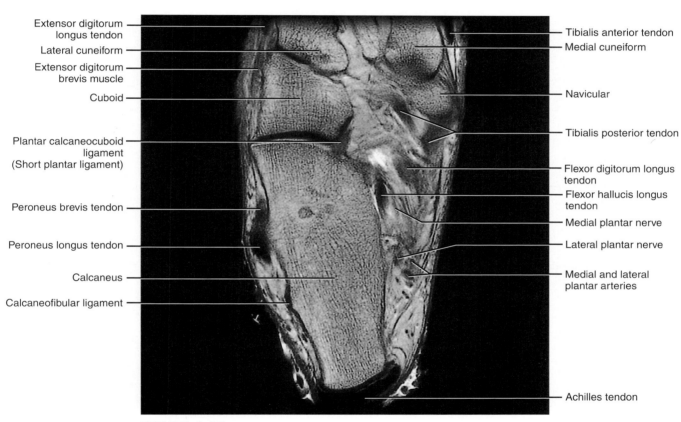

Extensor digitorum longus tendon

Lateral cuneiform

Extensor digitorum brevis muscle

Cuboid

Plantar calcaneocuboid ligament (Short plantar ligament)

Peroneus brevis tendon

Peroneus longus tendon

Calcaneus

Calcaneofibular ligament

Tibialis anterior tendon

Medial cuneiform

Navicular

Tibialis posterior tendon

Flexor digitorum longus tendon

Flexor hallucis longus tendon

Medial plantar nerve

Lateral plantar nerve

Medial and lateral plantar arteries

Achilles tendon

FIGURE 6-38

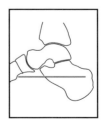

ANKLE: AXIAL

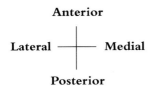

Anterior

Lateral ——|—— Medial

Posterior

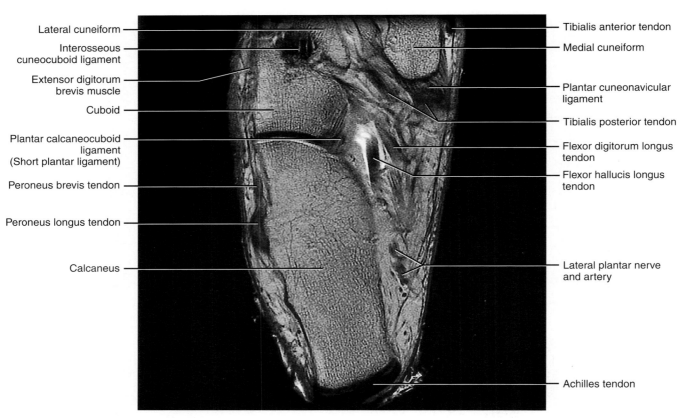

Lateral cuneiform

Interosseous cuneocuboid ligament

Extensor digitorum brevis muscle

Cuboid

Plantar calcaneocuboid ligament (Short plantar ligament)

Peroneus brevis tendon

Peroneus longus tendon

Calcaneus

Tibialis anterior tendon

Medial cuneiform

Plantar cuneonavicular ligament

Tibialis posterior tendon

Flexor digitorum longus tendon

Flexor hallucis longus tendon

Lateral plantar nerve and artery

Achilles tendon

FIGURE 6-39

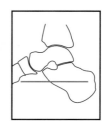

ANKLE: AXIAL

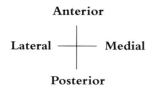

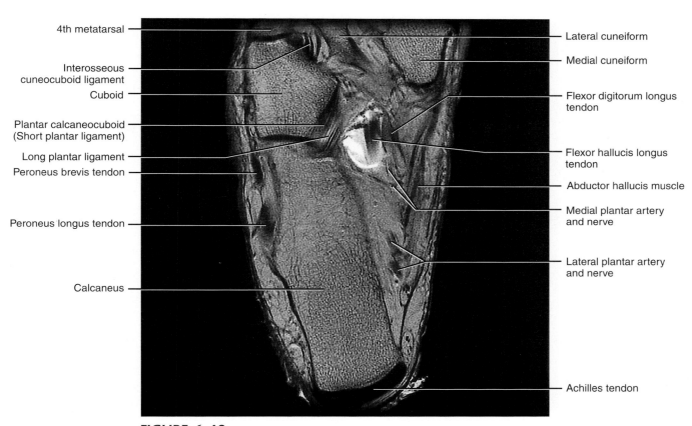

4th metatarsal

Interosseous cuneocuboid ligament

Cuboid

Plantar calcaneocuboid (Short plantar ligament)

Long plantar ligament

Peroneus brevis tendon

Peroneus longus tendon

Calcaneus

Lateral cuneiform

Medial cuneiform

Flexor digitorum longus tendon

Flexor hallucis longus tendon

Abductor hallucis muscle

Medial plantar artery and nerve

Lateral plantar artery and nerve

Achilles tendon

FIGURE 6-40

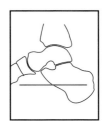

ANKLE: AXIAL

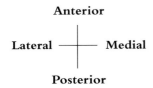

Anterior

Lateral ——|—— Medial

Posterior

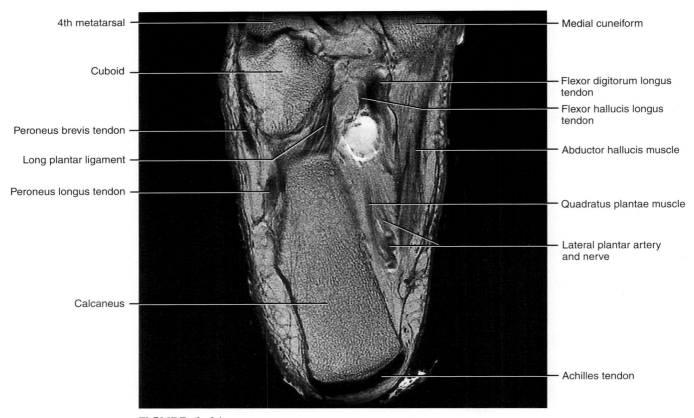

4th metatarsal

Cuboid

Peroneus brevis tendon

Long plantar ligament

Peroneus longus tendon

Calcaneus

Medial cuneiform

Flexor digitorum longus tendon

Flexor hallucis longus tendon

Abductor hallucis muscle

Quadratus plantae muscle

Lateral plantar artery and nerve

Achilles tendon

FIGURE 6-41

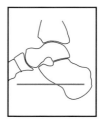

ANKLE: AXIAL

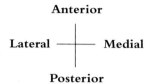

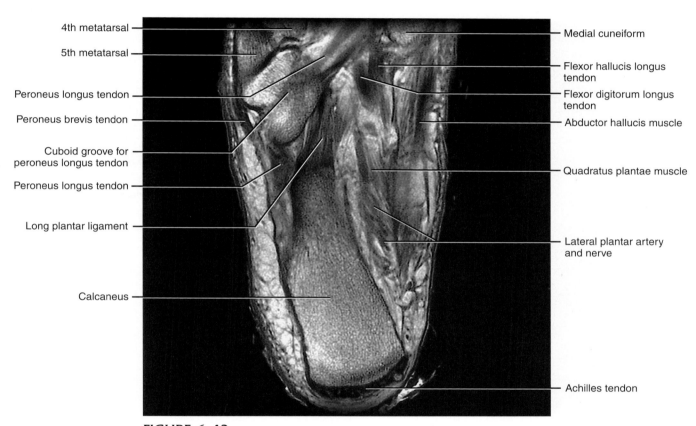

4th metatarsal

5th metatarsal

Peroneus longus tendon

Peroneus brevis tendon

Cuboid groove for
peroneus longus tendon

Peroneus longus tendon

Long plantar ligament

Calcaneus

Medial cuneiform

Flexor hallucis longus
tendon

Flexor digitorum longus
tendon

Abductor hallucis muscle

Quadratus plantae muscle

Lateral plantar artery
and nerve

Achilles tendon

FIGURE 6-42

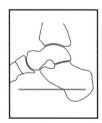

ANKLE: AXIAL

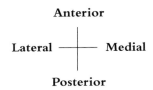

Anterior

Lateral —|— Medial

Posterior

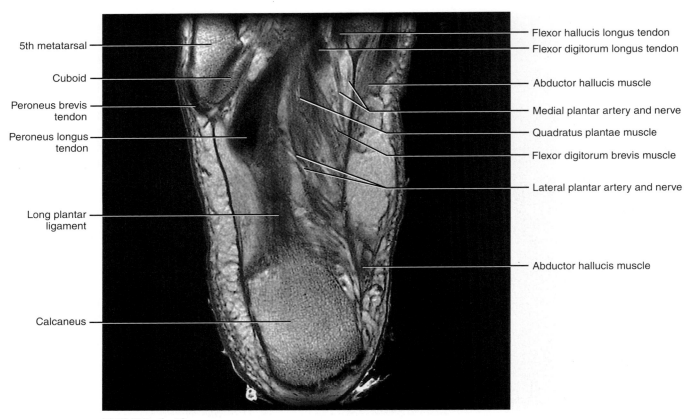

5th metatarsal

Cuboid

Peroneus brevis
tendon

Peroneus longus
tendon

Long plantar
ligament

Calcaneus

Flexor hallucis longus tendon

Flexor digitorum longus tendon

Abductor hallucis muscle

Medial plantar artery and nerve

Quadratus plantae muscle

Flexor digitorum brevis muscle

Lateral plantar artery and nerve

Abductor hallucis muscle

FIGURE 6-43

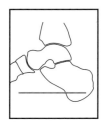

ANKLE: AXIAL

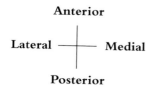

Anterior

Lateral ─┼─ Medial

Posterior

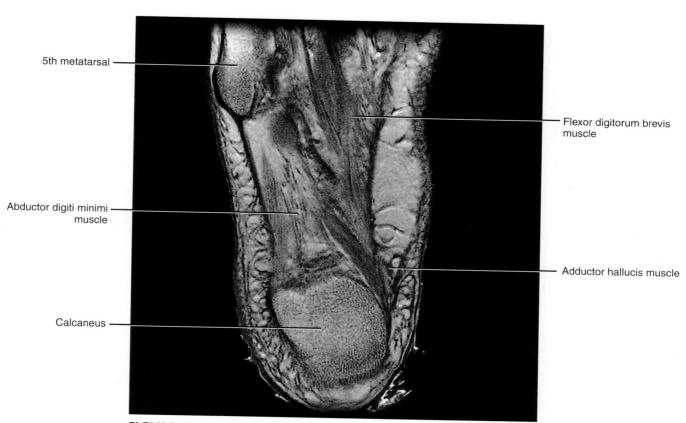

5th metatarsal

Flexor digitorum brevis muscle

Abductor digiti minimi muscle

Adductor hallucis muscle

Calcaneus

FIGURE 6-44

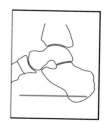

ANKLE: AXIAL

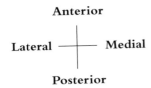

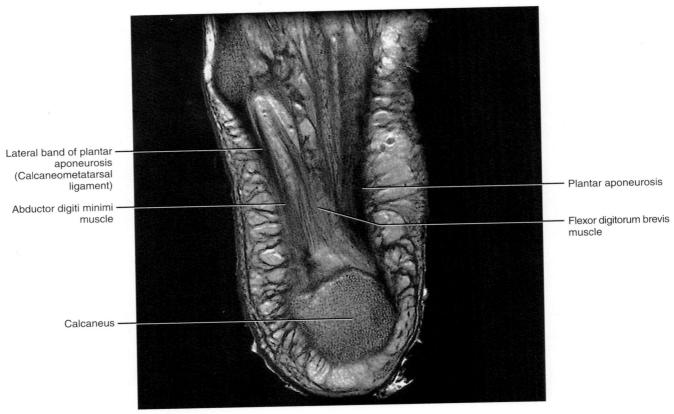

Lateral band of plantar aponeurosis (Calcaneometatarsal ligament)

Abductor digiti minimi muscle

Calcaneus

Plantar aponeurosis

Flexor digitorum brevis muscle

FIGURE 6-45

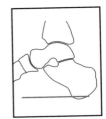

ANKLE: AXIAL

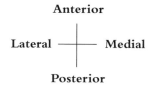

Anterior

Lateral ——+—— Medial

Posterior

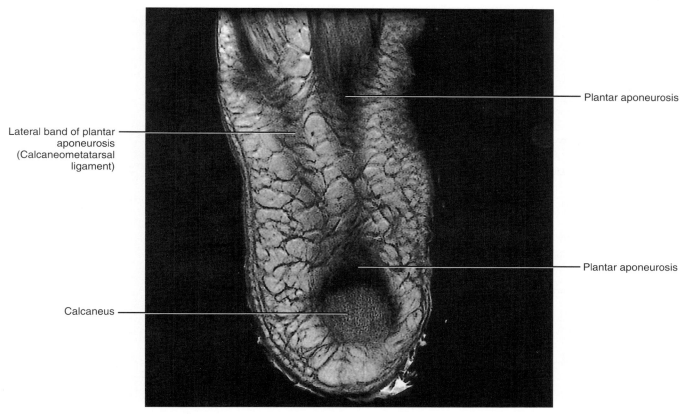

Plantar aponeurosis

Lateral band of plantar
aponeurosis
(Calcaneometatarsal
ligament)

Plantar aponeurosis

Calcaneus

FIGURE 6-46

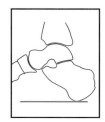

ANKLE: SAGITTAL

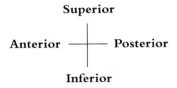

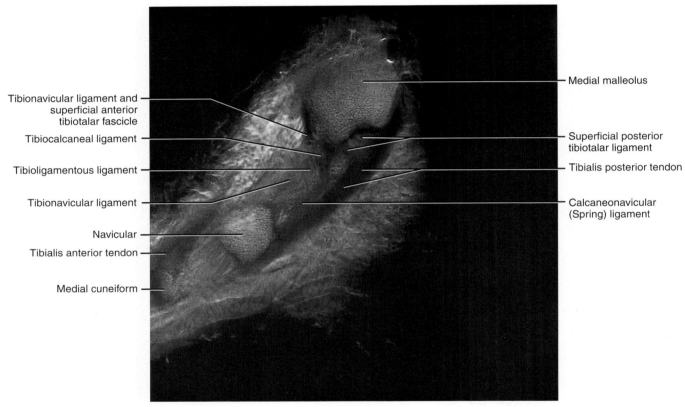

Tibionavicular ligament and
superficial anterior
tibiotalar fascicle

Tibiocalcaneal ligament

Tibioligamentous ligament

Tibionavicular ligament

Navicular

Tibialis anterior tendon

Medial cuneiform

Medial malleolus

Superficial posterior
tibiotalar ligament

Tibialis posterior tendon

Calcaneonavicular
(Spring) ligament

FIGURE 6-47

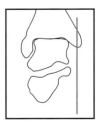

ANKLE: SAGITTAL

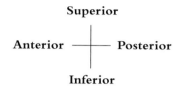

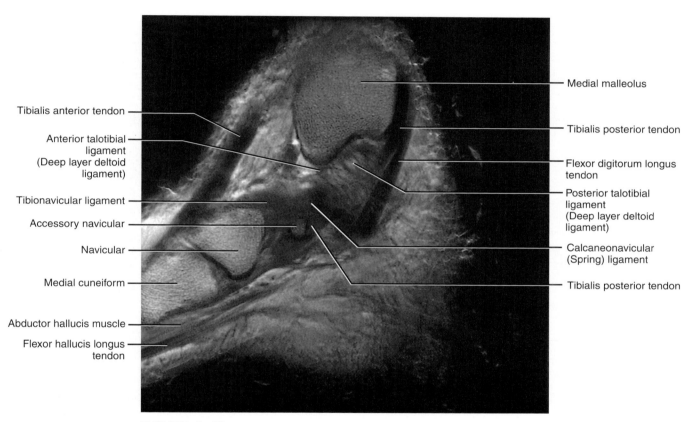

Tibialis anterior tendon

Anterior talotibial ligament (Deep layer deltoid ligament)

Tibionavicular ligament

Accessory navicular

Navicular

Medial cuneiform

Abductor hallucis muscle

Flexor hallucis longus tendon

Medial malleolus

Tibialis posterior tendon

Flexor digitorum longus tendon

Posterior talotibial ligament (Deep layer deltoid ligament)

Calcaneonavicular (Spring) ligament

Tibialis posterior tendon

FIGURE 6-48

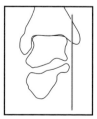

ANKLE: SAGITTAL

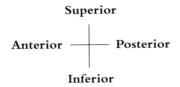

Superior

Anterior ——┼—— Posterior

Inferior

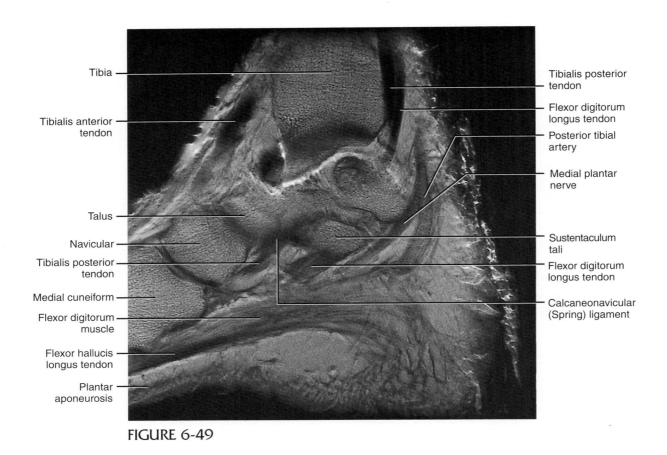

Tibia

Tibialis anterior tendon

Talus

Navicular

Tibialis posterior tendon

Medial cuneiform

Flexor digitorum muscle

Flexor hallucis longus tendon

Plantar aponeurosis

Tibialis posterior tendon

Flexor digitorum longus tendon

Posterior tibial artery

Medial plantar nerve

Sustentaculum tali

Flexor digitorum longus tendon

Calcaneonavicular (Spring) ligament

FIGURE 6-49

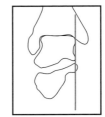

ANKLE: SAGITTAL

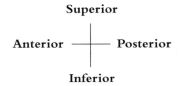

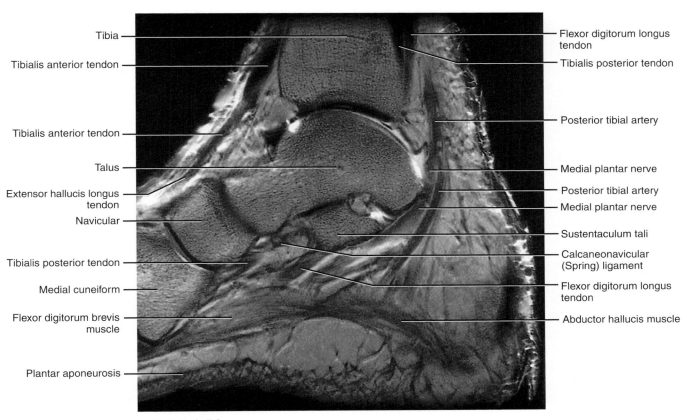

Tibia

Tibialis anterior tendon

Tibialis anterior tendon

Talus

Extensor hallucis longus tendon

Navicular

Tibialis posterior tendon

Medial cuneiform

Flexor digitorum brevis muscle

Plantar aponeurosis

Flexor digitorum longus tendon

Tibialis posterior tendon

Posterior tibial artery

Medial plantar nerve

Posterior tibial artery

Medial plantar nerve

Sustentaculum tali

Calcaneonavicular (Spring) ligament

Flexor digitorum longus tendon

Abductor hallucis muscle

FIGURE 6-50

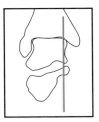

ANKLE: SAGITTAL

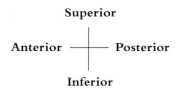

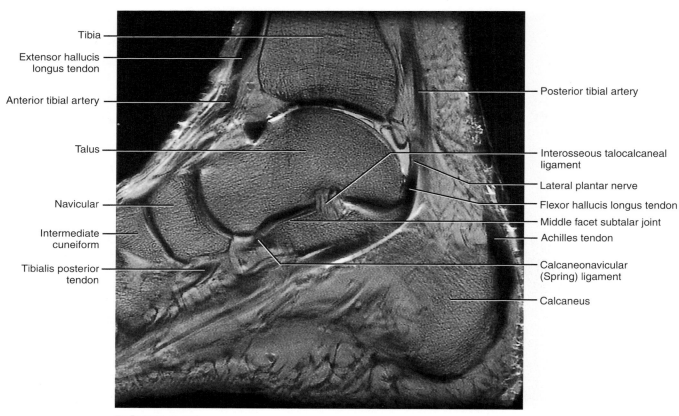

Tibia

Extensor hallucis longus tendon

Anterior tibial artery

Talus

Navicular

Intermediate cuneiform

Tibialis posterior tendon

Posterior tibial artery

Interosseous talocalcaneal ligament

Lateral plantar nerve

Flexor hallucis longus tendon

Middle facet subtalar joint

Achilles tendon

Calcaneonavicular (Spring) ligament

Calcaneus

FIGURE 6-51

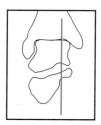

ANKLE: SAGITTAL

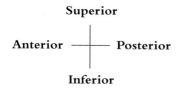

Superior

Anterior ——|—— Posterior

Inferior

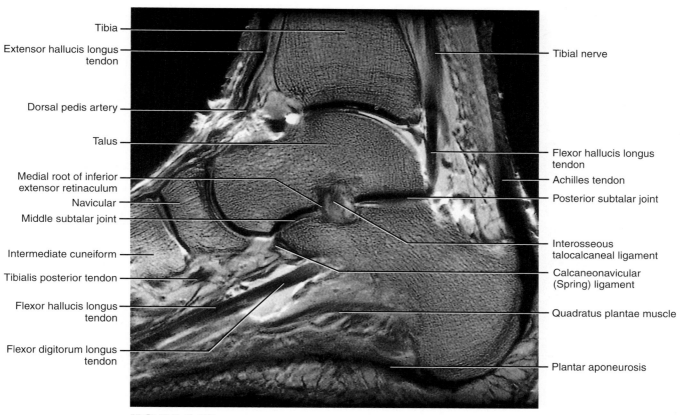

Tibia

Extensor hallucis longus tendon

Dorsal pedis artery

Talus

Medial root of inferior extensor retinaculum

Navicular

Middle subtalar joint

Intermediate cuneiform

Tibialis posterior tendon

Flexor hallucis longus tendon

Flexor digitorum longus tendon

Tibial nerve

Flexor hallucis longus tendon

Achilles tendon

Posterior subtalar joint

Interosseous talocalcaneal ligament

Calcaneonavicular (Spring) ligament

Quadratus plantae muscle

Plantar aponeurosis

FIGURE 6-52

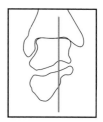

ANKLE: SAGITTAL

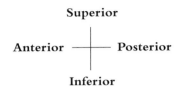

Extensor hallucis longus tendon

Anterior tibial artery

Tibia

Dorsal pedis artery

Talus

Navicular

Intermediate cuneiform

Tibialis posterior tendon

Flexor digitorum longus tendon

Flexor digitorum brevis muscle

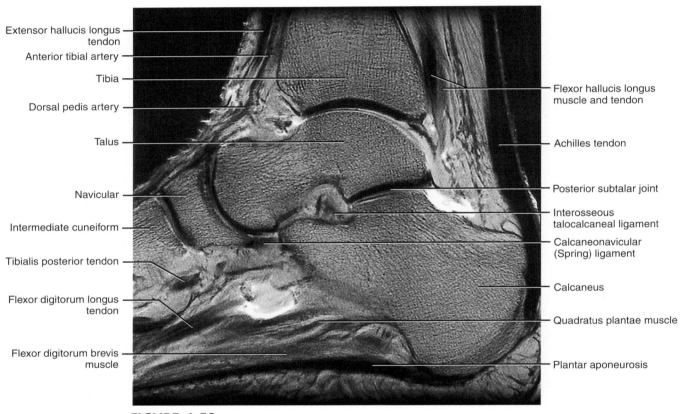

Flexor hallucis longus muscle and tendon

Achilles tendon

Posterior subtalar joint

Interosseous talocalcaneal ligament

Calcaneonavicular (Spring) ligament

Calcaneus

Quadratus plantae muscle

Plantar aponeurosis

FIGURE 6-53

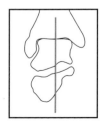

ANKLE: SAGITTAL

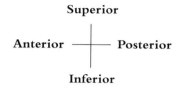

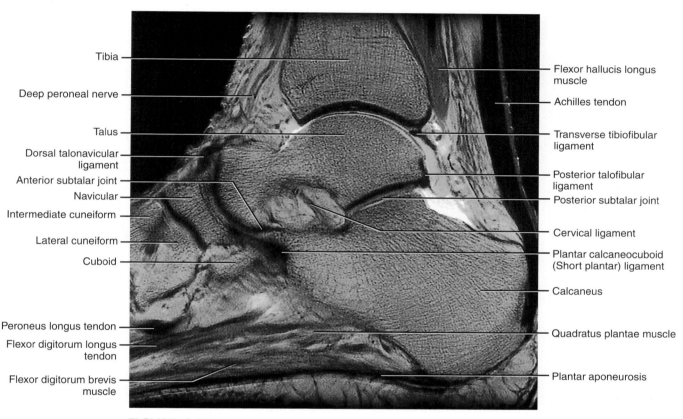

Tibia

Deep peroneal nerve

Talus

Dorsal talonavicular ligament

Anterior subtalar joint

Navicular

Intermediate cuneiform

Lateral cuneiform

Cuboid

Peroneus longus tendon

Flexor digitorum longus tendon

Flexor digitorum brevis muscle

Flexor hallucis longus muscle

Achilles tendon

Transverse tibiofibular ligament

Posterior talofibular ligament

Posterior subtalar joint

Cervical ligament

Plantar calcaneocuboid (Short plantar) ligament

Calcaneus

Quadratus plantae muscle

Plantar aponeurosis

FIGURE 6-54

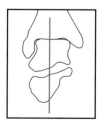

ANKLE: SAGITTAL

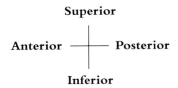

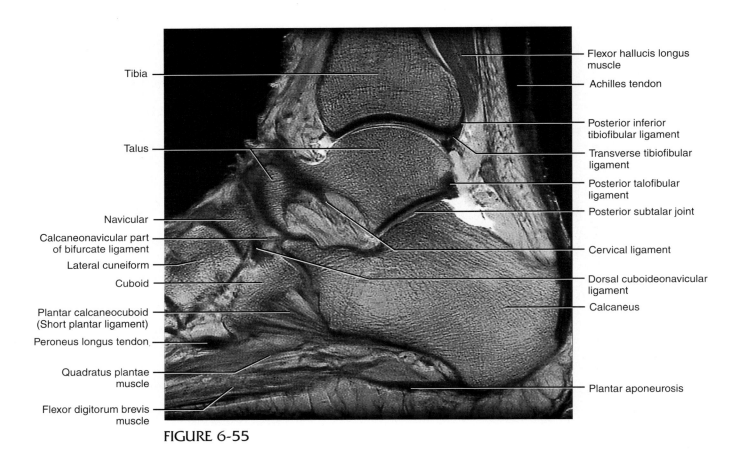

Tibia

Talus

Navicular

Calcaneonavicular part
of bifurcate ligament

Lateral cuneiform

Cuboid

Plantar calcaneocuboid
(Short plantar ligament)

Peroneus longus tendon

Quadratus plantae
muscle

Flexor digitorum brevis
muscle

Flexor hallucis longus
muscle

Achilles tendon

Posterior inferior
tibiofibular ligament

Transverse tibiofibular
ligament

Posterior talofibular
ligament

Posterior subtalar joint

Cervical ligament

Dorsal cuboideonavicular
ligament

Calcaneus

Plantar aponeurosis

FIGURE 6-55

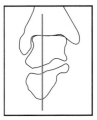

ANKLE: SAGITTAL

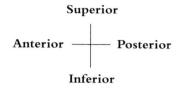

Superior

Anterior — Posterior

Inferior

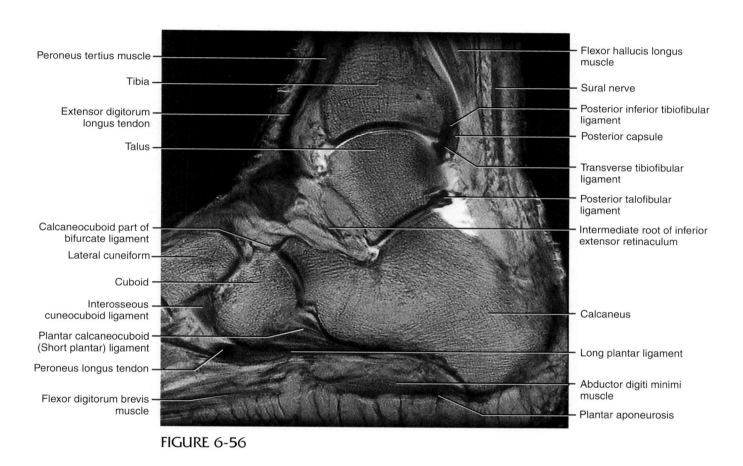

Peroneus tertius muscle

Tibia

Extensor digitorum longus tendon

Talus

Calcaneocuboid part of bifurcate ligament

Lateral cuneiform

Cuboid

Interosseous cuneocuboid ligament

Plantar calcaneocuboid (Short plantar) ligament

Peroneus longus tendon

Flexor digitorum brevis muscle

Flexor hallucis longus muscle

Sural nerve

Posterior inferior tibiofibular ligament

Posterior capsule

Transverse tibiofibular ligament

Posterior talofibular ligament

Intermediate root of inferior extensor retinaculum

Calcaneus

Long plantar ligament

Abductor digiti minimi muscle

Plantar aponeurosis

FIGURE 6-56

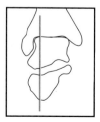

ANKLE: SAGITTAL

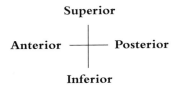

Superior

Anterior ——|—— Posterior

Inferior

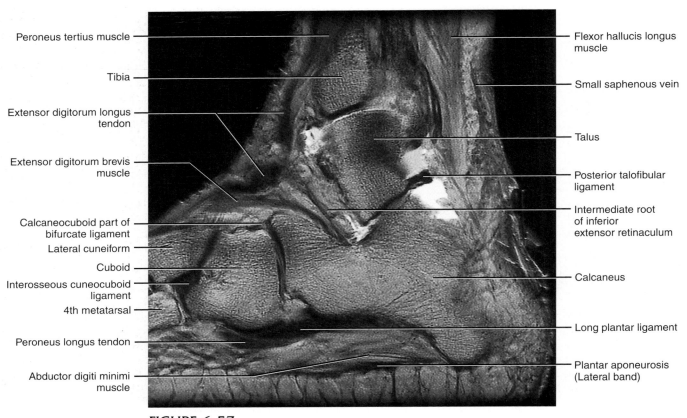

Peroneus tertius muscle	Flexor hallucis longus muscle
Tibia	Small saphenous vein
Extensor digitorum longus tendon	Talus
Extensor digitorum brevis muscle	Posterior talofibular ligament
Calcaneocuboid part of bifurcate ligament	Intermediate root of inferior extensor retinaculum
Lateral cuneiform	
Cuboid	Calcaneus
Interosseous cuneocuboid ligament	
4th metatarsal	Long plantar ligament
Peroneus longus tendon	Plantar aponeurosis (Lateral band)
Abductor digiti minimi muscle	

FIGURE 6-57

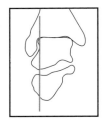

ANKLE: SAGITTAL

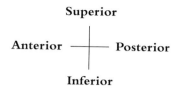

Superior

Anterior ——|—— Posterior

Inferior

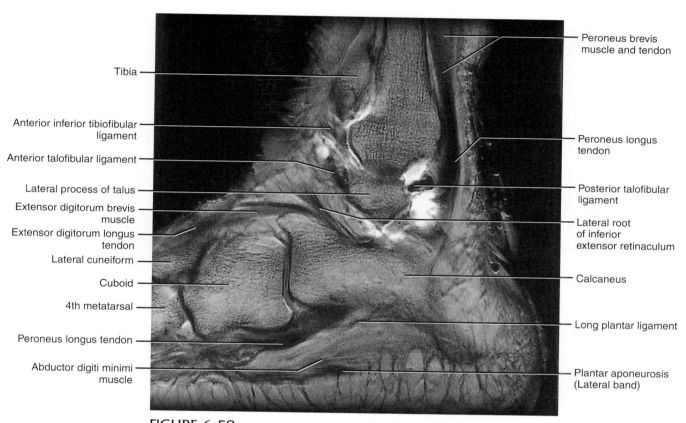

Peroneus brevis
muscle and tendon

Tibia

Anterior inferior tibiofibular
ligament

Anterior talofibular ligament

Peroneus longus
tendon

Lateral process of talus

Posterior talofibular
ligament

Extensor digitorum brevis
muscle

Lateral root
of inferior
extensor retinaculum

Extensor digitorum longus
tendon

Lateral cuneiform

Cuboid

Calcaneus

4th metatarsal

Long plantar ligament

Peroneus longus tendon

Abductor digiti minimi
muscle

Plantar aponeurosis
(Lateral band)

FIGURE 6-58

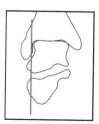

ANKLE: SAGITTAL

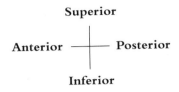

Superior

Anterior —┼— Posterior

Inferior

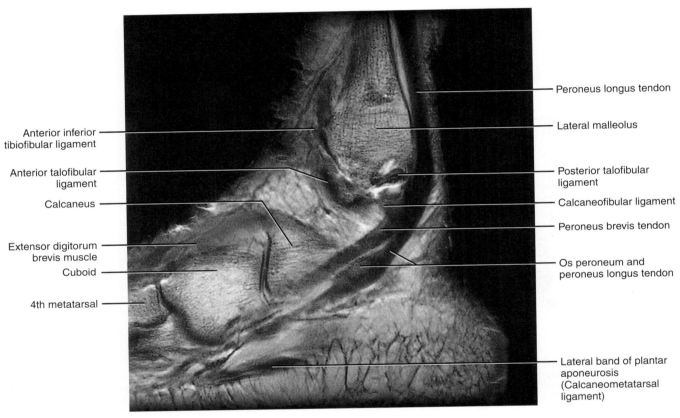

Anterior inferior tibiofibular ligament

Anterior talofibular ligament

Calcaneus

Extensor digitorum brevis muscle

Cuboid

4th metatarsal

Peroneus longus tendon

Lateral malleolus

Posterior talofibular ligament

Calcaneofibular ligament

Peroneus brevis tendon

Os peroneum and peroneus longus tendon

Lateral band of plantar aponeurosis (Calcaneometatarsal ligament)

FIGURE 6-59

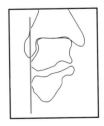

ANKLE: SAGITTAL

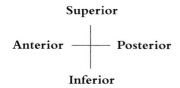

Superior

Anterior ——|—— Posterior

Inferior

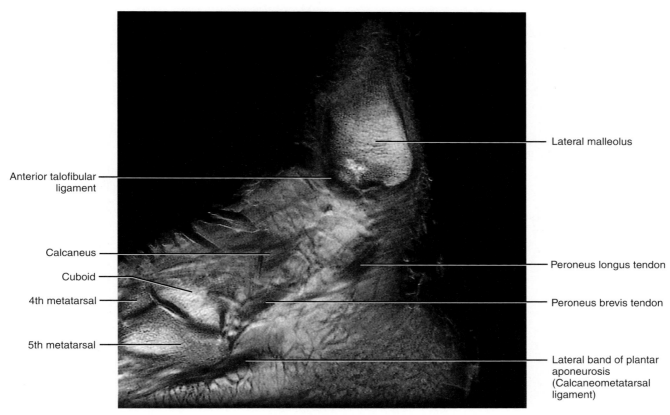

Lateral malleolus

Anterior talofibular
ligament

Calcaneus

Cuboid

4th metatarsal

5th metatarsal

Peroneus longus tendon

Peroneus brevis tendon

Lateral band of plantar
aponeurosis
(Calcaneometatarsal
ligament)

FIGURE 6-60

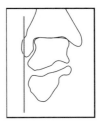

ANKLE: POSTERIOR LIGAMENTS, POSTERIOR VIEW

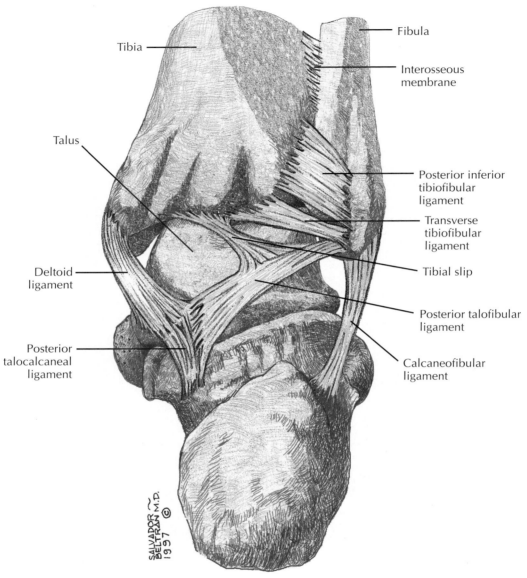

FIGURE 6-61

The tibiofibular syndesmosis consists of the anterior and posterior inferior tibiofibular ligaments, the transverse tibiofibular ligament, and the interosseous membrane. The transverse tibiofibular ligament lies deep and inferior to the posterior inferior tibiofibular ligament and is sometimes called the deep component of the posterior inferior tibiofibular ligament. The transverse tibiofibular ligament projects below the posterior tibial margin and constitutes a true posterior labrum, deepening the tibial articulating surface of the talus. During dorsiflexion, the posterior talofibular ligament moves distally to expose a synovial-lined cul–de–sac. The floor of this recess may demonstrate a thin band known as the "tibial slip." The tibial slip extends from the superior border of the posterior talofibular ligament and inserts on the posterior tibial margin, blending with the fibers of the transverse tibiofibular ligament. For related MR, arthroscopy, and surgical anatomy images see Figures 6-84 through 6-86.

ANKLE: LATERAL AND MEDIAL LIGAMENTS

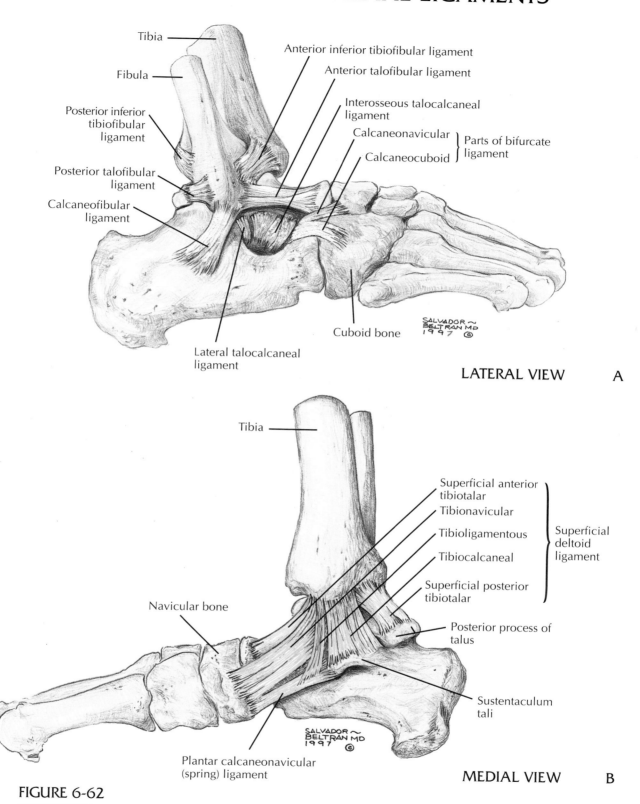

Tibia

Fibula

Posterior inferior tibiofibular ligament

Posterior talofibular ligament

Calcaneofibular ligament

Anterior inferior tibiofibular ligament

Anterior talofibular ligament

Interosseous talocalcaneal ligament

Calcaneonavicular

Calcaneocuboid

} Parts of bifurcate ligament

Cuboid bone

SALVADOR ~ BELTRAN MD 1997 ©

Lateral talocalcaneal ligament

LATERAL VIEW   **A**

Tibia

Navicular bone

Superficial anterior tibiotalar

Tibionavicular

Tibioligamentous

Tibiocalcaneal

Superficial posterior tibiotalar

} Superficial deltoid ligament

Posterior process of talus

Sustentaculum tali

Plantar calcaneonavicular (spring) ligament

SALVADOR ~ BELTRAN MD 1997 ©

MEDIAL VIEW   **B**

FIGURE 6-62

Ankle ligaments. **(A)** The lateral collateral ligamentous complex consists of three distinct structures: the anterior talofibular ligament, the calcaneofibular ligament, and the posterior talofibular ligament. **(B)** The thick deltoid ligament consists of superficial and deep fibers. The deep layer of the deltoid ligament consists of a small anterior component, the anterior talotibial ligament, and a strong posterior talotibial ligament. For related MR, arthroscopy, and surgical anatomy images see Figures 6-78, 6-79, and 6-81 through 6-83.

ANKLE: RETINACULA AND TENDONS, LATERAL VIEW

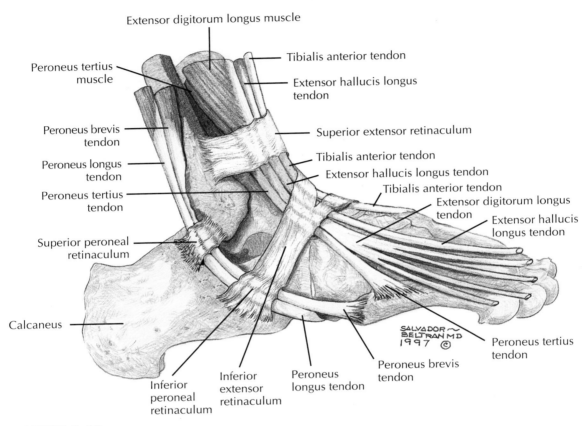

FIGURE 6-63

Lateral view of the retinacula and tendons. The superior extensor retinaculum attaches to the distal anterior fibula and tibia and invests the tibialis anterior tendon medially. The Y-shaped inferior extensor retinaculum attaches to the anterolateral part of the calcaneus (the stem) and extends to the medial malleolus (the upper limb) and the medial plantar fascia (the lower limb). The tibialis anterior, the extensor hallucis longus, the extensor digitorum longus, and the peroneus tertius tendons divide the upper limb of the retinaculum into superficial and deep layers. The superior peroneal retinaculum extends inferiorly and posteriorly from the lateral malleolus to the lateral calcaneal surface, binding the peroneus longus and brevis tendons. The inferior peroneal retinaculum is attached to the peroneal trochlea and calcaneus above and below the peroneal tendons. The lateral root of the inferior extensor retinaculum may be continuous with the inferior peroneal retinaculum. For related MR, arthroscopy, and surgical anatomy images see Figures 6-72 through 6-75.

ANKLE: RETINACULA AND TENDONS, MEDIAL VIEW

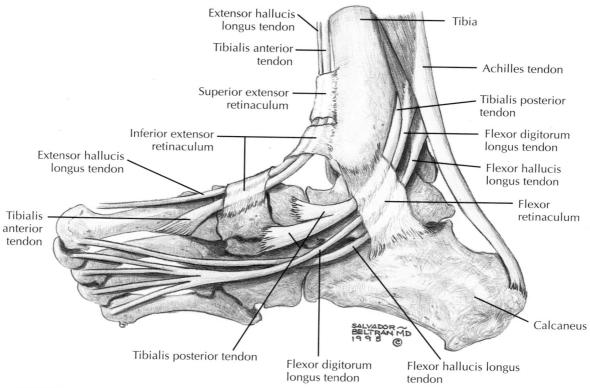

Extensor hallucis longus tendon

Tibialis anterior tendon

Superior extensor retinaculum

Inferior extensor retinaculum

Extensor hallucis longus tendon

Tibialis anterior tendon

Tibia

Achilles tendon

Tibialis posterior tendon

Flexor digitorum longus tendon

Flexor hallucis longus tendon

Flexor retinaculum

Calcaneus

SALVADOR ~ BELTRAN MD 1995 ©

Tibialis posterior tendon

Flexor digitorum longus tendon

Flexor hallucis longus tendon

FIGURE 6-64

Medial view of the retinacula and tendons. The flexor retinaculum extends inferiorly and posteriorly from the medial malleolus to the medial calcaneal surface. The tendons of the deep calf muscles (the flexor digitorum longus, the flexor hallucis longus, and the tibialis posterior) and the neurovascular structures in the posterior compartment pass underneath the flexor retinaculum before entering the foot. For related MR, arthroscopy, and surgical anatomy images see Figures 6-76 and 6-77.

DORSUM OF FOOT: SUPERFICIAL DISSECTION

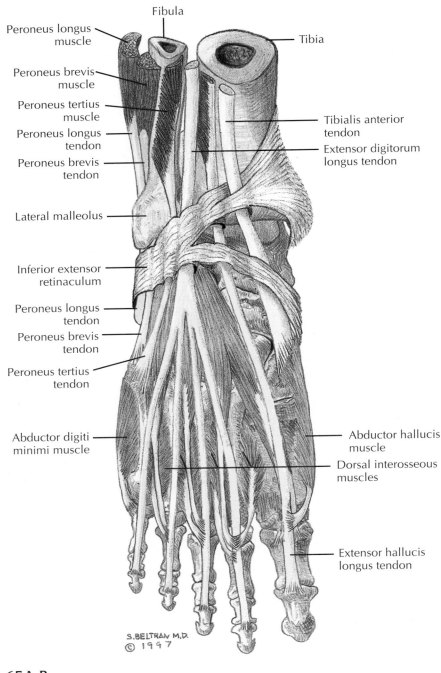

A

FIGURE 6-65A,B

(A) The superficial muscles and tendons are illustrated on the dorsum of the foot. The Y-shaped inferior extensor retinaculum binds the tibialis anterior, extensor hallucis longus, and extensor digitorum longus tendons as they pass to the dorsal aspect of the foot at the level of the tibiotalar joint. The peroneus tertius tendon inserts on the dorsal surface of the base of the fifth metatarsal. For related MR, arthroscopy, and surgical anatomy images see Figures 6-72 and 6-73.

DORSUM OF FOOT: SUPERFICIAL DISSECTION

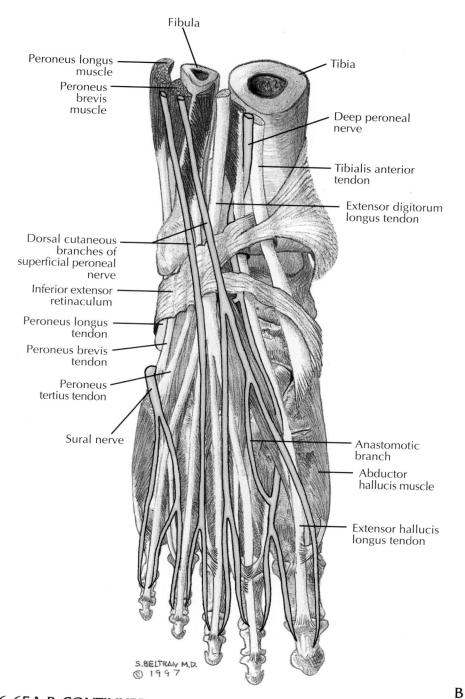

Fibula

Peroneus longus
muscle

Peroneus
brevis
muscle

Tibia

Deep peroneal
nerve

Tibialis anterior
tendon

Extensor digitorum
longus tendon

Dorsal cutaneous
branches of
superficial peroneal
nerve

Inferior extensor
retinaculum

Peroneus longus
tendon

Peroneus brevis
tendon

Peroneus
tertius tendon

Sural nerve

Anastomotic
branch

Abductor
hallucis muscle

Extensor hallucis
longus tendon

S.BELTRAN M.D.
© 1997

B

FIGURE 6-65A,B *CONTINUED*

(B) The superficial peroneal nerve with its dorsal cutaneous branches, the deep peroneal nerve, and the sural nerve are added to dorsal anatomy of the foot. For related MR, arthroscopy, and surgical anatomy images see Figures 6–72 and 6–73.

DORSUM OF FOOT: DEEP DISSECTION

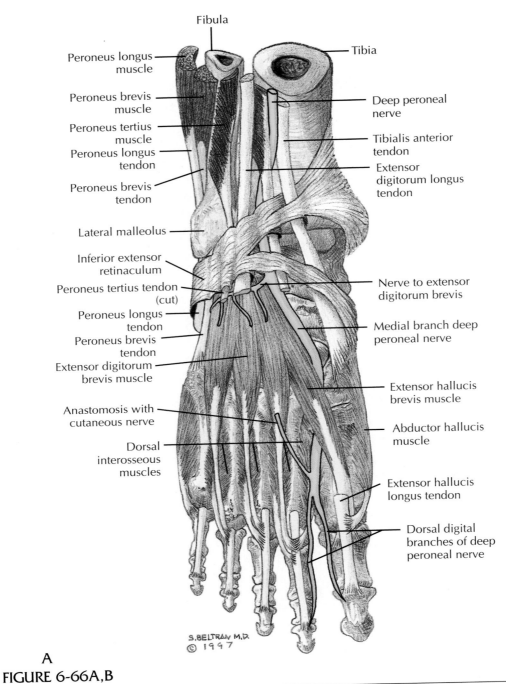

A

FIGURE 6-66A,B

(A and B) Deep dissection of the muscles and tendons of the dorsum of the foot with removal of overlying structures illustrates the branches of the deep peroneal nerve (A) and displays the extensor hallucis brevis and extensor digitorum brevis (B). The deep peroneal nerve arises from division of the common peroneal nerve between the fibula and the peroneus longus. The four dorsal interosseous muscles are also shown. For related MR, arthroscopy, and surgical anatomy images see Figures 6-72 and 6-73.

DORSUM OF FOOT: DEEP DISSECTION

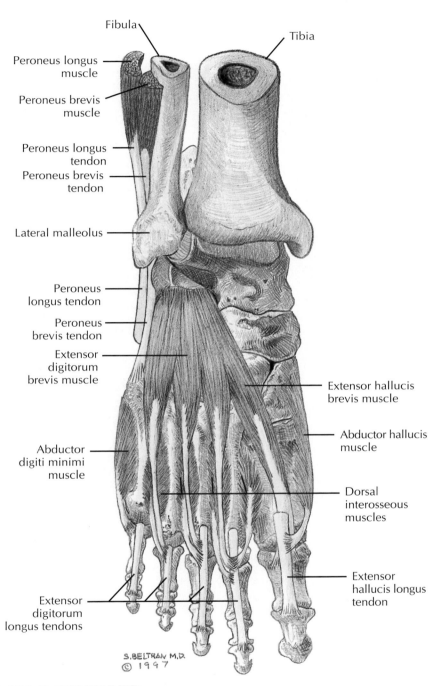

FIGURE 6-66A,B *CONTINUED*

For related MR, arthroscopy, and surgical anatomy images see Figures 6-72 and 6-73.

MUSCLES OF THE FOOT: FIRST LAYER

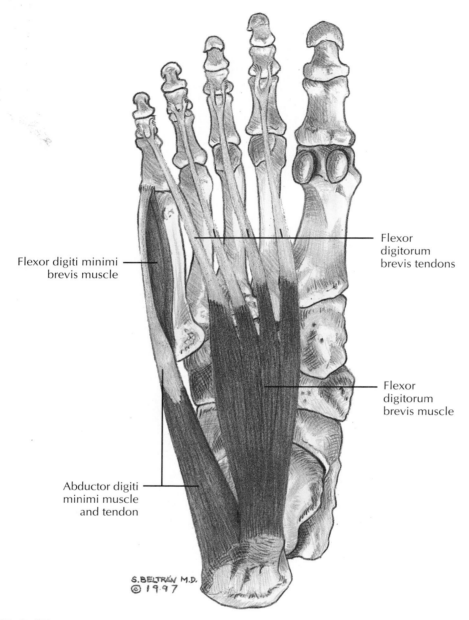

Flexor digiti minimi brevis muscle

Flexor digitorum brevis tendons

Flexor digitorum brevis muscle

Abductor digiti minimi muscle and tendon

S. BELTRÁN M.D.
© 1997

FIGURE 6-67

Muscles of the plantar aspect of the foot, first layer. The first layer consists of the abductor hallucis, the flexor digitorum brevis, and the abductor digiti minimi.

PLANTAR NERVES

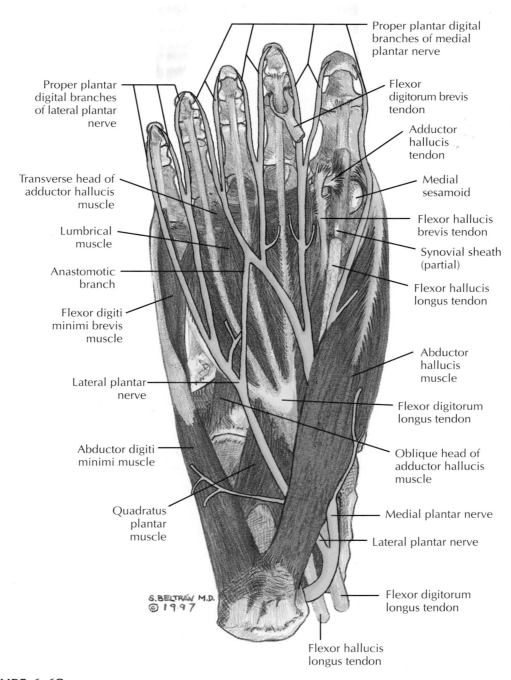

Proper plantar digital branches of medial plantar nerve

Flexor digitorum brevis tendon

Adductor hallucis tendon

Medial sesamoid

Flexor hallucis brevis tendon

Synovial sheath (partial)

Flexor hallucis longus tendon

Abductor hallucis muscle

Flexor digitorum longus tendon

Oblique head of adductor hallucis muscle

Medial plantar nerve

Lateral plantar nerve

Flexor digitorum longus tendon

Flexor hallucis longus tendon

Proper plantar digital branches of lateral plantar nerve

Transverse head of adductor hallucis muscle

Lumbrical muscle

Anastomotic branch

Flexor digiti minimi brevis muscle

Lateral plantar nerve

Abductor digiti minimi muscle

Quadratus plantar muscle

S. BELTRÁN M.D.
© 1997

FIGURE 6-68

Plantar nerves are illustrated by division of the tibial nerve into medial and lateral plantar nerves as well as their respective proper plantar digital branches.

MUSCLES OF THE FOOT: SECOND LAYER

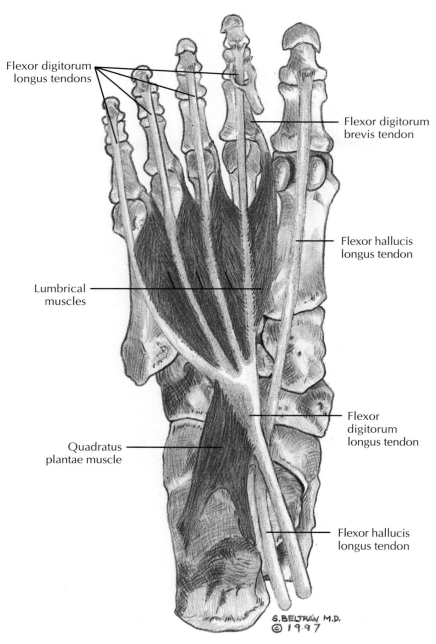

Flexor digitorum longus tendons

Flexor digitorum brevis tendon

Flexor hallucis longus tendon

Lumbrical muscles

Flexor digitorum longus tendon

Quadratus plantae muscle

Flexor hallucis longus tendon

S. BELTRAN M.D.
© 1997

FIGURE 6-69

Muscles of the plantar aspect of the foot, second layer. The second layer consists of the quadratus plantae, the lumbricals, the flexor digitorum longus tendon, and the flexor hallucis longus tendon.

MUSCLES OF THE FOOT: THIRD LAYER

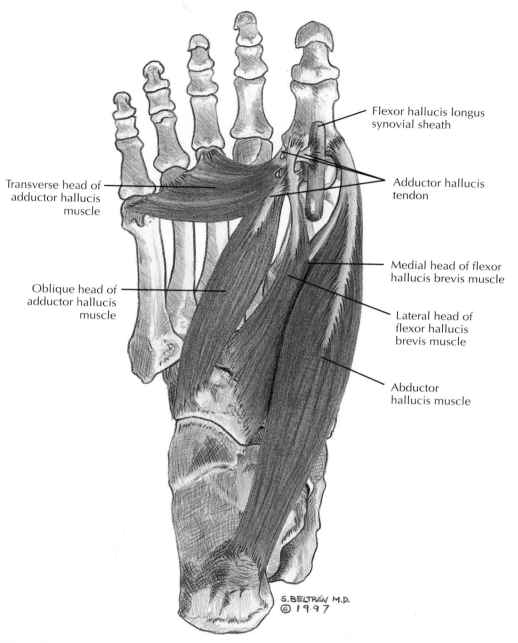

Flexor hallucis longus
synovial sheath

Transverse head of
adductor hallucis
muscle

Adductor hallucis
tendon

Medial head of flexor
hallucis brevis muscle

Oblique head of
adductor hallucis
muscle

Lateral head of
flexor hallucis
brevis muscle

Abductor
hallucis muscle

S. BELTRÁN M.D.
© 1997

FIGURE 6-70

Muscles of the plantar aspect of the foot, third layer. The third layer includes the flexor hallucis brevis, the adductor hallucis, and the flexor digiti minimi brevis (see Figure 6-68). The adductor hallucis muscle has a transverse and oblique head.

MUSCLES OF THE FOOT: FOURTH LAYER

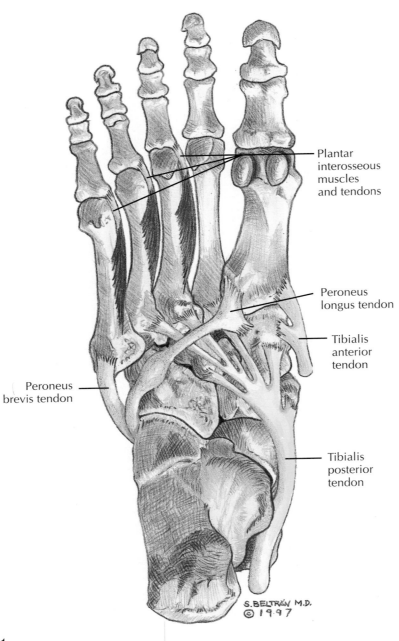

Plantar interosseous muscles and tendons

Peroneus longus tendon

Tibialis anterior tendon

Peroneus brevis tendon

Tibialis posterior tendon

S. BELTRÁN M.D.
© 1997

FIGURE 6-71

Muscles of the plantar aspect of the foot, fourth layer. The fourth layer is made up of the interosseous muscles. The attachments of the peroneus brevis, peroneus longus, tibialis anterior, and tibialis posterior are also illustrated. The peroneus brevis inserts on the lateral aspect of the fifth metatarsal. The peroneus longus inserts on the lateral aspect of the medial cuneiform and the base of the first metatarsal. The tibialis anterior inserts on the medial and plantar surfaces of the medial cuneiform and the base of the first metatarsal. The tibialis posterior inserts on the navicular tuberosity; the plantar surface of the three cuneiforms; and the plantar surface of the base of the second, third, and fourth metatarsals, the cuboid, and the sustentaculum tali.

ANKLE: TIBIALIS ANTERIOR
AND EXTENSOR HALLUCIS LONGUS

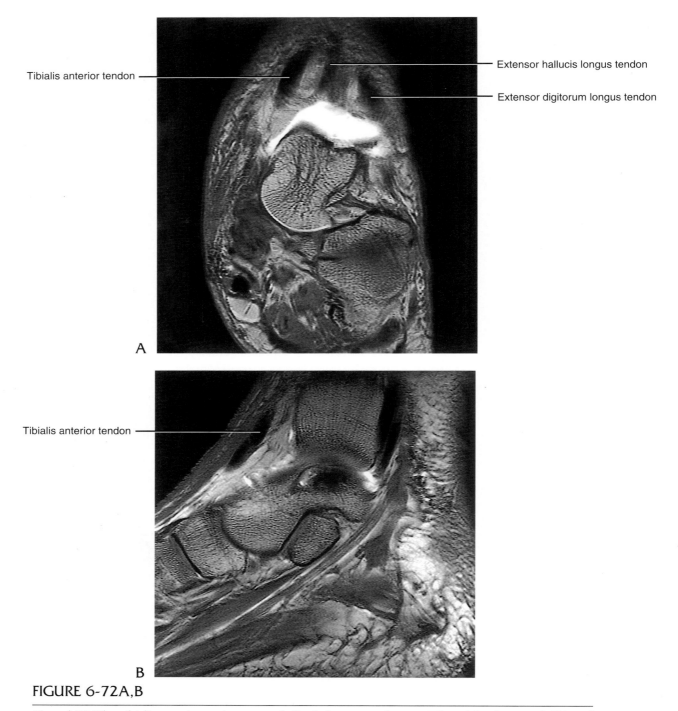

Tibialis anterior tendon —

Extensor hallucis longus tendon

Extensor digitorum longus tendon

A

Tibialis anterior tendon —

B

FIGURE 6-72A,B

(A and B) The tibialis anterior and extensor hallucis longus tendons on T1-weighted coronal (A) and sagittal (B) MR arthrograms. Rupture of the tibialis anterior tendon can occur between the extensor retinaculum and the insertion onto the medial cuneiform and adjacent base of the first metatarsal.

ANKLE: TIBIALIS ANTERIOR
AND EXTENSOR HALLUCIS LONGUS

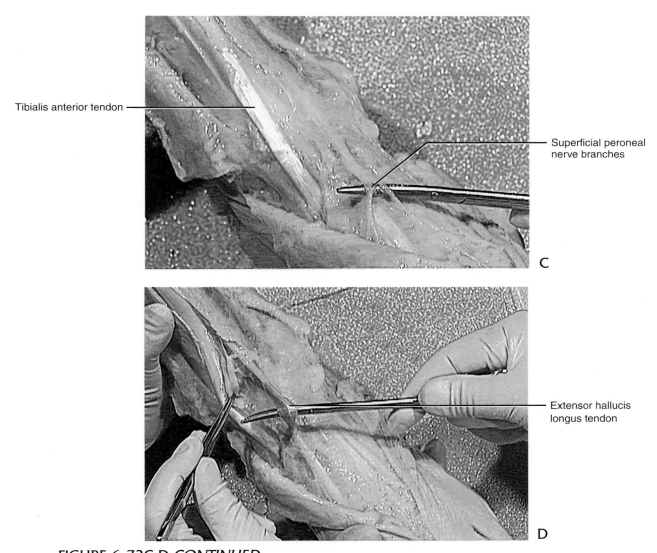

Tibialis anterior tendon

Superficial peroneal nerve branches

Extensor hallucis longus tendon

FIGURE 6-72C,D *CONTINUED*

(**C** and **D**) Corresponding dissections of the tibialis anterior (**C**) and extensor hallucis longus (**D**) tendons. Anatomic dissection of the superficial peroneal nerve and its branches is shown in part **C**.

ANKLE: EXTENSOR HALLUCIS LONGUS AND EXTENSOR DIGITORUM LONGUS

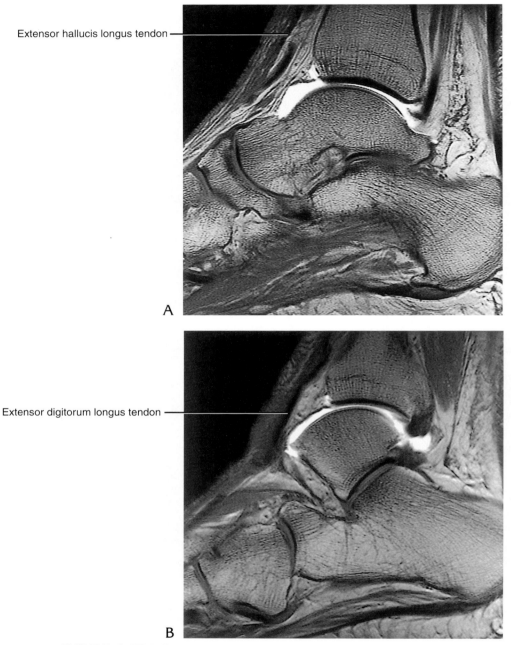

Extensor hallucis longus tendon —

A

Extensor digitorum longus tendon —

B

FIGURE 6-73A,B

(**A** and **B**) T1-weighted sagittal MR arthrograms depicting the extensor hallucis longus tendon (**A**) and extensor digitorum longus tendon (**B**) (the image in part **A** is medial to the image in part **B**). The extensor hallucis longus muscle is located between the tibialis anterior and the extensor digitorum longus, and its tendon crosses the anterior tibial vessels in a lateral to medial direction at the ankle.

ANKLE: EXTENSOR HALLUCIS LONGUS AND EXTENSOR DIGITORUM LONGUS

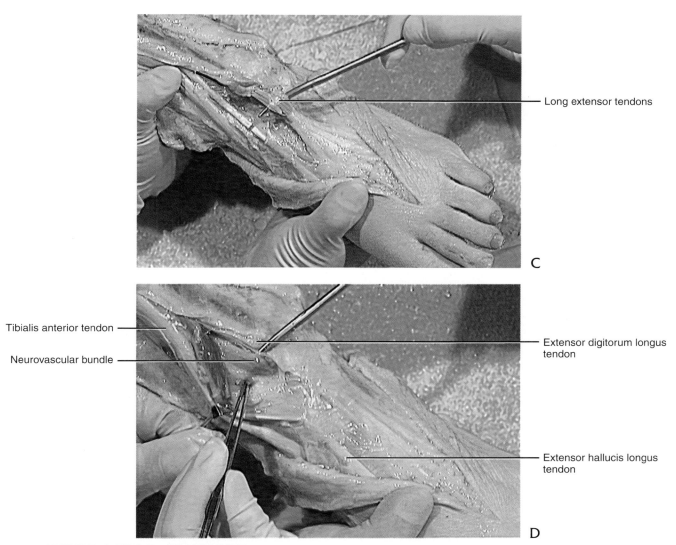

— Long extensor tendons

C

Tibialis anterior tendon —

Neurovascular bundle —

Extensor digitorum longus tendon

Extensor hallucis longus tendon

D

FIGURE 6-73C,D *CONTINUED*

(C) Corresponding gross dissection of the extensor hallucis longus tendon and extensor digitorum longus tendon. **(D)** In a separate specimen, the neurovascular bundle (the proximal portions of the anterior tibial vessels and deep peroneal nerve) is shown between the extensor digitorum and the tibialis anterior.

ANKLE: PERONEUS BREVIS AND LONGUS

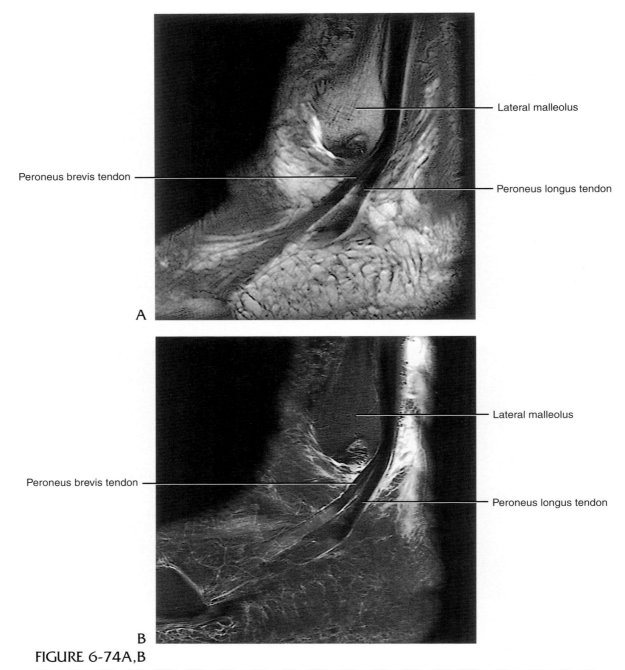

FIGURE 6-74A,B

(A and B) The peroneus brevis and peroneus longus on a T1-weighted MR arthrogram (A) and a fat-suppressed T2-weighted sagittal MR arthrogram (B). The peroneus brevis grooves the lateral malleolus and lies close to the bone. The peroneus longus lies just posterior to the peroneus brevis.

ANKLE: PERONEUS BREVIS AND LONGUS

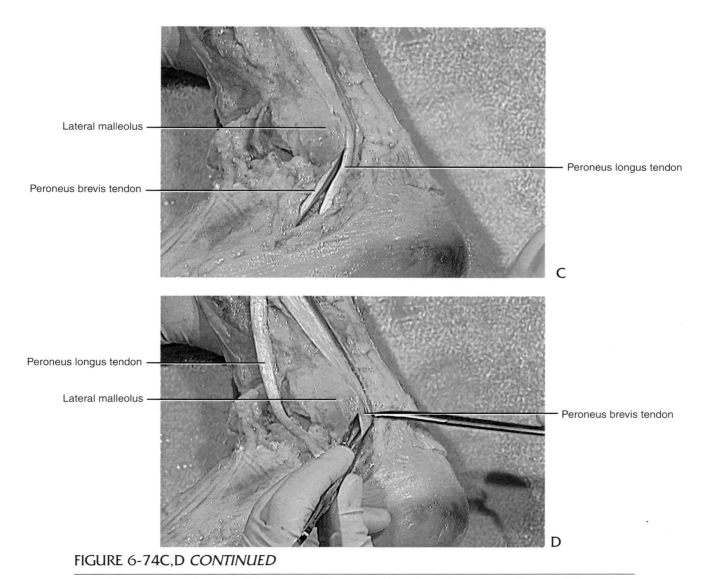

Lateral malleolus

Peroneus brevis tendon

Peroneus longus tendon

C

Peroneus longus tendon

Lateral malleolus

Peroneus brevis tendon

D

FIGURE 6-74C,D *CONTINUED*

(**C** and **D**) Corresponding lateral dissections of the peroneal tendons. The peroneus brevis is dislocated out of the fibular groove in part **D**.

ANKLE: SUPERIOR PERONEAL RETINACULUM AND FIBULAR GROOVE

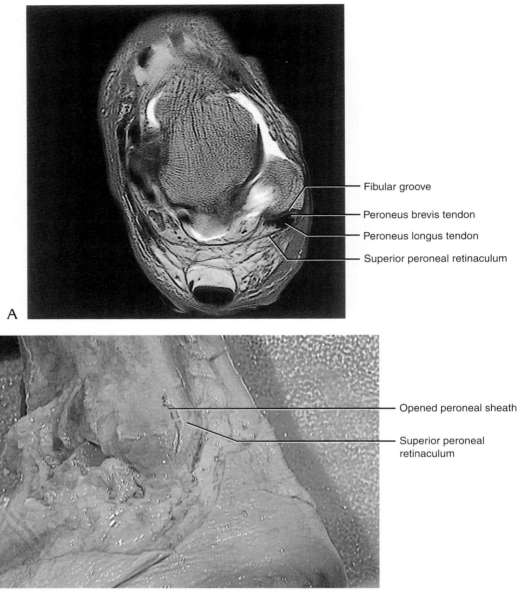

A

Fibular groove

Peroneus brevis tendon

Peroneus longus tendon

Superior peroneal retinaculum

Opened peroneal sheath

Superior peroneal retinaculum

B

FIGURE 6-75A,B

(A) T1-weighted axial image showing the superior peroneal retinaculum and fibular groove. (B) The superior retinaculum and opened peroneal sheath are demonstrated. The superior peroneal retinaculum represents the inferior part of the peroneal sheath.

ANKLE: SUPERIOR PERONEAL RETINACULUM AND FIBULAR GROOVE

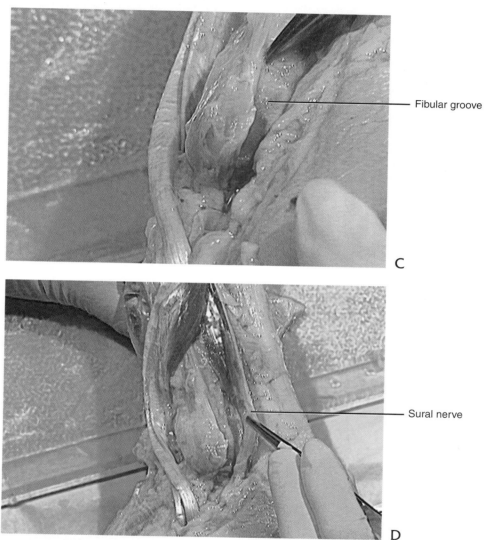

FIGURE 6-75C,D *CONTINUED*

(C) Posterior view of the fibular groove. (D) Posterolaterally, the sural nerve and short saphenous venous plexus lie in the subcutaneous tissue posterior to the peroneal tendons behind the lateral malleolus.

ANKLE: TIBIALIS POSTERIOR AND FLEXOR DIGITORUM LONGUS

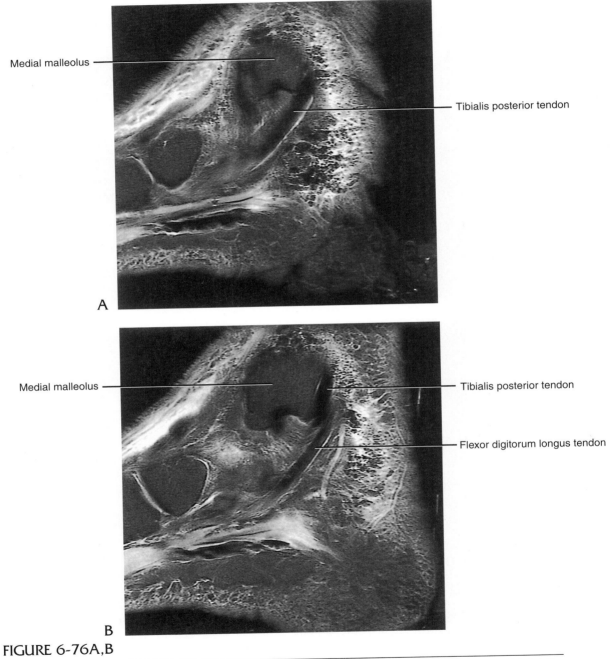

Medial malleolus —

— Tibialis posterior tendon

A

Medial malleolus —

— Tibialis posterior tendon

— Flexor digitorum longus tendon

B

FIGURE 6-76A,B

(**A** and **B**) The tibialis posterior and flexor digitorum longus tendons on fat-suppressed T2-weighted fast spin-echo MR arthrograms (the image in part **A** is medial to the image in part **B**).

ANKLE: TIBIALIS POSTERIOR
AND FLEXOR DIGITORUM LONGUS

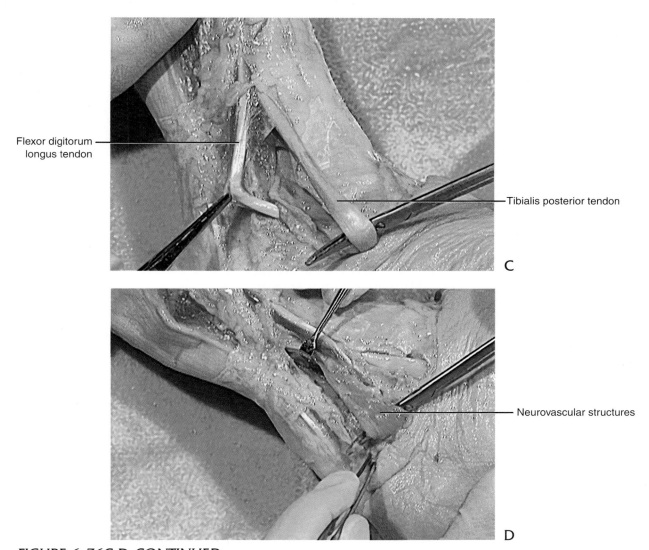

Flexor digitorum
longus tendon

Tibialis posterior tendon

C

Neurovascular structures

D

FIGURE 6-76C,D *CONTINUED*

(**C** and **D**) Corresponding medial dissections of the tibialis posterior (**C**) and flexor digitorum longus tendons (**D**). The neurovascular bundle, including the posterior tibial artery and posterior tibial nerve, is identified. The posterior tibial nerve lies between the flexor digitorum longus and the flexor hallucis longus, divides into the medial and lateral plantar nerves, and gives off calcaneal branches. The tarsal tunnel contains—from anterior to posterior—the tibialis posterior tendon, the flexor digitorum longus tendon, the posterior tibial artery and venae comitantes, the tibial nerve, and the flexor hallucis longus tendon.

ANKLE: FLEXOR HALLUCIS LONGUS AND TIBIALIS POSTERIOR

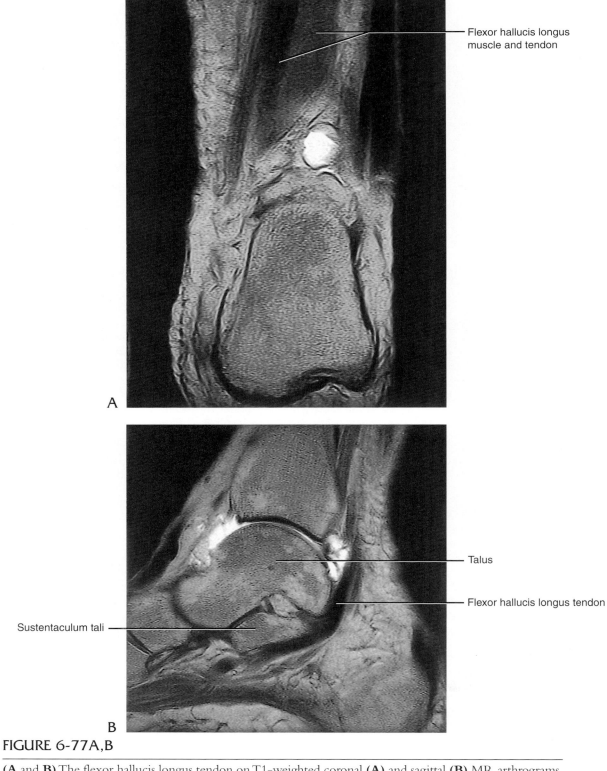

FIGURE 6-77A,B

(A and B) The flexor hallucis longus tendon on T1–weighted coronal (A) and sagittal (B) MR arthrograms.

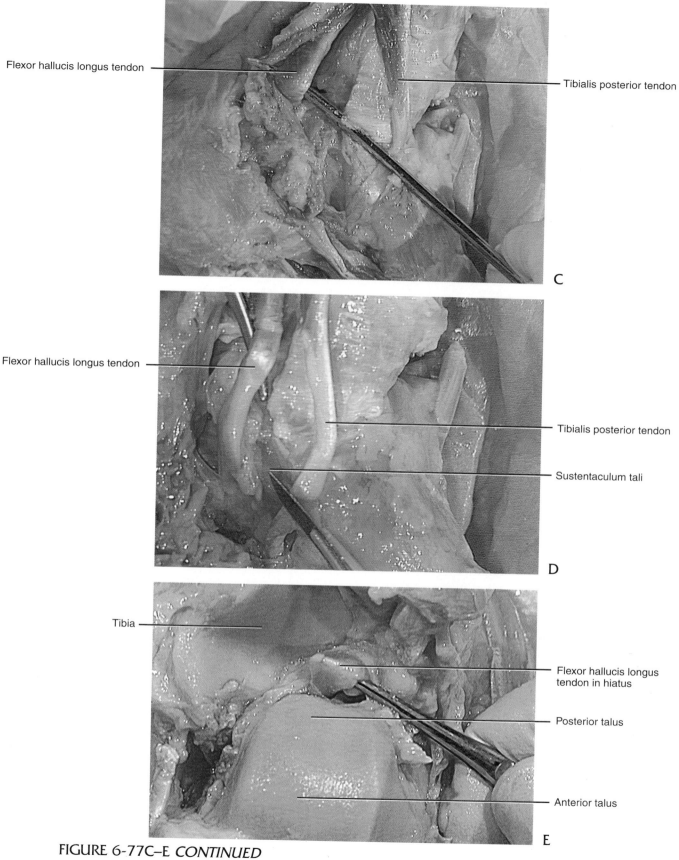

Flexor hallucis longus tendon

Tibialis posterior tendon

C

Flexor hallucis longus tendon

Tibialis posterior tendon

Sustentaculum tali

D

Tibia

Flexor hallucis longus tendon in hiatus

Posterior talus

Anterior talus

E

FIGURE 6-77C–E *CONTINUED*

(**C** and **D**) Corresponding dissections of the tibialis posterior tendon and flexor hallucis longus tendon. The flexor hallucis longus tendon grooves the posterior process of the talus and inferior surface of the sustentaculum tali. (**E**) The capsular reflection of the flexor hallucis longus tendon is medial to the transverse tibiofibular ligament. The tendon has been pulled through the hiatus in this anatomic dissection.

ANKLE: ANTEROLATERAL ANATOMY

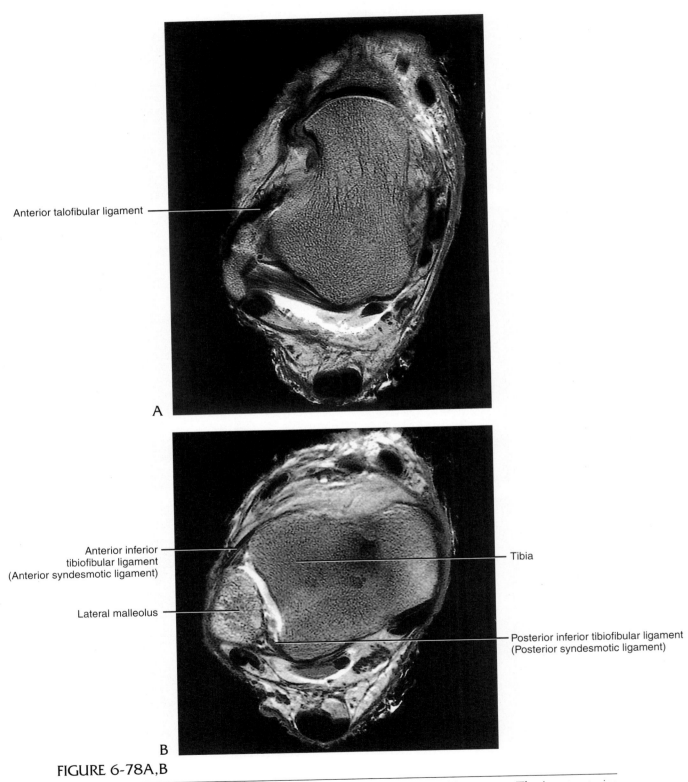

Anterior talofibular ligament

A

Anterior inferior
tibiofibular ligament
(Anterior syndesmotic ligament)

Tibia

Lateral malleolus

Posterior inferior tibiofibular ligament
(Posterior syndesmotic ligament)

B

FIGURE 6-78A,B

(A and B) T1–weighted axial MR arthrograms depicting anterolateral ankle anatomy. The intact anterior talofibular ligament is seen in part A and the anterior syndesmotic ligament is seen in part B (the image in part A is distal to the image in part B).

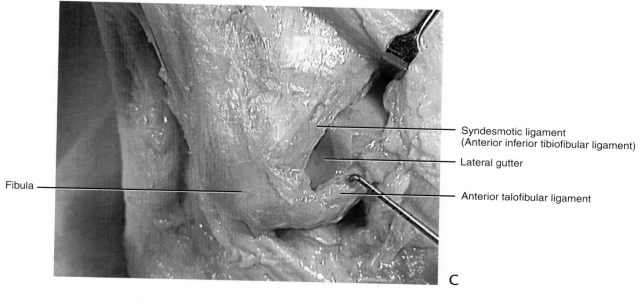

Syndesmotic ligament
(Anterior inferior tibiofibular ligament)

Lateral gutter

Fibula

Anterior talofibular ligament

C

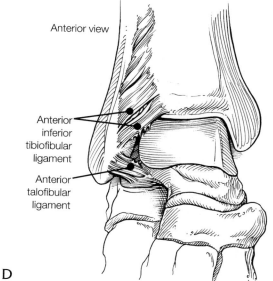

Anterior view

Anterior inferior tibiofibular ligament

Anterior talofibular ligament

D

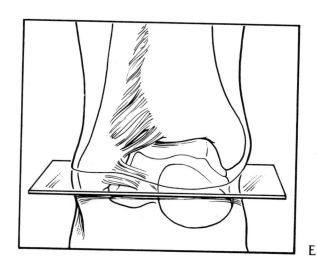

E

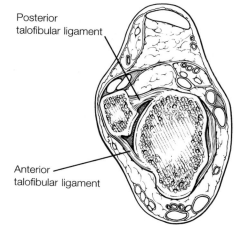

Posterior talofibular ligament

Anterior talofibular ligament

F

FIGURE 6-78C–F *CONTINUED*

(C) Corresponding anatomic dissection with anterolateral exposure of the anterior inferior tibiofibular ligament (anterior syndesmotic ligament), the anterior talofibular ligament, and the lateral gutter. (D) Potential soft tissue impingement sites are shown. The accessory fascicle of the anterior inferior tibiofibular ligament can impinge across the lateral talar dome. (E) Plane of cross-section through the lateral gutter. (F) Cross-sectional illustration of the lateral gutter. The boundaries of the lateral gutter are the talus medially, the fibula laterally, and the anterior and posterior talofibular ligaments.

ANKLE: LATERAL GUTTER
AND ANTEROLATERAL IMPINGEMENT

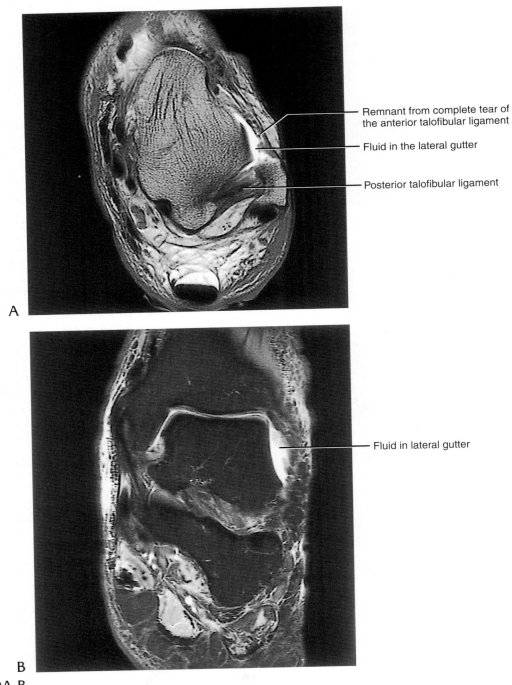

— Remnant from complete tear of
the anterior talofibular ligament

— Fluid in the lateral gutter

— Posterior talofibular ligament

A

— Fluid in lateral gutter

B

FIGURE 6-79A,B

(**A** and **B**) A tear of the anterior talofibular ligament as seen on a T1-weighted axial image (**A**) and a fat-suppressed T2-weighted fast spin-echo coronal image (**B**). Hyperintense fluid is seen within the lateral gutter.

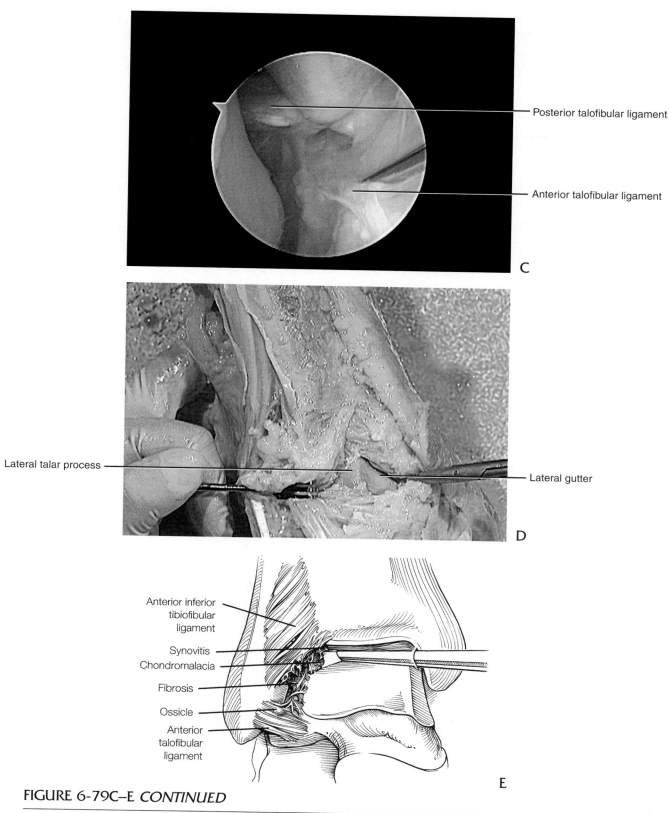

Posterior talofibular ligament

Anterior talofibular ligament

C

Lateral talar process

Lateral gutter

D

Anterior inferior tibiofibular ligament

Synovitis

Chondromalacia

Fibrosis

Ossicle

Anterior talofibular ligament

E

FIGURE 6-79C–E *CONTINUED*

(**C** and **D**) Arthroscopic view (**C**) and corresponding dissection (**D**) of the lateral gutter with a torn anterior talofibular ligament. (**E**) Anterolateral soft tissue impingement can occur at the anterior inferior tibiofibular ligament, the lateral gutter, and the anterior talofibular ligament. The arthroscopic appearance of anterolateral impingement is associated with synovitis, fibrosis, and chondromalacia in the anterolateral gutter. The finding of an adhesive thick scar band (a "meniscoid" lesion) is rare.

ANKLE: CENTRAL OVERHANG AND NOTCH OF HARTY

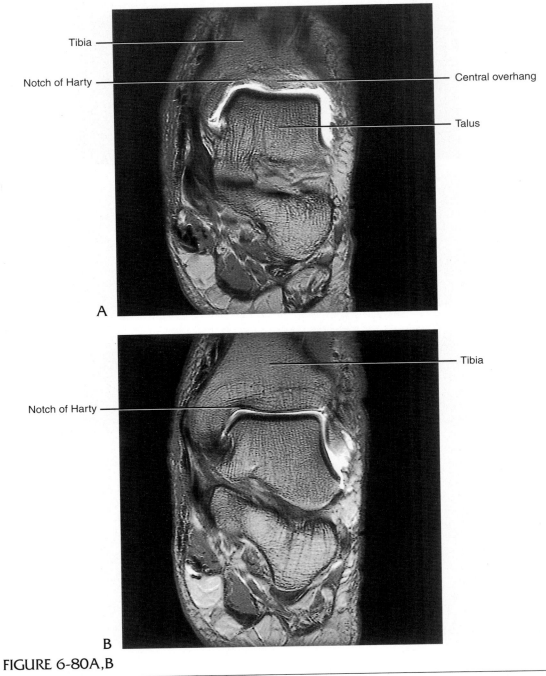

FIGURE 6-80A,B

(A and B) T1-weighted coronal MR arthrographic images showing the central overhang (ridge) **(A)** and the notch of Harty **(B)** (the image in part **A** is more anterior than the image in part **B**).

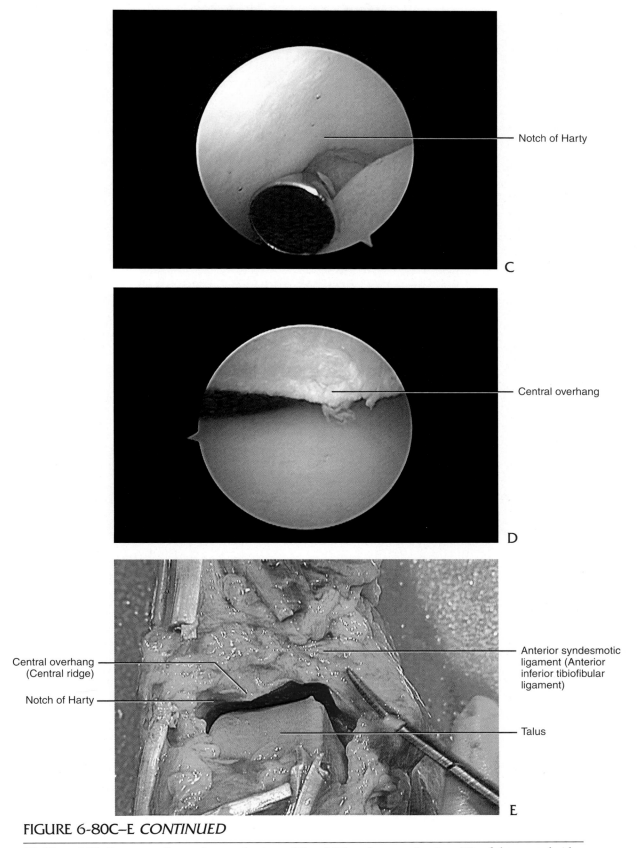

— Notch of Harty

— Central overhang

C

D

Central overhang
(Central ridge)

Notch of Harty

Anterior syndesmotic
ligament (Anterior
inferior tibiofibular
ligament)

Talus

E

FIGURE 6-80C–E *CONTINUED*

(**C, D,** and **E**) Corresponding arthroscopic views (**C** and **D**) and anatomic view (**E**) of the central ridge and notch of Harty. In establishing the anteromedial portal, the arthroscope is maneuvered through the notch of Harty to visualize the posterior structures. The central overhang represents a potential site for the formation of bone spurs.

ANKLE: SYNDESMOTIC LIGAMENT

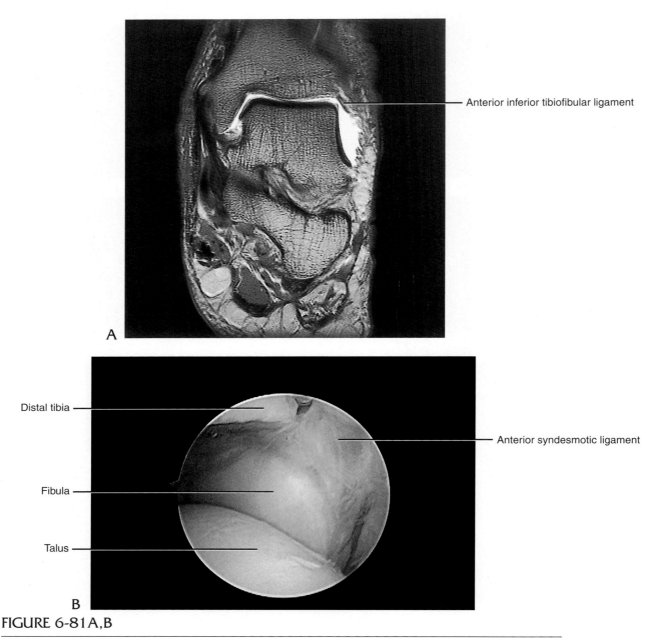

FIGURE 6-81A,B

(A) The anterior inferior tibiofibular ligament (anterior syndesmotic ligament) on a T1-weighted coronal MR arthrogram. **(B** and **C)** Corresponding arthroscopic view **(B)** and anatomic view **(C)** of the anterior inferior tibiofibular ligament. The synovial fringe is seen in the recess between the tibia and fibula. **(D)** Plane of cross-section through the syndesmosis. **(E)** A cross-sectional view through the syndesmosis demonstrates that impingement can occur anteriorly, centrally, or posteriorly.

ANKLE: SYNDESMOTIC LIGAMENT

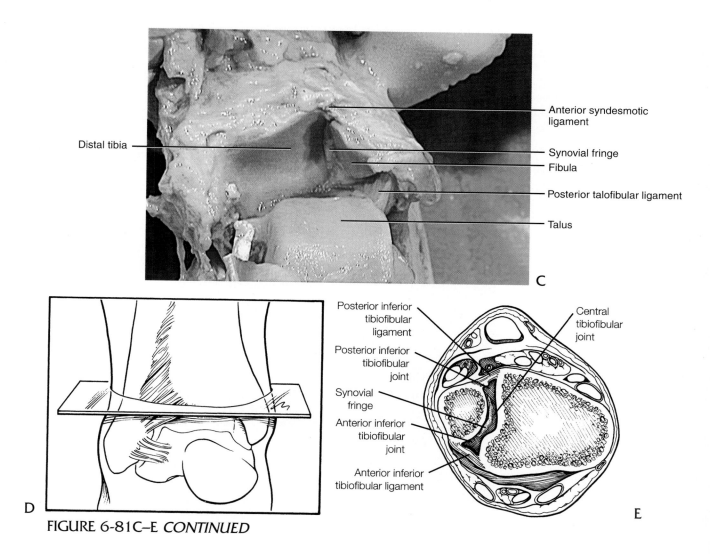

Distal tibia

Anterior syndesmotic ligament

Synovial fringe

Fibula

Posterior talofibular ligament

Talus

C

Posterior inferior tibiofibular ligament

Posterior inferior tibiofibular joint

Synovial fringe

Anterior inferior tibiofibular joint

Anterior inferior tibiofibular ligament

Central tibiofibular joint

D

E

FIGURE 6-81C–E *CONTINUED*

ANKLE: DELTOID LIGAMENT

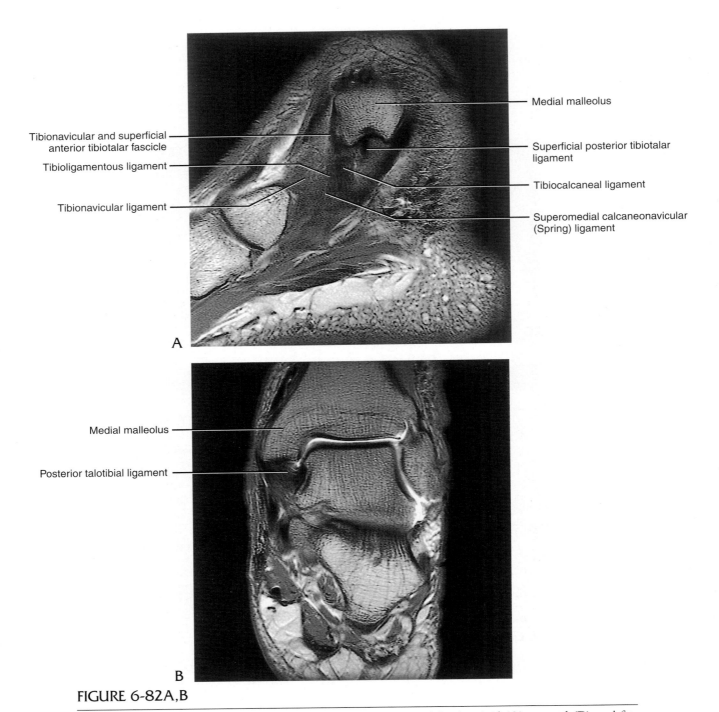

FIGURE 6-82A,B

(**A, B,** and **C**) The fibers of the deltoid ligament as seen on T1-weighted sagittal (**A**), coronal (**B**), and fat-suppressed T2-weighted fast spin-echo coronal (**C**) images. The superficial deltoid ligament fibers consist of the superficial anterior tibiotalar, tibionavicular, tibioligamentous, tibiocalcaneal, and superficial posterior tibiotalar components. (**D**) Corresponding arthroscopic view of an anterior examination as seen from the anteromedial portal shows the deep portion of the deltoid ligament. The deep layer of the deltoid ligament includes a small anterior talotibial ligament and a substantial posterior talotibial ligament. The posterior talotibial ligament runs obliquely inferiorly and posteriorly to insert on the medial surface of the talus as far as the posteromedial talar tubercle. The deep portion of the deltoid ligament is intraarticular and covered only by synovium. (**E**) The posterior fibers of the deltoid ligament form the floor of the tibialis posterior tendon sheath.

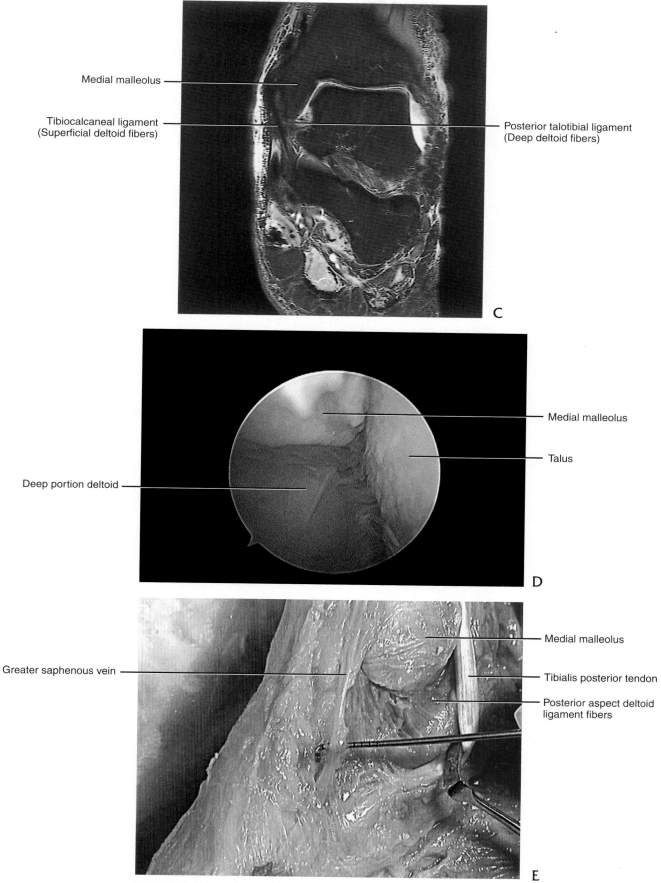

Medial malleolus

Tibiocalcaneal ligament
(Superficial deltoid fibers)

Posterior talotibial ligament
(Deep deltoid fibers)

C

Medial malleolus

Talus

Deep portion deltoid

D

Greater saphenous vein

Medial malleolus

Tibialis posterior tendon

Posterior aspect deltoid
ligament fibers

E

FIGURE 6-82C–E *CONTINUED*

ANKLE: CALCANEOFIBULAR LIGAMENT

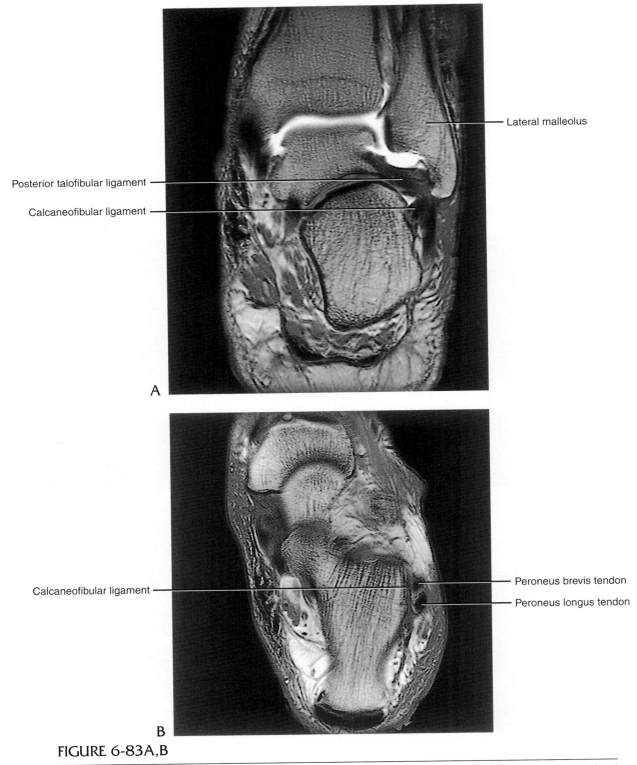

FIGURE 6-83A,B

(A, B, and **C)** The calcaneofibular ligament on a T1-weighted coronal MR arthrogram **(A)**, a T1-weighted axial image **(B)**, and a fat-suppressed T2-weighted fast spin-echo axial image **(C)**.

ANKLE: CALCANEOFIBULAR LIGAMENT

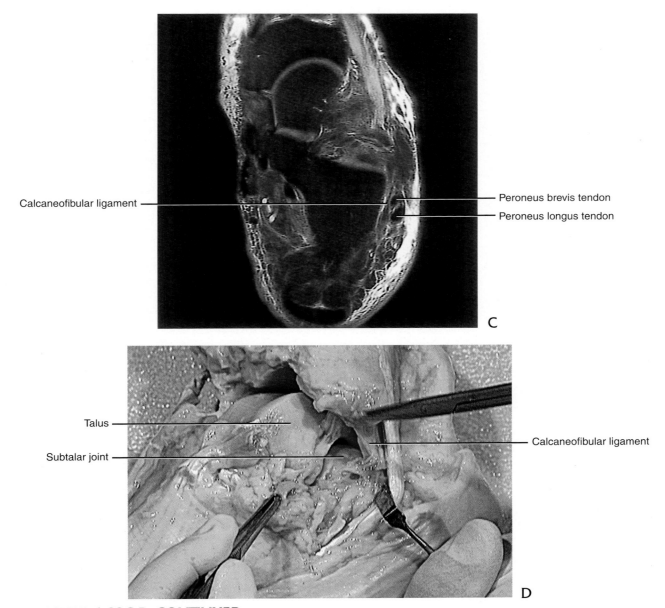

Calcaneofibular ligament —

— Peroneus brevis tendon
— Peroneus longus tendon

C

Talus —

Subtalar joint —

— Calcaneofibular ligament

D

FIGURE 6-83C,D *CONTINUED*

The calcaneofibular ligament originates from the lower segment of the anterior border of the lateral malleolus and courses inferiorly and slightly posteriorly to its insertion onto a small tubercle at the upper part of
the lateral surface of the calcaneus. The calcaneofibular ligament is crossed superficially by the peroneal tendons and their sheaths. **(D)** Corresponding anatomic dissection of the calcaneofibular ligament. This strong,
cordlike ligament is the largest of the three lateral collateral ligaments.

ANKLE: POSTERIOR ANKLE LIGAMENTS

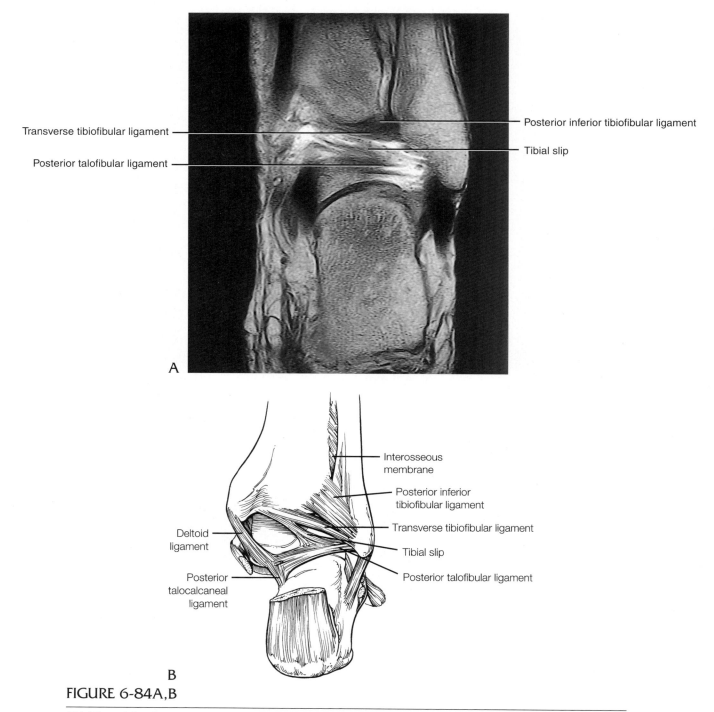

FIGURE 6-84A,B

(A) T1-weighted posterior coronal MR arthrogram depicting the posterior ankle ligaments including the posterior inferior tibiofibular ligament, the transverse tibiofibular ligament, and the separate tibial slip, attaching directly to the posterior talofibular ligament. **(B)** Corresponding illustration of the posterior ankle ligaments. These ligaments may be involved in posterior impingement. Posterior impingement can occur alone or in combination with anterolateral and syndesmosis impingement.

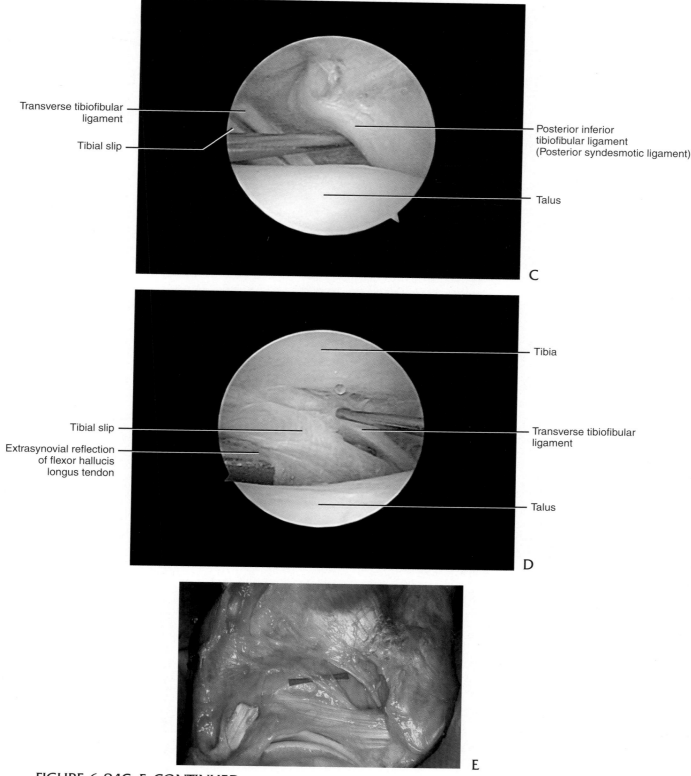

Transverse tibiofibular ligament

Tibial slip

Posterior inferior tibiofibular ligament (Posterior syndesmotic ligament)

Talus

C

Tibial slip

Extrasynovial reflection of flexor hallucis longus tendon

Tibia

Transverse tibiofibular ligament

Talus

D

E

FIGURE 6-84C–E *CONTINUED*

(**C** and **D**) Correlative arthroscopic images of the posterior inferior tibiofibular ligament (**C**) and the transverse tibiofibular ligament and tibial slip (**D**). The tibial slip is also referred to as the posterior intermalleolar ligament. The transverse ligament forms a labrum inferior to the posterior tibial margin. Hypertrophy of the synovial covering of the transverse ligament may result in painful hindfoot impingement. (**E**) The tibial slip (marker) courses from the posterior talofibular ligament and inserts on the posterior tibial margin, blending with the fibers of the transverse tibiofibular ligament.

ANKLE: POSTERIOR SYNDESMOTIC AND TRANSVERSE TIBIOFIBULAR LIGAMENTS

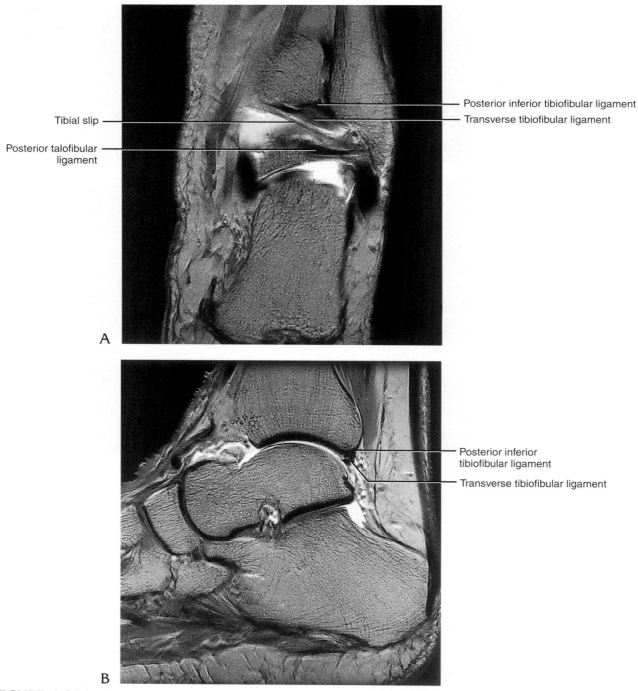

FIGURE 6-85A,B

(**A** and **B**) T1–weighted posterior coronal (**A**) and T1–weighted sagittal (**B**) MR arthrograms showing the normal posterior inferior tibiofibular ligament (posterior syndesmotic ligament), transverse tibiofibular ligament and tibial slip.

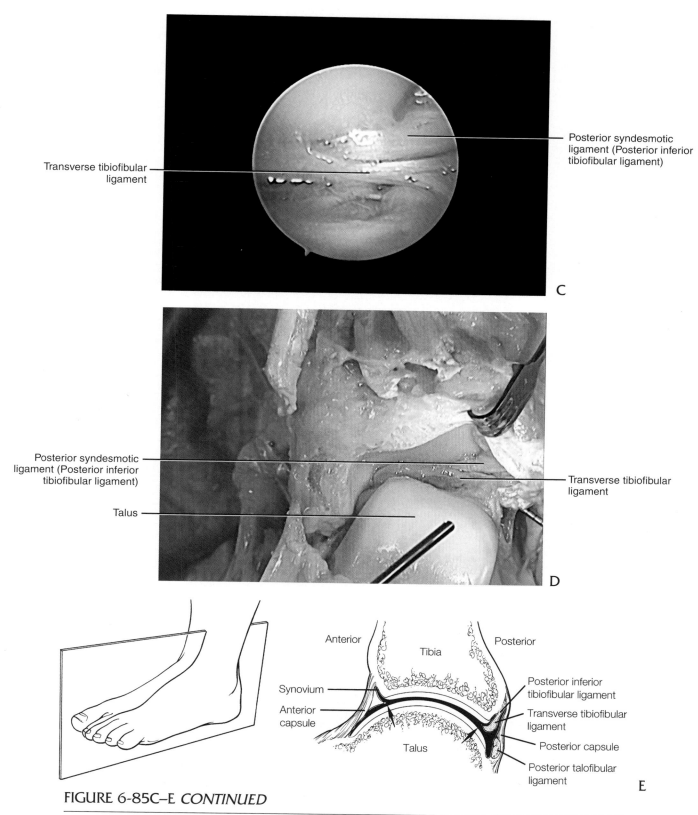

Posterior syndesmotic ligament (Posterior inferior tibiofibular ligament)

Transverse tibiofibular ligament

C

Posterior syndesmotic ligament (Posterior inferior tibiofibular ligament)

Talus

Transverse tibiofibular ligament

D

Anterior

Tibia

Posterior

Synovium

Anterior capsule

Talus

Posterior inferior tibiofibular ligament

Transverse tibiofibular ligament

Posterior capsule

Posterior talofibular ligament

E

FIGURE 6-85C–E *CONTINUED*

(**C** and **D**) Corresponding arthroscopic (**C**) and anatomic (**D**) views of the posterior inferior tibiofibular ligament (posterior syndesmotic ligament) and transverse tibiofibular ligament. (**E**) Sagittal plane of section through the tibiotalar joint showing corresponding anterior and posterior synovial folds. The location of the posterior inferior tibiofibular ligament and transverse tibiofibular ligament correlates with the MR image in part **B**.

ANKLE: POSTERIOR SYNDESMOTIC LIGAMENT AND TIBIAL SLIP

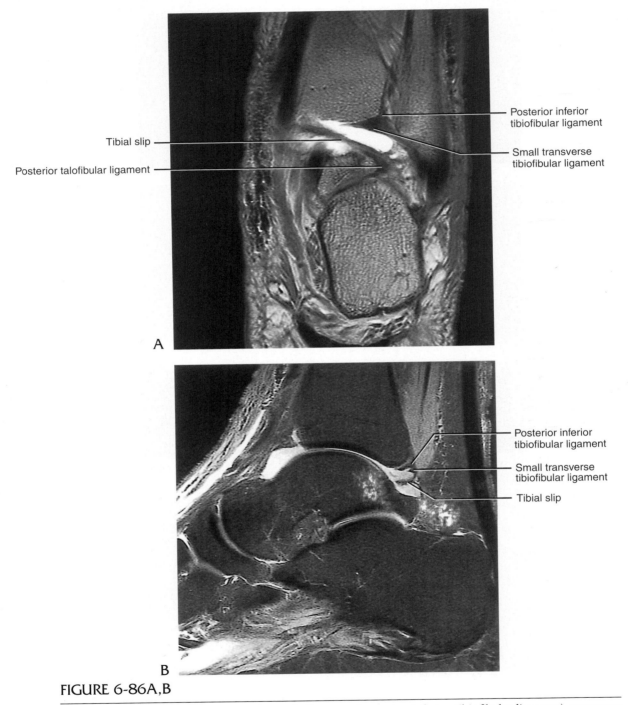

FIGURE 6-86A,B

(**A, B, C,** and **D**) The posterior syndesmotic ligament (posterior inferior tibiofibular ligament), transverse tibiofibular ligament and tibial slip can be seen. The small transverse tibiofibular ligament is a normal variant. (**A**) T1-weighted coronal MR arthrogram; (**B**) fat-suppressed T2 fast spin-echo sagittal MR arthrogram.

ANKLE: POSTERIOR SYNDESMOTIC LIGAMENT AND TIBIAL SLIP

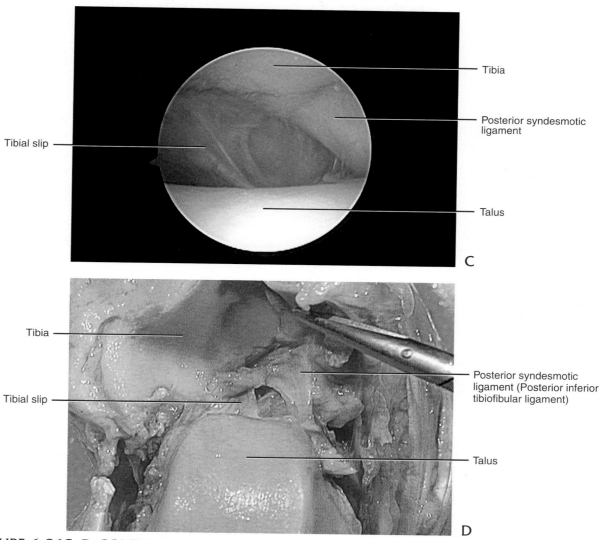

FIGURE 6-86C, D *CONTINUED*

(C) Posterolateral corner arthroscopic view; and **(D)** corresponding anatomic dissection. The transverse tibiofibular ligament should not be termed the tibial slip. Instead, the tibial slip extends from the posterior talofibular ligament to the transverse ligament. Its insertion on the posterior tibial margin may reach the posterior surface of the medial malleolus.

ANKLE: OSTEOCHONDRAL LESIONS

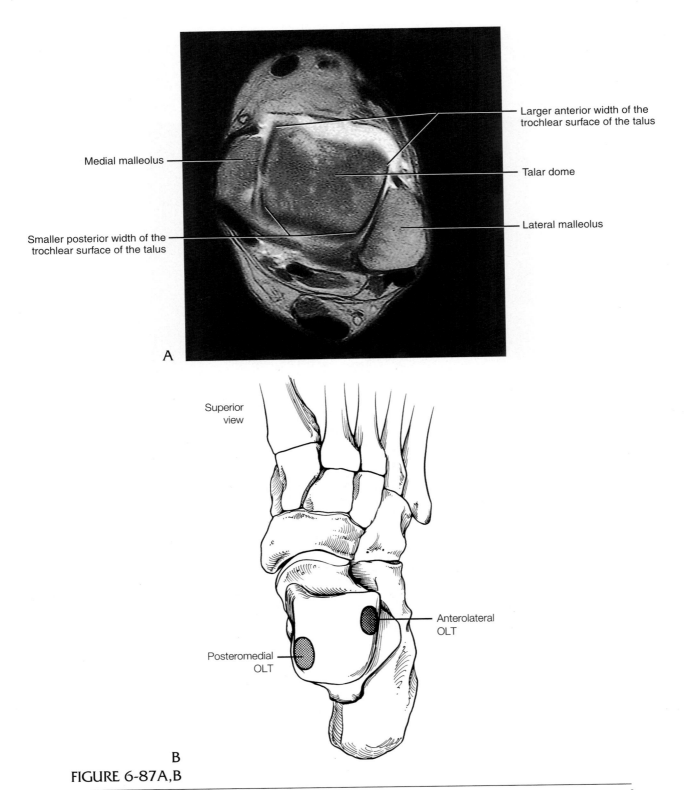

FIGURE 6-87A,B

(A) T1-weighted axial image of an intact talar dome. **(B)** Superior axial view depicting the location of osteochondral lesions of the talus (OLT). Most lesions are posteromedial or anterolateral. Lateral lesions tend to be shallower and wafer-shaped; medial lesions deeper and cup-shaped.

ANKLE: OSTEOCHONDRAL LESIONS

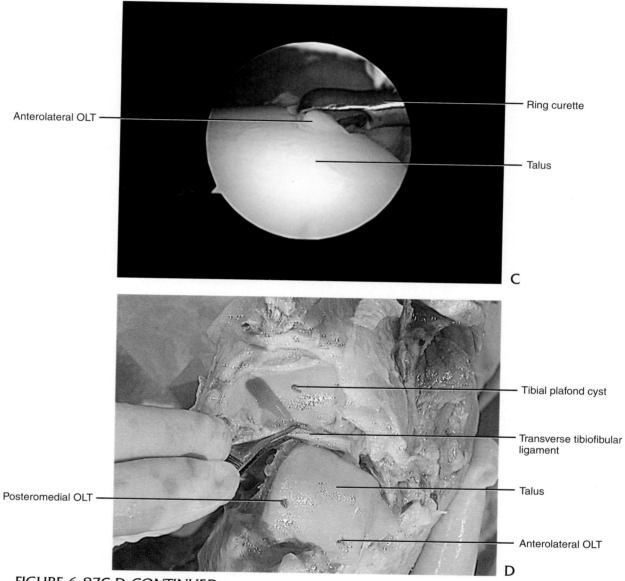

Anterolateral OLT

Ring curette

Talus

C

Tibial plafond cyst

Transverse tibiofibular ligament

Talus

Posteromedial OLT

Anterolateral OLT

D

FIGURE 6-87C,D *CONTINUED*

(C) Arthroscopic demonstration of the location of an anterolateral osteochondral lesion using a ring curette. **(D)** Anatomic dissection of the tibial plafond and talar dome with surgically created anterolateral and posteromedial osteochondral lesions and a distal tibial cyst.

ANKLE: INTEROSSEOUS TALOCALCANEAL LIGAMENT

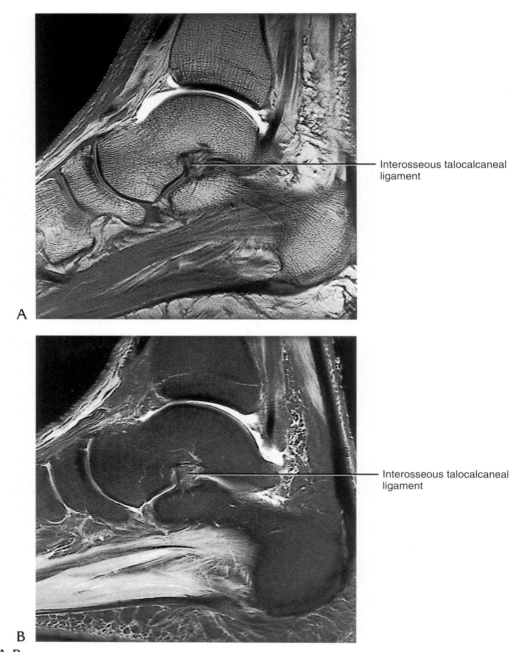

Interosseous talocalcaneal
ligament

Interosseous talocalcaneal
ligament

FIGURE 6-88A,B

(A, B, C, and **D)** The interosseous talocalcaneal ligament. The most important ligament connecting the talus and calcaneus, the interosseous talocalcaneal prevents eversion, heel valgus, and depression of the longitudinal arch. The interosseous talocalcaneal ligament and medial root of the inferior extensor retinaculum represent the deep layer of the lateral ligamentous support of the subtalar joint. **(A)** T1-weighted sagittal image; **(B)** fat-suppressed T2-weighted fast spin-echo sagittal image; **(C)** subtalar arthroscopic view; and **(D)** anatomic dissection.

ANKLE: INTEROSSEOUS TALOCALCANEAL LIGAMENT

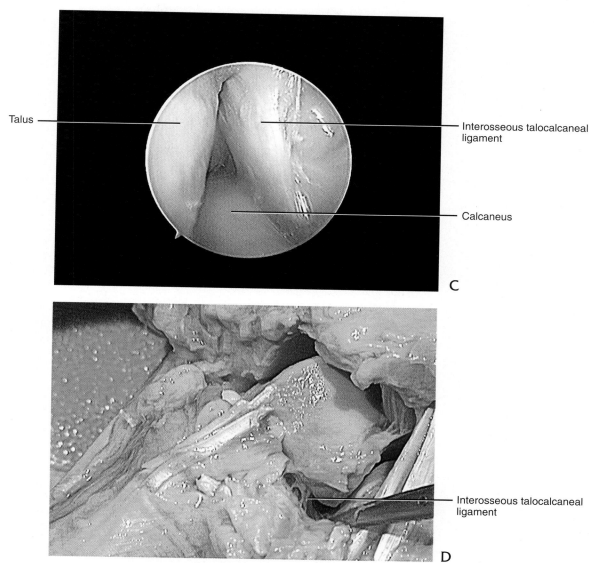

Talus — Interosseous talocalcaneal ligament

Calcaneus

C

Interosseous talocalcaneal ligament

D

FIGURE 6-88C,D *CONTINUED*

ANKLE: LIGAMENTS OF THE SUBTALAR JOINT

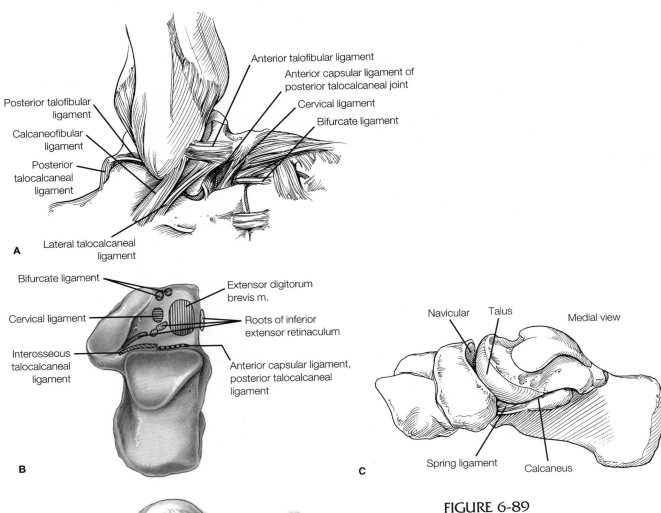

A

Anterior talofibular ligament

Anterior capsular ligament of posterior talocalcaneal joint

Cervical ligament

Bifurcate ligament

Posterior talofibular ligament

Calcaneofibular ligament

Posterior talocalcaneal ligament

Lateral talocalcaneal ligament

B

Bifurcate ligament

Cervical ligament

Interosseous talocalcaneal ligament

Extensor digitorum brevis m.

Roots of inferior extensor retinaculum

Anterior capsular ligament, posterior talocalcaneal ligament

C

Navicular　Talus　Medial view

Spring ligament　Calcaneus

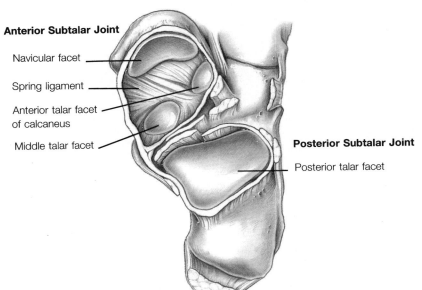

D

Anterior Subtalar Joint

Navicular facet

Spring ligament

Anterior talar facet of calcaneus

Middle talar facet

Posterior Subtalar Joint

Posterior talar facet

FIGURE 6-89

Ligaments of the subtalar joint. **(A)** Superficial lateral view of the subtalar joint with bones and ligaments. From this position, the interosseous ligament cannot be seen. **(B)** Superior view of the insertion sites on the calcaneus with the talus removed. **(C)** Anteromedial subtalar joint and talonavicular joint, demonstrating the important location of the spring ligament. The calcaneonavicular, or spring ligament, helps form the anterior subtalar joint (talocalcaneal navicular joint). **(D)** Anterior subtalar joint with the talus opened away from the calcaneus. The subtalar joint is divided into anterior and posterior articulations, separated by the sinus tarsi and the tarsal canal.

ANKLE: SINUS TARSI

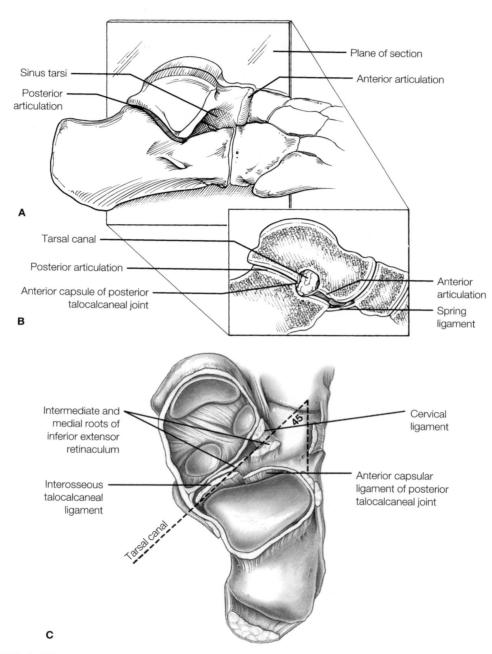

FIGURE 6-90

(A) Lateral view of the sinus tarsi. The sinus tarsi and tarsal canal separate the anterior and posterior articulations of the subtalar joint. **(B)** Corresponding sagittal section showing the tarsal canal and subtalar articulations. **(C)** Axial view of the tarsal canal. Note the location of the interosseous talocalcaneal and cervical ligaments. There is a 45° angle of orientation of the long axis of the sinus tarsi to the lateral aspect of the calcaneus.

ANKLE: SUBTALAR JOINT, PERIPHERAL LIGAMENTS

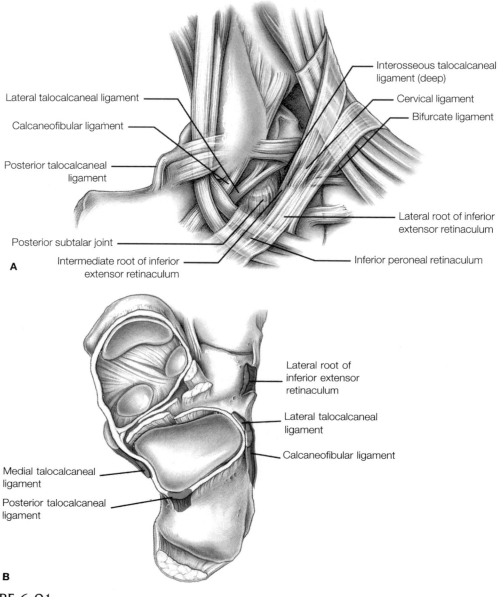

Lateral talocalcaneal ligament

Calcaneofibular ligament

Posterior talocalcaneal ligament

Posterior subtalar joint

Intermediate root of inferior extensor retinaculum

Interosseous talocalcaneal ligament (deep)

Cervical ligament

Bifurcate ligament

Lateral root of inferior extensor retinaculum

Inferior peroneal retinaculum

A

Lateral root of inferior extensor retinaculum

Lateral talocalcaneal ligament

Calcaneofibular ligament

Medial talocalcaneal ligament

Posterior talocalcaneal ligament

B

FIGURE 6-91

(A and **B)** Peripheral (superficial) ligaments shown on a lateral view of the right ankle **(A)** and an axial view **(B)**. The lateral talocalcaneal and calcaneofibular ligaments can be seen arthroscopically. The peripheral ligaments or superficial layer which supports the subtalar joint consists of the lateral root of the inferior extensor retinaculum, lateral talocalcaneal ligament, calcaneofibular ligament, posterior talocalcaneal ligament, and medial talocalcaneal ligament.

ANKLE: SUBTALAR JOINT, DEEP LIGAMENTS

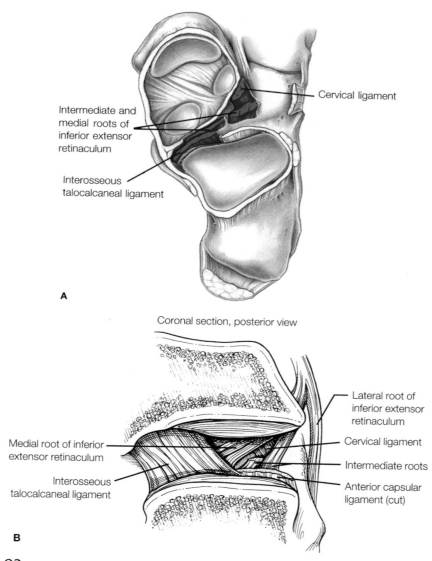

Cervical ligament

Intermediate and
medial roots of
inferior extensor
retinaculum

Interosseous
talocalcaneal ligament

A

Coronal section, posterior view

Lateral root of
inferior extensor
retinaculum

Medial root of inferior
extensor retinaculum

Cervical ligament

Intermediate roots

Interosseous
talocalcaneal ligament

Anterior capsular
ligament (cut)

B

FIGURE 6-92

Deep ligaments. **(A)** Axial view of the subtalar joint demonstrating the deep ligaments. **(B)** Coronal section of the subtalar joint showing the course of the interosseous talocalcaneal ligament in relation to the cervical ligament and surrounding roots. The intermediate layer of ligaments (intermediate root of the inferior extensor retinaculum and cervical ligament) and the deep layer of ligaments (medial root of the inferior extensor retinaculum and interosseous talocalcaneal ligament) are shown.

REFERENCES

1. Aichroth PM, Cannon WD Jr, Patel DV. *Knee Surgery: Current Practice.* 1992. Martin Dunitz, London.
2. Altchek DW (ed). Shoulder Instability. *Clinics in Sports Medicine.* 1995, volume 14 (no 4). W.B. Saunders Company, Philadelphia.
3. Andrews JR, Timmerman LA. *Diagnostic and Operative Arthroscopy.* 1997. W.B. Saunders Company, Philadelphia.
4. Clancy WG, Jr (ed). The Posterior Cruciate Ligament. *Clinics in Sports Medicine.* 1994, volume 13 (no 3). W.B. Saunders Company, Philadelphia.
5. Clemente CD. *Anatomy: A Regional Atlas of the Human Body,* 4th ed. 1997. Williams and Wilkins, Baltimore.
6. DePalma AF. *Surgery of the Shoulder,* 2nd ed. 1983. J.B. Lippincott Company, Philadelphia.
7. Detrisac DA, Johnson LL. *Arthroscopic Shoulder Anatomy: Pathologic and Surgical Implications.* 1986. Slack Publishing, Thorofare.
8. Ferkel RD. *Arthroscopic Surgery: The Foot and Ankle.* 1996. Lippincott-Raven Publishers, Philadelphia and New York.
9. Fu FH (ed). The Anterior Cruciate Ligament. *Clinics in Sports Medicine.* 1993, volume 12 (no 4). W.B. Saunders Company, Philadelphia.
10. Fulkerson JP (ed). Arthroscopic Surgery, Part I. *Clinics in Sports Medicine.* 1996, volume 15 (no 4). W.B. Saunders Company, Philadelphia.
11. Fulkerson JP (ed). Arthroscopic Surgery, Part II: The Knee. *Clinics in Sports Medicine.* 1997, volume 16 (no 1). W.B. Saunders Company, Philadelphia.
12. Golimbu CN. The Hand and Wrist. *Magnetic Resonance Imaging Clinics of North America.* 1995, volume 3 (no 2). W.B. Saunders Company, Philadelphia.
13. Guyot J. *Atlas of Human Limb Joints.* 1980. Springer-Verlag, Berlin, Heidelberg, New York.
14. Hawkins RJ, Misamore GW (eds). *Shoulder Injuries in the Athlete.* 1996. Churchill Livingstone, Edinburgh and New York.
15. Kang HS, Resnick D. *MRI of the Extremities: An Anatomic Atlas.* 1991. W.B. Saunders Company, Philadelphia.
16. Lichtman DM, Alexander AH. *The Wrist and its Disorders,* 2nd ed. 1997. W.B. Saunders Company, Philadelphia.
17. McMinn RMH. *Last's Anatomy: Regional and Applied,* 8th ed. 1980. Churchill Livingstone, Edinburgh and New York.
18. Miller MD, Osborne JR, Warner JJP, Fu FH. *MRI—Arthroscopy Correlative Atlas.* 1997. W.B. Saunders Company, Philadelphia.
19. Morrey BF (ed). *The Elbow.* 1994. Raven Press, New York.
20. Netter FH. The Musculoskeletal System. Part I: Anatomy, Physiology, and Metabolic Disorders. *The CIBA Collection of Medical Illustrations.* 1987. CIBA-GEIGY Corporation, Summit.
21. Rafii M (ed). Update on the Shoulder. *Magnetic Resonance Imaging Clinics of North America.* 1997, volume 5 (no 4). W.B. Saunders Company, Philadelphia.
22. Rayan GM. Compression Neuropathies, Including Carpal Tunnel Syndrome. *Clinical Symposia.* 1997, volume 49 (no. 2). Novartis Pharmaceuticals Corporation, Summit.

23. Rosenberg ZS (ed). The Elbow. *Magnetic Resonance Imaging Clinics of North America.* 1997, volume 5 (no 3). W.B. Saunders Company, Philadelphia.
24. Steinberg ME. *The Hip and its Disorders.* 1991. W.B. Saunders Company, Philadelphia.
25. Stoller DW. *Magnetic Resonance Imaging in Orthopaedics and Sports Medicine,* 2nd ed. 1997. Lippincott-Raven Publishers, Philadelphia and New York.
26. Strobel M, Stedfeld H-W. *Diagnostic Evaluation of the Knee.* 1990. Springer-Verlag, Berlin, Heidelberg, New York.

SUBJECT INDEX